Spirituality in Healthcare: Perspectives for Innovative Practice

Fiona Timmins • Sílvia Caldeira
Editors

Spirituality in Healthcare: Perspectives for Innovative Practice

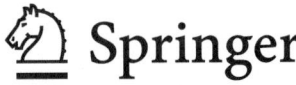

Editors
Fiona Timmins ⓘ
School of Nursing and Midwifery
Trinity College Dublin
Dublin
Ireland

Sílvia Caldeira ⓘ
Institute of Health Sciences
Catholic University of Portugal
Lisbon
Portugal

ISBN 978-3-030-04419-0   ISBN 978-3-030-04420-6   (eBook)
https://doi.org/10.1007/978-3-030-04420-6

© Springer Nature Switzerland AG 2019
This work is subject to copyright. All rights are reserved by the Publisher, whether the whole or part of the material is concerned, specifically the rights of translation, reprinting, reuse of illustrations, recitation, broadcasting, reproduction on microfilms or in any other physical way, and transmission or information storage and retrieval, electronic adaptation, computer software, or by similar or dissimilar methodology now known or hereafter developed.
The use of general descriptive names, registered names, trademarks, service marks, etc. in this publication does not imply, even in the absence of a specific statement, that such names are exempt from the relevant protective laws and regulations and therefore free for general use.
The publisher, the authors and the editors are safe to assume that the advice and information in this book are believed to be true and accurate at the date of publication. Neither the publisher nor the authors or the editors give a warranty, expressed or implied, with respect to the material contained herein or for any errors or omissions that may have been made. The publisher remains neutral with regard to jurisdictional claims in published maps and institutional affiliations.

This Springer imprint is published by the registered company Springer Nature Switzerland AG
The registered company address is: Gewerbestrasse 11, 6330 Cham, Switzerland

Contents

1. **What Is Spirituality?** 1
   Elizabeth Weathers

2. **The Psychology of Spirituality and Religion in Health Care** 23
   Jan M. A. de Vries

3. **Spiritual Assessment in Healthcare: An Overview of Comprehensive, Sensitive Approaches to Spiritual Assessment for Use Within the Interdisciplinary Healthcare Team** 39
   Wilfred McSherry, Linda Ross, Karnsunaphat Balthip, Natasha Ross, and Sadie Young

4. **Spirituality as a Public Health Issue: The Potential Role of Spirituality in Promoting Health** 55
   Richard Egan and Fiona Timmins

5. **Health Outcomes of Religious and Spiritual Belief, Behavior, and Belonging: Implications for Healthcare Professionals** 67
   Elizabeth Johnston Taylor

6. **Spirituality and Childbirth** 83
   Colm OBoyle and Vivienne Brady

7. **Providing Spiritual Care: An Exploration of Required Spiritual Care Competencies in Healthcare and Their Impact on Healthcare Provision** 97
   René van Leeuwen

8. **The Role of the Nurse in Providing Spiritual Care: A Case Study Approach to Exploring Specific Care Provision by Healthcare Workers in the Context of an Interdisciplinary Healthcare Team** 117
   Sílvia Caldeira, Joana Romeiro, and Helga Martins

9. **Loss and Grief in People with Intellectual Disability** 143
   Joy Powell

10	**The Role of the Healthcare Chaplain: A Summary of the Contribution of Healthcare Chaplains to Modern Healthcare Practice**... 151 Chris Swift	
11	**Teaching and Learning About Spirituality in Healthcare Practice Settings** .... 165 Jacqueline Whelan	
12	**Working with Diversity: An Overview of Diversity in Contemporary Society and the Effect of This on Healthcare Situations** .... 193 Gayatri Nambiar-Greenwood	
13	**Being Human: Cultivating Mindfulness and Compassion for Daily Living**... 211 Kathleen Neenan	

What Is Spirituality?

Elizabeth Weathers

Abstract

This introductory chapter explores contemporary understandings of spirituality and introduces the reader to spirituality and related concepts. It defines spirituality, spiritual distress and related concepts and describes associated key attributes. It gives the reader an understanding of the difficulties encountered with defining spirituality. The importance of spirituality is emphasised and expanded within a modern healthcare context. Practical resources, including websites and case studies, are provided to help the reader to explore their own spirituality and understand spiritual assessment and how to address the spiritual needs of others.

Abbreviations

JCAHO	Joint Commission on Accreditation of Healthcare Organisations
NANDA	North American Nursing Diagnosis Association
RCN	Royal College of Nursing
UTI	Urinary tract infection

1.1 Introduction

Since the mid-1990s, there has been an increase in the amount of literature published on the topic of spirituality across several disciplines including healthcare [1–4], psychology [5, 6], social work [7–10], counselling [11, 12] and

E. Weathers (✉)
Ion Beam Applications (IBA), Ottignies-Louvain-la-Neuve, Belgium
e-mail: elizabeth.weathers@iba-group.com

© Springer Nature Switzerland AG 2019
F. Timmins, S. Caldeira (eds.), *Spirituality in Healthcare: Perspectives for Innovative Practice*, https://doi.org/10.1007/978-3-030-04420-6_1

organisational and employment literature [13–17]. Spirituality can affect all aspects of a person's life highlighting the importance of the topic. It is particularly prominent during stressful life events, such as illness, suffering and bereavement and during the dying phase. Healthcare professionals such as nurses, doctors, social workers, etc. are present with people during all of these experiences illustrating the importance of spirituality to these professions [18]. Addressing spiritual needs can result in alleviation of suffering, a sense of well-being, enhanced ability to adapt and cope with adversity and a sense of peace and inner strength [19]. This chapter introduces the concept of spirituality and discusses the importance of spirituality from a clinical perspective. Furthermore, the concept of spiritual distress is introduced, and suggestions for addressing spiritual needs in clinical practice are proposed.

1.2 What Is Spirituality?

Spirituality is deemed to be that which gives life meaning, purpose and connection with others; is distinguished from religiosity but may incorporate religious beliefs for some people; and may comprise a religious system of beliefs and values or a nonreligious system of beliefs and values. It can be a metaphysical or transcendental phenomenon that relates to connectedness, transcendence and meaning and purpose in life [19].

1.2.1 Difficulties with Defining Spirituality

Conceptual and methodological inconsistencies have made it difficult to compare research findings and draw significant conclusions. Spirituality is an ambiguous concept, and few theoretical frameworks exist which aim to provide a deeper understanding of the concept. Therefore, much of the empirical research on spirituality has not been guided by a theoretical framework. There is disagreement amongst researchers in relation to both conceptual and operational definitions of spirituality with some researchers suggesting that spirituality in its essence may not be measureable. Conversely other researchers propose that spirituality is just as measureable as other subjective variables such as hope, adaptation or coping, all of which are well-established in the literature [20, 21]. Irrespective of these contrasting opinions, Breitbart [22] emphasises that spirituality and spiritual needs are of major concern for future research particularly in relation to the illness experience. According to Sessanna et al. [23], amongst the confusion and complexity, it remains that spirituality is a complex and abstract concept.

1.2.2 Useful Definitions of Spirituality

The Royal College of Nursing (RCN) [24] surveyed 4054 nurses to establish their understanding and attitudes towards spirituality and the provision of spiritual care. An online resource was created based on the findings to educate and create awareness about the concept of spirituality and spiritual care. Spirituality was stated as being difficult to define (see Fig. 1.1 and Boxes 1.1, 1.2, and 1.3).

According to Swinton [25], illnesses are deeply meaningful events that can challenge people to take a different perspective on their lives. Spirituality offers ways in which people can explain and cope with their illness experiences and in so doing discover and maintain a sense of hope, inner harmony and peacefulness despite the challenges that arise when a person is ill. Swinton concludes that the experience of

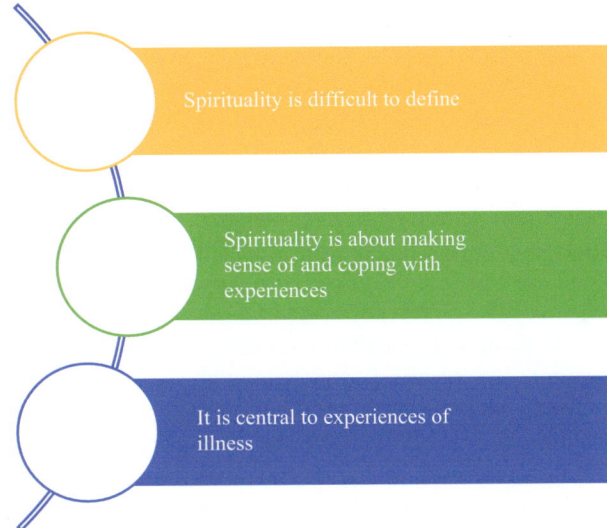

Fig. 1.1 What do we know about spirituality?

- Spirituality is difficult to define
- Spirituality is about making sense of and coping with experiences
- It is central to experiences of illness

Box 1.1: Spirituality is complex
Spirituality is difficult to define but very important. It is complex—however it is no more complex than other commonly used terms within healthcare. Think how difficult it is to define everyday terms such as care, community, love, attention and affection. The fact that spirituality is difficult to define and that people tend to define it in different ways is not unusual in terms of the language we use as healthcare professionals (RCN) [24].

Box 1.2: Spirituality is important in healthcare
All illnesses are first and foremost deeply meaningful human experiences. Professionals may offer diagnoses—cancer, schizophrenia, appendicitis, depression, anxiety, influenza, etc. Yet, behind the diagnostic label is a real person experiencing their illness within a specific context, accompanied by emotions and understandings. Spirituality can help people make sense of and cope better with experiences of illness and other difficult experiences (RCN) [24].

> **Box 1.3: Spirituality is as important as physical care**
> A person's spirituality, whether religious or nonreligious, provides belief structures and ways of coping through which people begin to rebuild and make sense of their lives in times of trauma and distress. These experiences are not secondary to the 'real' process of clinical diagnosis and technical care (RCN) [24].

illness is essential to a person's movement towards health and fullness of life even in the face of the most traumatic illness or life event [25]. Other theorists have also expressed this idea of personal growth and spiritual enlightenment in the face of illness and suffering. For example, Viktor Frankl was an Austrian psychologist and a psychiatrist who was captured during World War II and kept as a prisoner in the concentration camps. Frankl developed a theory of meaning, which he called 'Logotheory' derived from the word 'logos', which, in Greek philosophy, means purpose or meaning. According to Frankl, everyone will endure suffering at some stage of their life—it might be physical, psychological or spiritual. If a person is able to deal with this suffering in a positive way, by changing their attitude towards the situation, it can lead to a sense of inner peace and connection with others and, for some, an enhanced connection with God or a Higher Power [26].

Many authors have tried to clarify and define the concept of spirituality. Steinhauser et al. [27] stated that some clarity regarding a definition of spirituality can be established when one considers the difference between defining spirituality for the purpose of clinical practice as opposed to a definition that is used for research purposes. The focus in clinical practice is on individuality, promoting conversations and capturing the breadth of the experience of spirituality. Furthermore, in clinical practice, psychological or emotional concepts overlap with spirituality. Meanwhile, in research the focus is on measurement and generalising findings to large samples. Therefore, the concept needs to be clearly defined and differentiated from other related concepts, and specific dimensions of the concept under investigation need to be clearly delineated.

Spirituality can mean different things to different people. Figure 1.2 was developed by the authors and outlines some of the words used to describe what spirituality means to different people.

Given the complexity of the concept of spirituality and the difficulties with defining it, it is often useful to identify what spirituality is not. The RCN have outlined what spirituality is not [24]. Firstly, spirituality is not something that has no connection with clinical practice. Spirituality has clinical significance. In order to care for people, it is crucial to know and be able to recognise what the meaning of the illness is at the personal level. Secondly, spirituality is not just about religious beliefs and practices. It applies to people of all faiths and no faith. Spirituality is increasingly being recognised as something separate to religion but inclusive of religious beliefs and values depending on a person's belief system. Thus, people can be spiritual but not necessarily religious. Thirdly, spirituality is not only important for chaplains.

1 What Is Spirituality?

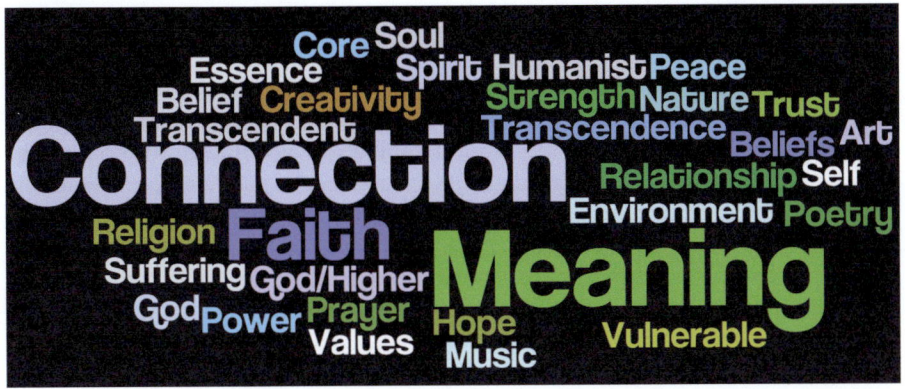

Fig. 1.2 Words used to describe spirituality

Chaplaincy is central to the delivery of spiritual care. However, chaplaincy is not the only discipline that benefits from understanding and recognising what spirituality is and how it functions in the lives of people experiencing illness and distress. Spirituality is important for all healthcare professionals. However, chaplains should be recognised as experts in the provision of spiritual care and also provide expertise and education to other healthcare professionals. Fourthly, spirituality is not only important for patients – it is important for all persons. Healthcare professionals are spiritual people, and learning to work with one's own spirituality within a caring context is a vital tool for the delivery of holistic care; to care well, one needs to be cared for well. Finally, spirituality is not about imposing your own beliefs and values on another. Although the spirituality of carers is important and needs to be considered, this does not mean that it is in any way appropriate for carers to impose their values and beliefs on patients in situations where they are clearly vulnerable.

> **Personal Reflection Activity**
> Read the following paper: Weathers, E., McCarthy, G., & Coffey, A. (2016). Concept analysis of spirituality: an evolutionary approach. *Nursing Forum* 51 (2) 79–96.
> After reading the paper, answer and reflect on the following questions:
>
> 1. What are the defining attributes of spirituality?
> 2. What are the antecedents and consequences of spirituality?
> 3. What is the conceptual definition of spirituality presented in the paper?
> 4. What are the implications of the findings for healthcare practitioners and your own practice?
> 5. Now consider your understanding of spirituality. Does this differ from the understanding offered in the paper?

1.3 Why Is Spirituality Important?

Spirituality is important for physical and psychological health as proven in prior research [4, 28–32]. Spirituality is becoming increasingly recognised as an important part of healthcare as reflected in global initiatives undertaken to promote the inclusion of spiritual care into healthcare [1]. A number of guidance documents and professional standards internationally have referred to the provision of spiritual care, further emphasising its importance in clinical practice (see Box 1.4). It is clear that the assessment of spirituality, and the provision of spiritual care, is being increasingly acknowledged within health policy and standards. Yet, the best way of implementing these recommendations in practice has yet to be fully discerned. Koenig [33] emphasised the importance of creating awareness amongst physicians with regard to conducting spiritual assessment and taking a spiritual history. It is equally important that nurses and other healthcare professionals are aware of spirituality and the spiritual needs of patients.

> **Box 1.4: Useful Resources**
> **Example of policies and guidelines that make reference to spiritual care:**
>
> - NMBI Requirements for Nurse Registration Education Programmes (2005), http://www.nursingboard.ie/en/publications_current.aspx?page=3 (*see p14, 17, 21, 26, 27, 32 & 33*).
> - Nursing and Midwifery Board of Ireland (NMBI) Scope of Nursing and Midwifery Practice Framework (2015), Available at: https://www.nmbi.ie/nmbi/media/NMBI/Publications/Scope-of-Nursing-Midwifery-Practice-Framework.pdf?ext=.pdf (*see p10 & 16*).
> - Nursing and Midwifery Council (NMC) Standards for Pre-Registration Nursing Education, UK (2010), Available at: https://www.nmc.org.uk/globalassets/sitedocuments/standards/nmc-standards-for-pre-registration-nursing-education.pdf (*see p18, 27, 36, 38, 45, 108, 113, 114, 148 & 149*).
> - NMC Standards for Competence for Registered Nurses, UK (2010), Available at: https://www.nmc.org.uk/globalassets/sitedocuments/standards/nmc-standards-for-competence-for-registered-nurses.pdf (*see p8 & 16*).
> - International Council of Nurses Code of ethics (2012), available at: http://www.icn.ch/images/stories/documents/about/icncode_english.pdf (*see p2 & 10*).
>
> **Example of practice resources for the provision of spiritual care:**
>
> - Spiritual Care Matters: An Introductory Resource for all NHS Scotland Staff (2009), UK. Available at: http://www.nes.scot.nhs.uk/media/3723/spiritualcaremattersfinal.pdf
> - Royal College of Nursing (RCN) (2010) Spirituality in Nursing Care: Online Resource. Available at: https://my.rcn.org.uk/__data/assets/pdf_file/0008/395864/Sprituality_online_resource_Final.pdf

- Manitoba's Spiritual Health Care Partners (2017) Core Competencies for Spiritual Health Care Practitioners. Available at: https://www.gov.mb.ca/health/mh/spiritualhealth/docs/core_competencies.pdf

Example of published government reports on spirituality:

- Department of Health (2009) Religion or Belief: A Practical Guide for the National Health Service, UK. Available at: http://webarchive.nationalarchives.gov.uk/20130107105354/http:/www.dh.gov.uk/en/Publicationsandstatistics/Publications/PublicationsPolicyAndGuidance/DH_093133
- Health Service Executive (2011) A Question of Faith: the Relevance of Faith and Spirituality in Health Care. Available at: http://www.hse.ie/eng/services/publications/corporate/Your_Service,_Your_Say_Consumer_Affairs/Reports/questionoffaith.pdf
- Health Service Executive/Trinity College Dublin (2016) An Exploration of Current in-Hospital Spiritual Care Resources in the Republic of Ireland and Review of International Chaplaincy Standards: A Preliminary Scoping Exercise to Inform Practice Development: Available at: https://www.researchgate.net/profile/Silvia_Caldeira/publication/313876297_An_Exploration_of_Current_Spiritual_Care_Resources_in_Health_Care_in_the_Republic_of_Ireland_ROI

1.4 Challenges with Terminology

There has been much societal change in recent years in relation to religion and spirituality. Gray [34] describes a 'mood of uncertainty' in modern society which has been marked by the decline of mainstream religion and the emergence of new forms of spiritual expression (p. 178). This societal shift has caused a loss of tradition and shared meanings, resulting in many people raising questions about the relevance of religion and its importance in people's lives. Society appears to be moving away from institutionalised religion towards a more individualised religion, which involves a personal search for meaning [26, 35]. Also, many people now draw on Eastern philosophy or New Age thinking to emphasise the importance of values such as loyalty, respect and responsibility [34]. As a consequence of these societal changes, the terminology and meaning of the word spirituality has changed. Historically, spirituality was considered a concept that develops within a religious context and usually within established institutions designed to facilitate spirituality [27]. Nowadays, spirituality and religion are considered separate concepts that can be interrelated for some people, depending on their belief system [19, 27]. Healthcare professionals need to be aware of this diversity in meaning when caring for patients, especially given that healthcare professionals are now caring for more and more people from diverse cultural backgrounds, with different beliefs and rituals. Additionally, healthcare professionals themselves in turn hold different religious beliefs and come from different cultural backgrounds. An overview of some strategies that can be used by healthcare professionals to enhance self-awareness and create a better understanding of individual spirituality is provided in Table 1.1.

Table 1.1 Strategies for enhancing self-awareness and understanding of one's own spirituality

Personal reflection	Taking time to mentally reflect on experiences in practice is a vital part of personal and professional development. There are many different models that can be used to guide a personal reflection. For example, Gibb's model (1988) outlines six stages: Description, feelings, evaluation, analysis, conclusion and action plan. Other models include John's model (1994) and Rolfe's reflective model (2001)
Reflective diary	Keeping a reflective diary is a written form of reflection that can help healthcare professionals to document their experiences in clinical practice. Any of the above-mentioned models could be used to guide this process. Or alternatively the healthcare professional may prefer to use an ad hoc or verbatim process of documenting their experience. This form of reflection also allows the professional to gather their thoughts on any given clinical experience and to make sense of it
Meditation	Meditation is a very useful method of enhancing a person's awareness of self and their spirituality. Meditation is useful because, like the above methods, it can be practised alone. Healthcare professionals wishing to adopt this strategy should try to identify a quiet space where they can sit and meditate. Some people prefer to have music playing in the background or to have some candles lighting also. The aim is to create a space in which the healthcare professional can dissociate from the experience in clinical practice and truly reflect on it

This evolution has been described as moving from underlying constructs that are theistic (belief in a supreme being) to religious (including shared customs and practices) through phenomenological (based on lessons learned from life experience) and existential (the search for meaning and purpose) to the mystical (relationship between the transcendent, interpersonal and transpersonal) [27], p. 429.

> This evolution has been described as moving from underlying constructs that are theistic (belief in a supreme being) to religious (including shared customs and practices) through phenomenological (based on lessons learned from life experience) and existential (the search for meaning and purpose) to the mystical (relationship between the transcendent, interpersonal and transpersonal) [27], p. 429.

1.4.1 Differentiating Religion and Spirituality

As described in the former section, there has been a societal shift that has led to difficulties and challenges in relation to the terminology to describe spirituality. This evolution has also led to a differentiation between the concepts of spirituality and religion. The word 'religion' was derived from the Latin word meaning that which 'binds together' inferring connections to a deity or Supreme Being, to other persons and to one's beliefs and values [27]. In light of the earlier described evolution, the word religion now increasingly refers to institutional, social, doctrinal and denominational practices or experiences [27]. Meanwhile, the word spirituality is considered to denote a broader search for meaning and purpose and connection with self, others and the transcendent [19]. From a clinical practice perspective, it is important to not assume anything in relation to a person's spiritual or religious beliefs or practices. Implementing reflective techniques as described earlier can be useful to enhance a person's ability to remain non-judgemental and to avoid making any assumptions.

1.5 Spirituality, Religion and Nursing

Of all the healthcare professions, nursing has the strongest spiritual and religious heritage [36–38]. Spirituality has been embedded within the nursing profession dating back to the pre-Christian era [38, 39]. In pre-Christian times, nursing was considered a noble act, and nursing care was concerned with nourishment of the human spirit including prayer to the Gods during illness [38, 39]. In ancient Celtic writings, a nurse was referred to as an '*anam cara*' or a *soul friend* illustrating the embodiment of spirituality within nursing from a very early stage [40]. During the Christian era, nurses continued to nourish the human spirit but in accordance with a religious (Christian) framework. The mission of these Christian groups (e.g. the Béguines and the Sisters of Charity) was to care for the sick in the same manner that Jesus had cared for the sick [38, 39]. 'Compassionate accompaniment' was the driving force of nursing at the time [41, 42].

During the twentieth century, the rise of modern science resulted in the introduction of university-affiliated nursing programmes, which focused on the professionalisation of nursing, striving to establish a universal system of nursing education and regulation of nursing practice [37, 42–44]. Nursing curricula reduced the content on spirituality and spiritual care to knowledge of major religions and associated dietary practices or rituals [45, 46]. The nursing profession was said to be inadvertently led into adopting the biological, reductionist approach to healthcare [47]. However, from the 1970s onwards, the concept of holistic nursing began to re-emerge, and with it came lots of literature on the meaning of spirituality and the spiritual needs of patients [3, 43, 48–51]. The scientific biomedical model that had encapsulated nursing was no longer sufficient and left many questions unanswered [45]. Timmins and McSherry [38] (p. 951) suggest that nursing had become 'disconnected from the spiritual dimension' with too much focus on the technical, scientific, medical and physiological aspects.

1.6 Spiritual Needs, Assessment and Spiritual Care

The predominance of the biomedical model of care with a focus on the physical dimension has impeded the provision of spiritual care in healthcare delivery [37, 39, 43, 52, 53]. The biomedical model has been criticised for not acknowledging the spiritual dimension even though healing traditions began with care of the spirit [54–56]. Nonetheless, according to Watson [51], nursing models and theories have extended beyond this limited view of physical care opting for a holistic approach to health. Nursing theories and models have conceptualised health as more than merely the absence of physical disease to include the psychological and spiritual dimensions of man [57]. There is a recent spiritual re-emergence in society, and the paternalistic, biomedical model is no longer considered adequate to address the diverse health-associated needs of human beings [51, 58]. Consequently, there has been an increase in the number of published research studies exploring the concept of spirituality.

1.6.1 Spiritual Needs

Studies have investigated whether patients considered it appropriate for healthcare professionals to ask about their spiritual needs and reported that 52–63% of patients considered it appropriate [59, 60]. Additionally, addressing spiritual needs of individuals with cancer has been associated with improved satisfaction with care, better quality of life, higher existential well-being and lower costs [61–64]. Other studies have examined the spiritual needs of individuals diagnosed with cancer (see Fig. 1.3).

The spiritual needs of individuals with cancer are similar irrespective of cultural background. For example, Hatamipour et al. [65] identified the spiritual needs of people with cancer ($n = 18$) in Iran (age range 22–72 years old). Participants emphasised the need for connection (i.e. social support and to be treated normally), seeking peace (i.e. inner peace, forgiveness and hope), meaning and purpose (i.e. accepting the reality, cause of disease, reliance on self and meaning of life) and transcendence (i.e. strengthening spiritual belief, communication with God and prayer).

> **Personal Reflection Activity**
> First think about your own clinical experience in caring for spiritual needs. Then use an online search engine or database to find articles that investigate spiritual needs. Now consider both your experience and the research that you found to answer the following questions:
>
> - What samples were included in this prior research (e.g. people with cancer, chronic pain, people with dementia, etc.)?
> - Were other types of spiritual needs identified? If so, what were they?
> - What about individuals who are cognitively impaired—how might you address their spiritual needs?

1 What Is Spirituality?

> **Hocker et al. (2014)[65]**
> - Explored spiritual needs in patients with early and advanced cancer (n=285) in Germany
> - Mean age was 61.3 years and most were male
> - Almost all patients (94%) reported at least one spiritual need
> - The two most frequent needs were *'to plunge into the beauty of nature '*(77%) and *'to turn to someone in a loving attitude'* (77%)
>
> **Darby et al. (2014)[66]**
> - Explored the spiritual needs of young people (n=9) aged between 11 and 16 years
> - Spiritual needs were classified into three main themes:
> - *Personal issues*-fear of the unknown, loss (hobbies, attending school), boredome and loneliness
> - *Relationships and attitudes*-presence of family members and friends, anticipation of being discharged
> - *Environment*-importance of having a conducive emotional space, building a sesne of community and belonging especially with people who have survived cancer, building a sense of community and belonging especially with people who have survived cancer.
> - Spiritual needs were found to change over time and it was recomended that heatlhcare professionals should re-assess spiritual needs.

Fig. 1.3 Spotlight on oncology research

As identified earlier in this chapter, all individuals have spiritual needs, even those who are cognitively impaired (e.g. individuals with intellectual disability or dementia). Frankl [26] identifies three dimensions to every person: the soma (body), the psyche (mind) and the noos (the soul or spirit). For individuals who are cognitively impaired, this tridimensional core of the person does not change, and they still have physical, psychological and spiritual needs. However, it is more difficult to establish their care needs, especially their spiritual needs.

In terms of assessing spiritual needs of patient who are cognitively impaired, it is best to assess the person as early as possible in the disease trajectory and develop a plan for spiritual care for both the individual and their caregiver [66]. Remarkably, some studies have found that spirituality can slow cognitive decline in people with dementia [67] and even protect against cognitive decline in middle-aged and older adults [68]. This emphasises the importance of addressing spiritual needs in all individuals.

1.6.2 Spiritual Assessment

As discussed earlier in the chapter, many governmental and professional bodies and organisations recommend the inclusion of spiritual assessment in healthcare. For example, the Joint Commission on Accreditation of Healthcare Organisations (JCAHO) mandates that all patients must be assessed for spiritual beliefs and practices. Thus, it is essential for healthcare professionals to understand how to efficiently and effectively assess cancer patients for spiritual distress. Many authors advocate a two-tiered approach (see Box 1.5) to spiritual assessment [69–72].

> **Box 1.5: A Two-Tiered Approach to Spiritual Assessment**
> - Tier 1 is a brief, superficial initial assessment that will obtain data to determine if there is any distress that requires further focused assessment. This assessment can be limited to asking the patient about general spiritual status (e.g. how are your spirits now?), spiritual needs (e.g. what spiritual concerns are bothering you most now?) and spiritual resources (e.g. what do you think might help you with these concerns?)
> - Tier 2 is a focused assessment that engages the patient to describe the specific type(s) of spiritual distress being experienced. For example, during the initial assessment, the healthcare professional may learn that the patient is wondering 'why?'. Tier 2 assessment questions would then reflect this specific problem of meaning. Follow-up questions could include 'Tell me more about your "why" questions' or 'What answers are you finding for why?'.

Healthcare professionals can craft original questions to reflect the patient's immediate concerns and language. Indeed, when talking with patients about their spiritual distress, it is important for healthcare professionals to be aware of the language utilised. To introduce the topic of spiritual distress, healthcare professionals can employ neutral phrases or use the language proffered by the patient. For example, if a patient remarks that it is *faith and family that are getting me through this*, the healthcare professional can create an assessment question using *faith*. Neutral phrases such as *matters of the heart* or *spiritual interests* may also be helpful. Other aspects of spiritual assessment are also important to consider. First, the quality of the data collected during a spiritual assessment will be determined by the rapport and trust the healthcare professional has established with the patient. Patients will more likely speak freely of their spiritual concerns to a healthcare professional whom they perceive as warm, kind and respectful and personally interested. Rapport can be developed rapidly by a healthcare professional who is genuinely caring. A healthcare professional presence, nonverbal messages and behaviours can convey readily the qualities a patient needs to talk openly about spirituality. Assessment data can be collected not only from the verbal interactions with patients. Healthcare professionals must also consider the nonverbal messages a patient sends. Objects such as religious jewellery or spiritually oriented books in the patient's environment can signal information about a patient's spirituality. This is particularly important for people with cognitive impairment.

Having read the previous sections on spiritual needs and spiritual assessment, consider the following case study activity:

1 What Is Spirituality?

1.6.3 Case Study Activity

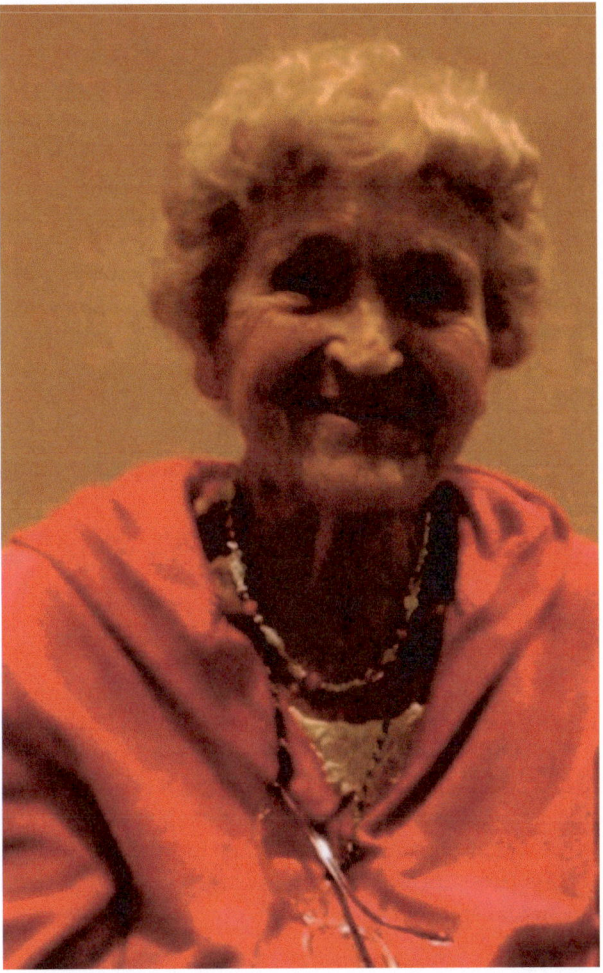

Joan is 82 years old and attended the emergency department last night accompanied by her daughter, Shauna. Joan was complaining of difficulty passing urine for 3 days, and her daughter informed staff that she had also observed Joan to be disorientated for the previous 2 days. A short while later, Joan was admitted to the ward with a diagnosis of a urinary tract infection (UTI).

You are asked to assess Joan on admission to the unit. In your assessment, you discover that Joan is widowed for the past 4 years, and since then, she has lived with her eldest daughter, Shauna. Shauna has a family of her own, but she can manage well as Joan is usually semi-independent with mobilising, hygiene, toileting and dressing. However, with the past 3 days, Shauna has noticed that her mother has been quite disorientated and has required more assistance with some of these tasks. You continue to ask Shauna questions about Joan's disorientation, and you discover that Joan's memory has actually been deteriorating over the past year. Shauna reveals to you that Joan has noticed a change herself but is reluctant to discuss it with anyone. She says that the family are very worried about Joan especially over the past 2 months when they have noticed that Joan does not attend any social events anymore. Shauna tells you that ever since she can remember, Joan would go to the local church every Sunday for mass and would meet all her friends afterwards in the village coffee shop, next to the church. Shauna says that Joan really enjoyed this every week and looked forward to it. However, over the past 2 months, Joan has refused to attend mass and has had no interaction with her friends.

As part of Joan's care plan, you need to consider spiritual needs and spiritual care. Reflect on the following questions:

- What kind of terms would you use to discuss spirituality and spiritual needs with Joan?
- How would you introduce the topic?
- Who would you involve in the discussion?
- What specific spiritual needs might arise in Joan's case?
- How would you ensure that Joan's spiritual needs are prioritised along with other needs?
- Which departments/disciplines would you consider referring Joan's case to?

1.6.4 Spiritual Care

Spiritual care should be considered as an approach to care [73]. In other words, spiritual care is not an addition to what nurses and other healthcare professionals already do, but rather it is a natural part of compassionate care, which shouldn't present an extra ambiguous burden to deal with [73]. The importance of communication within the healthcare professional-patient relationship is emphasised and numerous ways in which physical care or other biomedical interventions can be made spiritual [73]. Box 1.6 provides an overview of therapeutic approaches to spiritual assessment and spiritual care.

> **Box 1.6: Approaches to Spiritual Assessment and Spiritual Care**
> - Allowing person to discuss concerns
> - Active listening
> - Using full or transcendence presence
> - Offering spiritually nurturing books, videos or other resources
> - Educating about and supporting spiritually healing nonreligious rituals
> - Facilitating the expression of the spirit through art (e.g. painting, sculpting, music, quilting)
> - Supporting religious practices
> - Introducing journal writing
> - Prayer
> - Meditation
> - Guided spiritual imagery
> - Making appropriate referrals

One way in which healthcare professionals can help people towards wholeness and finding meaning in their illness is by referral to other multidisciplinary team services or sometimes external support services. For example, referrals can be made to the following team members:

Chaplains (trained in clinical pastoral education, pastoral counselling and fusion of theological and psychological knowledge)
Clergy (depending on the religious denomination)
Mental health professionals (counselling experience)
Parish nurses (have some pastoral counselling training and understand the varieties of spiritual distress amidst illness)
Spiritual directors (clergy or lay persons with some training in becoming 'holy listeners')
Spiritual healers (shamans, medicine men, folk healers considered to be spiritual care experts)

> **Personal Reflection Activity**
> Think about your clinical experience and your clinical setting. Now consider the following questions:
>
> - What spiritual support services are available for patients?
> - What spiritual support services are available for staff?
> - Is there a need to implement further support services and education on spiritual care in your clinical setting?

1.7 Spiritual Distress

Research studies have shown that spiritual distress or spiritual pain (e.g. feeling abandoned by God) is associated with worse outcomes for patients with diverse conditions. For example, spiritual distress has been associated with increased depressive symptoms, poorer quality of life, more functional limitations, increased risk of mortality, emotional adjustment and quality of life [74–76]. Spiritual distress has been defined as a disturbance in the belief or value system that provides strength, hope and meaning to life [77]. Spiritual distress has been accepted as a nursing diagnosis in the NANDA International (formerly, North American Nursing Diagnosis Association) since 1978 [78]. According to Caldeira et al. [79], spiritual distress may be diagnosed if the patient is in a state of suffering associated with the meaning of his/her life, related to a connection to self, others, world or a Superior Being. A list of manifestations of spiritual distress has been identified by NANDA International (see Fig. 1.4).

Spiritual distress is said to arise from unmet needs, and the greater the degree that a spiritual need remains unmet, the greater the level of spiritual distress experienced by the patient [79]. All humans have a spirit that deeply yearns for

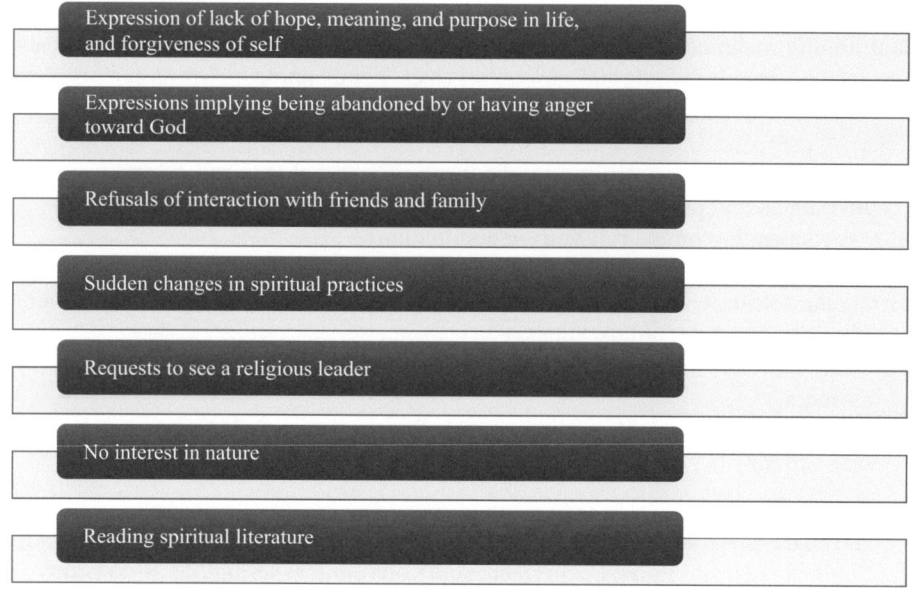

Fig. 1.4 NANDA list of manifestations of spiritual distress

meaningfulness, inner peace, love and connection with a transcendent. This is magnified during the experience of illness or a traumatic life event due to feelings of loss and change, which can also initiate a search for meaning and raise existential questions [71]. Furthermore, individuals can experience a realisation of mortality; a feeling of powerlessness and vulnerability; an isolation and loneliness; and feelings of guilt or shame [71]. Thus, losses and changes to which a patient cannot assign meaning or reconcile with basic beliefs about the world will contribute to spiritual distress. Being unable to sense that one's existence will continue in some manner after death may also exacerbate spiritual distress. Unanswered existential questions, a continued sense of vulnerability, loneliness, and guilt may have the same effect [71]. Unlike physical or psychological symptoms, spiritual distress may not always

> **Online Activity: Part I**
> Watch this TedTalk by Debra Jarvis, who describes her experience as a healthcare chaplain and cancer survivor:
> https://www.youtube.com/watch?v=4n8qT0vQbWk
>
> No one can tell us what our experience means…we have to decide what it means.
>
> Reflecting on your clinical practice, consider how meaning can be fostered in the patients you care for who are ill.

be a symptom to avoid. However, healthcare professionals need to be aware that spiritual distress can lead to negative religious coping as a result of poor adjustment to illness [79]. Examples of negative religious coping include believing that God is punishing the individual, feeling abandoned by God, viewing cancer as an act of the devil and passive deferring of decisions to the divine. Yet, spiritual distress may be a necessary and vital part of the spiritual journey, as alluded to by Debra in the YouTube clip. Although the experience will still be experienced as painful, it can produce new spiritual growth. Spiritual distress may be a natural part of a process that can lead to spiritual transformation. Although some persons may get 'stuck', those who embrace and learn from inwardly painful spiritual distress may experience transformation.

> **Online Activity: Part II**
> Remembering the words of Debra Jarvis:
>
> Claim your experience…don't let it claim you.
>
> Consider Debra's message about suffering and how people can interpret and deal with it in different ways. What are your experiences from your clinical practice?

1.8 Spotlight on Spirituality Research

Some researchers claim that the study of spirituality is fragmented and in the early stages [80, 81]. The progress of spirituality research has been challenged by a lack of consensus on definitions and measures [48, 57, 58, 81–83]. The ambiguity surrounding the conceptualisation of spirituality has been exacerbated by a lack of acceptable measurement instruments that address spirituality in a patient-centred, theoretically integrative and comprehensive manner [84, 85]. The majority of quantitative research conducted to date uses instruments measuring spiritual well-being [86, 87], spiritual experiences [88, 89] and spiritual practices [90], to operationalise spirituality. In some instances, measurement of spirituality has been simplified to religious practices [91, 92] or religiosity [93–95]. This may be due to poor differentiation between the concepts of spirituality and religiosity, which are often used interchangeably in the literature [3, 96, 97]. Nonetheless, the link between spirituality and health outcomes is well-established in the literature [98, 99].

1.9 Conclusion

The recent spiritual re-emergence in society has resulted in the paternalistic, biomedical model no longer being considered adequate to address the diverse health-associated needs of human beings [52, 58]. Spirituality is a highly personal and individualised concept; thus many definitions of spirituality exist. Spirituality is essential to healthcare and is increasingly recognised in healthcare policies, standards and guidelines. Spirituality can help people cope with difficult life events including a cancer diagnosis. Previous research has illustrated the prevalence and diversity of spiritual needs amongst individuals diagnosed with illness [65, 100, 101]. Spirituality can be helpful to the health and well-being of individuals; however, a person can also experience spiritual distress. Spiritual distress may manifest in many different ways depending on the person's situation and their belief system. Yet, spiritual distress may not always be a symptom to avoid. Rather, it may be a necessary part of the spiritual journey that can lead to transformation in the individual.

With regard to spiritual assessment, a two-tiered approach is recommended. This involves an initial brief spiritual screening assessment to identify any evidence of spiritual distress. This could be performed by any healthcare professional and used to make appropriate and timely referral to spiritual support services such as the chaplaincy service. There are many different modes of assessment including surveys and interview questions. For a spiritual assessment to be successful, there must be a strong rapport developed between the nurse and the patient, and the nurse should be aware of the importance of the language utilised. Spiritual assessment also includes nonverbal and behavioural observation, e.g. looking for signals in the patient's environment and observing their body language closely when opening a conversation with them about spirituality. Finally, spiritual care is an integral part of nursing care and should not be regarded as an 'added extra'. Rather spiritual care is an approach to care and should be at the core of everyday nursing care provided to people with cancer [73].

Acknowledgements Thanks to Fiona Timmins and Silvia Caldeira for the opportunity to author a chapter for this exciting new book. I also wish to acknowledge James Collins for his support of everything I try to achieve in life (the big things and the little things).

References

1. Cockell N, McSherry W. Spiritual care in nursing: an overview of published international research. J Nurs Manag. 2012;20(8):958–69.
2. Monod S, Brennan M, Rochat E, Martin E, Rochat S, Büla CJ. Instruments measuring spirituality in clinical research: a systematic review. J Gen Intern Med. 2011;26(11):1345.
3. Pike J. Spirituality in nursing: a systematic review of the literature from 2006-10. Br J Nurs. 2011;20(12):743–9.
4. Williams DR, Sternthal MJ. Spirituality, religion and health: evidence and research directions. Med J Aust. 2007;186(10):S47.
5. Leach MM, Sato T. A content analysis of the psychology of religion and spirituality journal: the initial four years. Psychol Relig Spiritual. 2013;5(2):61.
6. Saslow LR, John OP, Piff PK, Willer R, Wong E, Impett EA, Kogan A, Antonenko O, Clark K, Feinberg M, Keltner D. The social significance of spirituality: new perspectives on the compassion–altruism relationship. Psychol Relig Spiritual. 2013;5(3):201.
7. Bullis RK. Spirituality in social work practice. Washington, DC: Taylor & Francis; 2013.

8. Canda ER, Smith ED. Transpersonal perspectives on spirituality in social work. Abingdon: Routledge; 2013.
9. Crisp BR. Spirituality and social work. Abingdon: Routledge; 2016.
10. Moody HR. Religion, spirituality, and aging: a social work perspective. Hove: Psychology Press; 2005.
11. Daniels C, Fitzpatrick M. Integrating spirituality into counselling and psychotherapy: theoretical and clinical perspectives. Can J Couns Psychother (Online). 2013;47(3):315.
12. Rowan J. The transpersonal: spirituality in psychotherapy and counselling. Abingdon: Taylor & Francis; 2005.
13. Crossman J. Conceptualising spiritual leadership in secular organizational contexts and its relation to transformational, servant and environmental leadership. Leadersh Organ Dev J. 2010;31(7):596–608.
14. Crossman J. Environmental and spiritual leadership: tracing the synergies from an organizational perspective. J Bus Ethics. 2011;103(4):553–65.
15. Karakas F. Spirituality and performance in organizations: a literature review. J Bus Ethics. 2010;94(1):89–106.
16. Phipps KA. Spirituality and strategic leadership: the influence of spiritual beliefs on strategic decision making. J Bus Ethics. 2012;106(2):177–89.
17. Pawar BS. Workplace spirituality facilitation: a comprehensive model. J Bus Ethics. 2009;90(3):375–86.
18. Malinski VM. Developing a nursing perspective on spirituality and healing. Nurs Sci Q. 2002;15(4):281–7.
19. Weathers E, McCarthy G, Coffey A. Concept analysis of spirituality: an evolutionary approach. Nurs Forum. 2016;51(2):79–96.
20. Cohen MZ, Holley LM, Wengel SP, Katzman RM. A platform for nursing research on spirituality and religiosity: definitions and measures. West J Nurs Res. 2012;34(6):795–817.
21. Miller WR, Thoresen CE. Spirituality, religion, and health: an emerging research field. Am Psychol. 2003;58(1):24.
22. Breitbart W. Who needs the concept of spirituality? Human beings seem to! Palliat Support Care. 2007;5(2):105–6.
23. Sessanna L, Finnell D, Jezewski MA. Spirituality in nursing and health-related literature: a concept analysis. J Holist Nurs. 2007;25(4):252–62.
24. Royal College of Nursing. Spirituality in nursing care: online resource. 2010. Available from https://my.rcn.org.uk/__data/assets/pdf_file/0008/395864/Sprituality_online_resource_Final.pdf.
25. Swinton J. In: Cobb M, editor. The hospital chaplain's handbook: a guide for good practice. Norwich: Canterbury Press; 2005.
26. Frankl VE. Man's search for meaning. New York: Simon and Schuster; 1985.
27. Steinhauser KE, Fitchett G, Handzo GF, Johnson KS, Koenig HG, Pargament KI, Puchalski CM, Sinclair S, Taylor EJ, Balboni TA. State of the science of spirituality and palliative care research part I: definitions, measurement, and outcomes. J Pain Symptom Manag. 2017;54(3):428–40.
28. Dalmida SG. Spirituality, mental health, physical health, and health-related quality of life among women with HIV/AIDS: integrating spirituality into mental health care. Issues Ment Health Nurs. 2006;27(2):185–98.
29. Koenig HG. Religion, spirituality and medicine: the beginning of a new era. South Med J. 2005;98(12):1235–7.
30. Moreira-Almeida A, Koenig HG, Lucchetti G. Clinical implications of spirituality to mental health: review of evidence and practical guidelines. Rev Bras Psiquiatr. 2014;36(2):176–82.
31. Powell LH, Shahabi L, Thoresen CE. Religion and spirituality: linkages to physical health. Am Psychol. 2003;58(1):36.
32. Rippentrop AE, Altmaier EM, Chen JJ, Found EM, Keffala VJ. The relationship between religion/spirituality and physical health, mental health, and pain in a chronic pain population. Pain. 2005;116(3):311–21.

33. Koenig HG. Taking a spiritual history. JAMA. 2004;291(23):2881–2.
34. Gray M. Viewing spirituality in social work through the lens of contemporary social theory. Br J Soc Work. 2006;38(1):175–96.
35. Holden A. Jehovah's witnesses: portrait of a contemporary religious movement. Hove: Psychology Press; 2002.
36. Reed PG. Demystifying self-transcendence for mental health nursing practice and research. Arch Psychiatr Nurs. 2009;23(5):397–400.
37. Connell Meehan T. Spirituality and spiritual care from a careful nursing perspective. J Nurs Manag. 2012;20(8):990–1001.
38. Timmins F, McSherry W. Spirituality: the holy grail of contemporary nursing practice. J Nurs Manag. 2012;20(8):951–7.
39. Johnson RW, Tilghman JS, Davis-Dick LR, Hamilton-Faison B. A historical overview of spirituality in nursing. ABNF J. 2006;17(2):60.
40. Groves RF, Klauser HA. The American book of dying: lessons in healing spiritual pain. Berkeley: Celestial Arts; 2005.
41. Donley R. Nursing's mission: spiritual dimensions of health care. J Contemp Health Law Policy. 1991;7:207.
42. Fealy GA. History of apprenticeship nurse training in Ireland. Abingdon: Routledge; 2006.
43. O'Brien ME. Spirituality in nursing: standing on holy ground. Sudbury, MA: Jones and Bartlett Publishers; 2010.
44. Scanlan P. The Irish nurse: a study of nursing in Ireland: history and education, 1718–1981. Manorhamilton: Drumlin; 1991.
45. Barnum BS. Spirituality in nursing: from traditional to new age. New York: Springer; 2006.
46. Barnum BS. Spirituality in nursing: the challenges of complexity. New York: Springer; 2010.
47. McSherry W, Draper P. The debates emerging from the literature surrounding the concept of spirituality as applied to nursing. J Adv Nurs. 1998;27(4):683–91.
48. McSherry W, Cash K. The language of spirituality: an emerging taxonomy. Int J Nurs Stud. 2004;41(2):151–61.
49. Paley J. Spirituality and secularization: nursing and the sociology of religion. J Clin Nurs. 2008;17(2):175–86.
50. Pesut B. Ontologies of nursing in an age of spiritual pluralism: closed or open worldview? Nurs Philos. 2010;11(1):15–23.
51. Watson J. The philosophy and science of caring, revised edition. Boulder: University of Colorado; 2008.
52. Bradshaw A. Lighting the lamp: the covenant as an encompassing framework for the spiritual dimension of nursing care. In: Farmer E, editor. Exploring the spiritual dimension of care; 1996. p. 1–28.
53. Burkhardt MA, Nagai-Jacobson MG. Re-awakening spirit in clinical practice. J Holist Nurs. 1994;12(1):9–21.
54. Kimble MA. Beyond the biomedical paradigm: generating a spiritual vision of ageing. J Relig Gerontol. 2002;12(3–4):31–41.
55. Wilson D. The nurse's role in improving indigenous health. Contemp Nurse. 2003;15(3):232–40.
56. McSherry W. Making sense of spirituality in nursing and health care practice: an interactive approach. London: Jessica Kingsley Publishers; 2006.
57. Berry D. Methodological pitfalls in the study of religiosity and spirituality. West J Nurs Res. 2005;27(5):628–47.
58. Young C, Koopsen C. Spirituality, health, and healing: an integrative approach. Sudbury, MA: Jones and Bartlett Publishers; 2010.
59. Astrow AB, Wexler A, Texeira K, He MK, Sulmasy DP. Is failure to meet spiritual needs associated with cancer patients' perceptions of quality of care and their satisfaction with care? J Clin Oncol. 2007;25(36):5753–7.
60. Kang J, Shin DW, Choi JY, Park CH, Baek YJ, Mo HN, Song MO, Park S, Moon DH, Son KY. Addressing the religious and spiritual needs of dying patients by healthcare

staff in Korea: patient perspectives in a multi-religious Asian country. Psycho-Oncology. 2012;21(4):374–81.
61. Balboni TA, Vanderwerker LC, Block SD, Paulk ME, Lathan CS, Peteet JR, Prigerson HG. Religiousness and spiritual support among advanced cancer patients and associations with end-of-life treatment preferences and quality of life. J Clin Oncol. 2007;25(5):555–60.
62. Balboni TA, Paulk ME, Balboni MJ, Phelps AC, Loggers ET, Wright AA, Block SD, Lewis EF, Peteet JR, Prigerson HG. Provision of spiritual care to patients with advanced cancer: associations with medical care and quality of life near death. J Clin Oncol. 2009;28(3):445–52.
63. Balboni T, Balboni M, Paulk ME, Phelps A, Wright A, Peteet J, Block S, Lathan C, VanderWeele T, Prigerson H. Support of cancer patients' spiritual needs and associations with medical care costs at the end of life. Cancer. 2011;117(23):5383–91.
64. Pearce MJ, Coan AD, Herndon JE, Koenig HG, Abernethy AP. Unmet spiritual care needs impact emotional and spiritual well-being in advanced cancer patients. Support Care Cancer. 2012;20(10):2269–76.
65. Hatamipour K, Rassouli M, Yaghmaie F, Zendedel K, Majd HA. Spiritual needs of cancer patients: a qualitative study. Ind J palliat Care. 2015;21(1):61.
66. Alzheimer's Care Today. Spirituality: Tips & Strategies. Alzheimer's Care Today. 2009;10(4):238–9.
67. Agli O, Bailly N, Ferrand C. Spirituality and religion in older adults with dementia: a systematic review. Int Psychogeriatr. 2015;27(5):715–25.
68. Hosseini S, Chaurasia A, Oremus M. The effect of religion and spirituality on cognitive function: a systematic review. The Gerontologist. 2017;12:gnx024.
69. Maddox M. Teaching spirituality to nurse practitioner students: the importance of the interconnection of mind, body, and spirit. J Am Assoc Nurse Pract. 2001;13(3):134–9.
70. McSherry W, Ross L. Dilemmas of spiritual assessment: considerations for nursing practice. J Adv Nurs. 2002;38(5):479–88.
71. Taylor EJ. Spiritual care: nursing theory, research, and practice. Upper Saddle River: Prentice Hall; 2002.
72. Mauk KL, Schmidt NA, editors. Spiritual care in nursing practice. Philadelphia: Lippincott Williams & Wilkins; 2004.
73. Clarke J. Spiritual care in everyday nursing practice: a new approach. Basingstoke: Palgrave Macmillan; 2013.
74. Pargament KI, Koenig HG, Tarakeshwar N, Hahn J. Religious coping methods as predictors of psychological, physical and spiritual outcomes among medically ill elderly patients: a two-year longitudinal study. J Health Psychol. 2004;9(6):713–30.
75. Sherman AC, Plante TG, Simonton S, Latif U, Anaissie EJ. Prospective study of religious coping among patients undergoing autologous stem cell transplantation. J Behav Med. 2009;32(1):118–28.
76. Winkelman WD, Lauderdale K, Balboni MJ, Phelps AC, Peteet JR, Block SD, Kachnic LA, VanderWeele TJ, Balboni TA. The relationship of spiritual concerns to the quality of life of advanced cancer patients: preliminary findings. J Palliat Med. 2011;14(9):1022–8.
77. Yarbro CH, Wujcik D, Gobel BH. Cancer symptom management. Burlington: Jones & Bartlett Learning; 2013.
78. Herdman TH, editor. Nursing diagnoses 2012–14: definitions and classification. Hoboken: Wiley; 2009.
79. Caldeira S, Carvalho EC, Vieira M. Spiritual distress—proposing a new definition and defining characteristics. Int J Nurs Knowl. 2013;24(2):77–84.
80. Ellor JW, editor. Methods in religion, spirituality & aging. Abingdon: Routledge; 2013.
81. Moberg DO. Spirituality and aging: research and implications∗: sociology. J Relig Spiritual Aging. 2008;20(1–2):95–134.
82. George LK, Larson DB, Koenig HG, McCullough ME. Spirituality and health: what we know, what we need to know. J Soc Clin Psychol. 2000;19(1):102–16.
83. Maj M. Foreword. In: Verhagen P, Van Praag HM, López-Ibor Jr JJ, Cox J, Moussaoui D, editors. Religion and psychiatry: beyond boundaries. Hoboken: Wiley; 2012.

84. Ho DY, Ho RT. Measuring spirituality and spiritual emptiness: toward ecumenicity and transcultural applicability. Rev Gen Psychol. 2007;11(1):62.
85. Stefanek M, McDonald PG, Hess SA. Religion, spirituality and cancer: current status and methodological challenges. Psycho-Oncology. 2005;14(6):450–63.
86. Ellison LL. The spiritual well-being scale. 2006. Available from http://mds.marshalledu/co_faculty.
87. McClain CS, Rosenfeld B, Breitbart W. Effect of spiritual Well-being on end-of-life despair in terminally-ill cancer patients. Lancet. 2003;361(9369):1603–7.
88. Campbell JD, Yoon DP, Johnstone B. Determining relationships between physical health and spiritual experience, religious practices, and congregational support in a heterogeneous medical sample. J Relig Health. 2010;49(1):3–17.
89. Underwood LG. The daily spiritual experience scale: overview and results. Religions. 2011;2(1):29–50.
90. Thomas JC, Burton M, Quinn Griffin MT, Fitzpatrick JJ. Self-transcendence, spiritual well-being, and spiritual practices of women with breast cancer. J Holist Nurs. 2010;28(2):115–22.
91. Shafranske EP, Cummings JP. Religious and spiritual beliefs, affiliations, and practices of psychologists. In: Pargament KI, Mahoney AE, Shafranske EP, editors. APA handbook of psychology, religion, and spirituality (Vol 2): an applied psychology of religion and spirituality. Washington, DC: American Psychological Association; 2013.
92. Urry HL, Roeser RW, Lazar SW, Poey AP, Warren AE, Lerner RM, Phelps E. Prefrontal cortical activation during emotion regulation: linking religious/spiritual practices with well-being. In: Thriving and spirituality among youth: research perspectives and future possibilities. Hoboken: Wiley; 2012. p. 17–31.
93. Lee E, Zahn A, Baumann K. "Religion in psychiatry and psychotherapy?" a pilot study: the meaning of religiosity/spirituality from staff's perspective in psychiatry and psychotherapy. Religions. 2011;2(4):525–35.
94. Lucchetti G, Lucchetti AL, Koenig HG. Impact of spirituality/religiosity on mortality: comparison with other health interventions. EXPLORE. 2011;7(4):234–8.
95. Weiss DH. Religiosity/Spirituality as a protective factor for posttraumatic stress disorder among African American students at Jackson State University [Unpublished thesis]. 2011. Available from https://etd.library.emory.edu/view/record/pid/emory:9471f.
96. Koenig HG. Religion, spirituality, and medicine: application to clinical practice. JAMA. 2000;284(13):1708.
97. Peres JF, Moreira-Almeida A, Nasello AG, Koenig HG. Spirituality and resilience in trauma victims. J Relig Health. 2007;46(3):343–50.
98. Beery TA, Baas LS, Fowler C, Allen G. Spirituality in persons with heart failure. J Holist Nurs. 2002;20(1):5–25.
99. Moberg DO. Spirituality research: measuring the immeasurable? Perspect Sci Christ Faith. 2010;62(2):99–114.
100. Höcker A, Krüll A, Koch U, Mehnert A. Exploring spiritual needs and their associated factors in an urban sample of early and advanced cancer patients. Eur J Cancer Care. 2014;23(6):786–94.
101. Darby K, Nash P, Nash S. Understanding and responding to spiritual and religious needs of young people with cancer: Kathryn Darby and colleagues explore ways to support this patient group by focusing on non-medical aspects of care. Cancer Nurs Pract. 2014;13(2):32–7.

The Psychology of Spirituality and Religion in Health Care

Jan M. A. de Vries

Abstract

This chapter explores psychological aspects of spirituality. After an introduction to the psychology of spirituality and religion, the evolutionary psychological basis of transcendent belief is explored. A novel model is proposed based on the idea that 'believing' information from trusted sources was advantageous and possibly adaptive in our evolutionary history, which has facilitated the development of spirituality within the human species across the globe. The essential elements of this model are (a) believing as knowledge transmission, (b) believing as motivation or drive and (c) spiritual and religious beliefs as the basis for community (beyond kinship). These factors are further examined in relation to their benefits in health care today.

2.1 Introduction

Spirituality and religion have been shown to have health benefits. In fact, the relationship between spirituality/religion and health and well-being has become a growing area of interest [1–3]. A positive relationship has been established between spirituality and well-being in the general population [4], in patients with chronic illness [5, 6], with mental health problems [7], in ageing [8] and in palliative care [9]. Research in health psychology has established that, regardless of whether a transcendent element is included, belief and search for meaning are salubrious aspects in health and illness [10]; most notably there are signs that a spiritual or religious element may be particularly supportive in stress management and avoiding burnout [11, 12].

J. M. A. de Vries (✉)
School of Nursing and Midwifery, Trinity College Dublin, Dublin, Ireland
e-mail: jan.devries@tcd.ie

How spirituality and religiosity lead to those health benefits can be explained in more than one way. Of course, those experiencing the benefits of such beliefs will highlight the transcendental element. For instance, when a person prays for recovery from an illness, he or she may believe that God heard the prayer and brought about the cure. Or, someone may believe to have received a sacred sign to maintain health by treating the body like a temple and thereby received a divine health blessing. Or, an individual with mental health problems may benefit from psychotherapy which explores previous lives and discovers the cause of the problems in an earlier reincarnation. In contrast, a medic, nurse or psychologist is expected to provide explanations within their fields of professional expertise, which requires a secular understanding.

A psychological approach to the impact of spirituality or religion does not require belief in actual transcendent, supernatural or divine intervention but instead emphasises how normal psychological processes mediate between spiritual or religious beliefs and health and well-being. A Dutch psychologist, who researched the use of reincarnation therapy with people suffering from phobias, was asked on television whether he believed in reincarnation, to which he answered 'that does not matter, as long as it works' [13]. It was not important that the psychologist believed in reincarnation, as long as the participants in the study were convinced that through regression to an earlier reincarnation, they could address their mental health problems. Without believing in its transcendental foundation, the therapy could not work. Like psychologists, health-care workers must be respectful of such beliefs, to ensure that the benefits occur, even if the mechanisms as understood by health-care workers are entirely different from what the patient/client believes. The effective handling of this duality is an essential aspect of health care.

Keeping this in mind, we can now embark on the main mission of this chapter. After a brief introduction to the psychology of spirituality and religion, the chapter will outline:

- A novel model for the evolution of spirituality and religion as central aspects in human psychological and communal functioning.
- An overview of health benefits of spirituality and religion based on elements put forward in the evolutionary model.

Implications for practice will be discussed specifically in three discussion and application sections.

2.2 Psychology of Spirituality and Religion

Psychology used to be seen as intrinsically incompatible with spirituality and religion. Psychology's efforts to uncover the mysteries of all things human based on empirical evidence were considered a threat to religion and spirituality. While early psychological theorists such as William James and Carl Jung have contributed important insights on spiritual and religious matters [14], indeed throughout the twentieth century, psychology as a field has been more concerned with observable behaviours and measurable cognitive and emotional phenomena. Even the contribution of humanistic psychology, which advocated focussing on self-development, meaning in life, hope, free will and empathy [15, 16], was considered contrary to a religious or spiritual perspective on life. The emphasis on individualism and the centrality of the 'self' have sometimes led to accusations of psychology as a dangerous 'cult of self-worship' [17].

But things have changed. The loosening grip of Christian religious dogma on Western society has facilitated the emergence of a spirituality that not only shares common ground but vividly relates to psychology, in particular to the humanistic aspects listed above. Moreover, enlightened religious leadership has generated a climate in which psychology is no longer frowned upon in many churches. At the same time, psychology has evolved to the acceptance of spirituality and religion as fields of scholarly interest. Social psychology, clinical psychology, personality theory, evolutionary psychology and even cognitive neuroscience have each contributed to this [3]. Interestingly, for a while, the study of parapsychology which focussed on extra-sensory perception, telekinesis, telepathy, clairvoyance and other paranormal claims opened the door for the study of spiritual experiences as part of controlled psychic experiments and case studies [18, 19]. However, robust empirical support remained elusive [20], and this effort has all but been abandoned in academic institutions. Perhaps most importantly, the new movement of positive psychology [21] which focusses on all that can contribute to optimal human functioning has ensured that the integrated study of psychology and spirituality remained on the agenda. Popular psychological themes, such as mindfulness [22] and stress management techniques, meditation and yoga, contain spiritual elements.

In addition to these developments, the establishment in 1976 of the Society for the Psychology of Religion and Spirituality (Division 36) of the APA (American Psychological Association) more or less galvanised the topic as a discrete area [23]. This spawned several journals, handbooks and ground-breaking publications to harness the progress in this area. Still, this does not mean that a coherent area with well-established questions and answers has been established yet. Even at the level of defining religion and spirituality, there is considerable disagreement [3]. Often the distinction has been between spirituality as encompassing more individual interpretations of soul, spirit or the supernatural, in contrast with religiosity which is generally defined as a communal interpretation and practice of divine beliefs [24]. However, most conceptualisations have met with considerable disagreement within the field. So much so, that authoritative recent texts suggest a pragmatic perspective which avoids artificial distinctions [25] and highlights the commonalities between religion and spirituality [26]. This approach is also taken in this chapter. In essence, organised religion and spirituality are understood to share *belief in* and *search for significant meaning* in transcendent, value-based and sacred aspects of existence and the actions motivated by it [27]. It is beyond the scope of this chapter to present a more detailed overview of the state of affairs (see for this [3]), but it is not hard to imagine the complexities. For one thing, the diversity of religion and spirituality across the world and a psychology that is mainly fuelled by Western thinking generate obstacles and compatibility issues. Be that as it may, how religion and spirituality may have evolved to be present all over the world is worth addressing in more detail, particularly because of how it relates to issues of health and well-being.

2.3 Psychological Perspectives on the Development of Religion and Spirituality

There are several notable psychological perspectives on the development of transcendent experience. Cultural psychology, like anthropological perspectives, would take a historical view which emphasises how culture, society and religion interact and have developed over time [28]. Within this field, the development of religion is often related to morality and ethics and their impact on culture and society [29]. In contrast, personality psychologists have looked at the individual side, with theorists advocating positions on either side of the nature-nurture debate. Saddling both sides of the debate, one of the most influential psychologists of the twenty-first century, Gordon Allport, suggested that religiosity is the result of natural maturation of personality in the individual [30]. A similar position has been taken by developmental psychologists who have proposed stage theories of religiosity [31].

Whether spiritual experiences are desirable or not has first and foremost been addressed by clinical psychologists, who have both identified it as a sign of mental health and mental illness [32]. Likewise social psychologists have studied prosocial interactions in religious communities as well as worrying developments in spiritual communities and cults [33]. An interesting critical cognitive perspective is based on the consideration that we are prone to misattribute the cause of events in transcendent, superstitious or religious fashion whenever we encounter occurrences we fail to understand in mechanistic ways [34]. If we don't understand why something happens, it must be of a transcendent nature. Boerenkamp's study of clairvoyants showed that they had developed this tendency in extremum [20].

The study of the development of religious thought [35] prompted cognitive neuroscientists to look for specific parts of the brain involved in the processing of transcendent experiences [36] and consider whether our brain is hardwired for religion [37]. Although we must be very cautious in interpreting these findings [38], this led to many considering a preparedness or adaptation for spirituality and religion in the brain. Perhaps evolutionary psychologists have come closest to providing an understanding of this. While most perspectives in the field address the functionality (does it serve a purpose and what is that purpose?) of psychological mechanisms and processes, evolutionary psychology takes a step further and seeks to understand humans from the perspective of how we have evolved through adapting to our environments. This process of adaptation has been affected by natural and reproductive selection. Humans with adaptive traits that made them more successful in surviving and reproducing will have produced more surviving offspring than those without those traits. Thus the genetic basis for such traits would have become more common with successive generations [39–41]. Evolutionary psychologists often relate their theories to the time when humans lived as hunter-gatherers (up to 20,000 years ago) when life was harsh and survival pressure immense. They hypothesise that many psychological features of our species have been shaped in this period and hence that to understand the development of religion and spirituality, we need to go back to this era.

Perceiving religion and spirituality through this lens has met with some trepidation. Buss's [42] seminal handbook of evolutionary psychology only devotes one page to it! Yet some interesting perspectives have been expressed. One is that religion and spirituality could be seen by-products of selection for other adaptive aspects of the human survival and reproduction apparatus, such as our propensity to seek attachment [43, 44]. Attachment is an adaptive process that benefits offspring of many animals by providing protection, nearness to sustenance, support and learning. While normally aimed at caregivers, it is hypothesised that religion is the result of projecting this on a deity [45], thus providing a broader and beneficial connectedness to community and the world in general. Others have argued that religion and spirituality have a myriad of survival and reproductive advantages through shared and coordinated social life and may be a complex adaptation in its own right [46, 47].

2.4 A Novel Evolutionary Model of Spirituality and Religion

Building on these evolutionary principles, other perspectives can be hypothesised. Forgive the audacity, but there is scope for a novel perspective, which hinges on the human propensity to make assumptions, 'believe' in information from trusted sources, and engage in actions based on them. Core to this perspective is the fact that our executive functions and working memory are limited in size [48] and therefore that we are restricted in the extent of our cognitive appraisal of complex events [49]. We simplify and make assumptions, often based on partial evidence. This helps us avoid lengthy inner deliberations in situations where fast decision-making and well-coordinated action are required. This cognitive tendency is an essential aspect of how not only humans, but many organisms, survive. The understanding of *believing (or making assumptions) as an adaptation*, or an instinct [50], is not entirely new, and how it pertains also to transcendent beliefs is only a small step. We act on beliefs about many aspects of the world that are either not verified or not verifiable. For our hunter-gatherer ancestors, much of the understanding of the world was hard to verify, regardless of whether it pertained to the natural or supernatural realm. In fact, differences between beliefs in natural and transcendent understanding may have been much less pronounced than they are today. Without the vast scientific understanding of our world, our hunter-gatherer would have been just as easily swayed by supernatural beliefs.

Let's take a leap back in time. Twenty thousand years ago or longer, our species roamed the planet in small groups, families, extended families and tribes. These groups were nomadic and lived from hunting and gathering whatever was edible (fruit, nuts, mushrooms, etc.). Life was full of hazards, and the knowledge base for survival contained many uncertainties, such as what to eat to remain healthy in the long term, how to prevent and treat illness and injuries, how to predict death or survival, etc. Very often our ancestors would have 'believed' rather than known things for sure. Believing was beneficial, regardless of whether transcendent aspects were included. There are three pervasive reasons to assume this: (a) believing is essential for sharing of vital information; (b) believing is a motivating factor with drive-like qualities; and (c) believing in the same things generates community.

So firstly, it was *beneficial to 'believe' in information provided by trusted sources*: where to find food, what to eat and what to avoid, the imminence of danger, whether to fight or flee, etc. To make up our minds, we needed to observe and believe others. Humans are not unique in this. Most animals are extremely responsive to the behaviours and signals of conspecifics as warnings or indications of opportunities. In addition, in humans, an essential knowledge to survive was transmitted verbally from generation to generation by elders. Their wisdom would have been unfathomable to a new generation, and therefore they would have had to believe the elders' judgement. Transcendent, spiritual wisdom or religious beliefs would have been transmitted in the same way. Perhaps this kind of knowledge, which could neither be confirmed nor falsified, may have been transmitted with particular conviction.

This brings us to the second benefit, which is the *motivational aspect of beliefs*. If you believe in something, you are more likely to succeed. Henry Ford's famous quote "Whether you think you can, or you think you can't: you're right" epitomises this. Believing has drive-like properties that trigger motivation and thus activate the brain and the sympathetic nervous system to facilitate energetic responses and action patterns to succeed in achieving a wide variety of goals [51]. Believing in a positive outcome will have motivated our ancestors in their daily efforts to find sustenance and protect themselves. It will have motivated them to devote energy to developing better shelters, weaponry, food preparation and medicine. In this sense, the quality to have strong beliefs may have been a survival benefit, and the inheritable element of it may have become more abundant with each generation. Some authors have argued that the motivational impact of transcendent beliefs may be particularly salient [52] and will have served as overarching motivating factors leading to extraordinary achievements.

Thirdly, *shared beliefs generate community*. Trust in others and what they tell us or promise is an essential element in the system of reciprocity in each community. Believing in the same perceptions and conceptions of the world and ourselves is also a great uniting factor. Beliefs most likely to unite people are the kinds that transcend what could be easily established or observed objectively. Typically the most enduring of such beliefs would be those that can neither be confirmed nor falsified by empirical evidence. Once refuted, a belief becomes meaningless, and the same is the case for a belief that is confirmed to be objectively true. It loses its fascination and power, and the special bond between believers evaporates. Hence, beliefs that retain a degree of mystery, such as those from the realm of the supernatural, religious or spiritual, could well be more effective at connecting communities than other factors. It is possible that in our evolutionary past, shared transcendent beliefs generated a special bond that exceeded tribal and familial bonds. With many tribes based on extended families, lack of reproductive opportunities and inbreeding were problematic. Shared transcendent beliefs would have created ties between different tribes that would have facilitated intermarriage and avoidance of inbreeding and therefore stronger offspring.

In sum, it is argued that the motivational and knowledge transmission advantages of 'believing' in general may have been adaptive in our hunter-gatherer ancestors but also that beliefs in the spiritual world may well have precipitated the formation of more intimate ties between non-kin individuals and groups, which because of avoiding inbreeding may have led to higher reproductive success.

A specific feature that would have made most forms of religion and spirituality attractive in our hunter-gatherer past, and still does, is the offering of a *transcendent meaning to life*, which may have the overarching motivating impact suggested in the above. Other important selling points of religion were the idea of an *afterlife*, which provides an answer to the most essential fear humans have. Believing that our spirit lives on after we die and we would be reunited with our loved ones in a heavenly afterlife with all suffering gone must be mood enhancing for most people and may have significantly reduced the inevitable suffering in what must have been difficult lives. While the functionality and benefits of each of these aspects are clear, more consideration is needed before we might attribute the qualities of evolutionary adaptations to it. This is for another publication.

Another word of caution also needs to be inserted here. The complexity of human behaviour and the varying and changing circumstances in which we live and have lived are such that it is very hard to establish whether spiritual and religious behaviours as an adaption would on balance outweigh the possible maladaptive aspects and risk factors. Bulbulia mentions several negative aspects of religion that require consideration, such as 'misperceiving reality as phantom infested, frequent prostrations before icons, the sacrifice of livestock, repetitive terrifying or painful rituals, investment in costly objects and architecture, celibacy, religious violence and non-reciprocal altruism, to name a few' ([53], p. 655). We may also question whether religion and spirituality as unifying factors compensate for their divisive potential, often leading to conflict and war. Talking of war, we might consider whether religious warfare was more effective than non-religious warfare and provided more benefits for the survival and reproductive fitness of those engaging in it and their progeny. Would plundering, pillaging and rape have been more effective under the banner of spreading a religion? Also, many religions have periods of fasting included in their yearly calendar. Evolutionary psychologists would be asking whether on balance fasting had survival and reproductive benefits or disadvantages. Of course, addressing these multifaceted questions is beyond the remit of this chapter, but it is important to appreciate the complexity of the issue of adaptiveness and health benefits and that we have to be cautious in our approach. Nonetheless, with the case for spirituality and religion as adaptations presented, it is worth establishing how survival advantages in our evolutionary past translate into benefits for health and wellness today.

2.5 Health Benefits of Spirituality and Religion

2.5.1 Health Beliefs and Transcendent Beliefs

The study of health beliefs is an important area in health psychology [10]. A fundamental principle is that with health information generally complex, overwhelming and ambiguous, the average patient tends to simplify their understanding often based on stereotypical health beliefs. For instance, while few people would contest the existence of transmittable illnesses, viruses or bacteria, the complex workings of the different systems in our bodies or the importance of medical interventions, the complexity of it all is such that it exceeds the layperson's powers of processing and verification. Just like we argued for our hunter-gatherer ancestors, it is therefore a matter of trusting and believing experts rather than that we can fathom or verify any of these ourselves. In many ways, believing in physical and health sciences requires the same leap of faith as believing in spirituality or religion.

And what we believe matters. In health care, believing in success of a treatment has been identified as an important additional factor in its potential effectiveness. Even without an established working ingredient in an intervention, expectations of a positive impact (the placebo effect) have often been shown to be effective [54–58]. This principle also applies to spiritual or religious beliefs that are in alignment with the information about and impact of treatment (see Fig. 2.1).

The belief in sacred support or that God cures can be equivalent or perhaps superior to the trust in a doctor or the intervention itself. In fact, the belief in transcendent or divine support, if it is firm, has the advantage that it is not subject to fluctuations in confidence in specific doctors or treatments, nor does it need

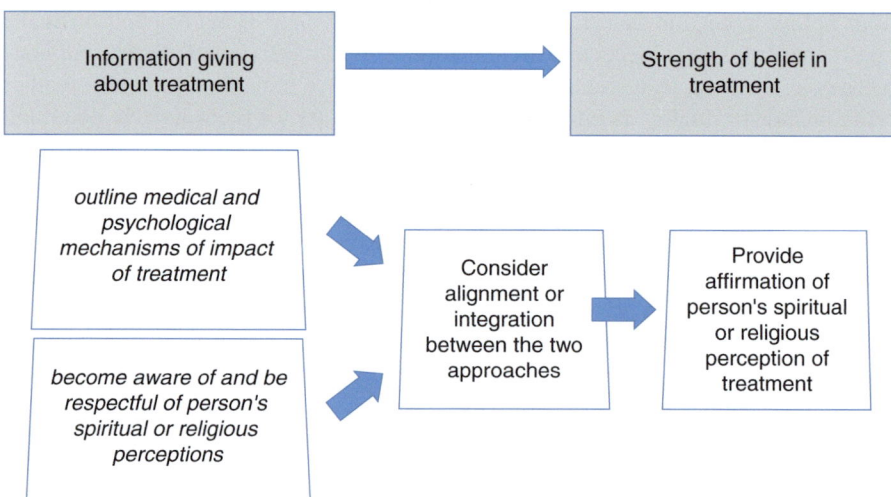

Fig. 2.1 Recommended approach to integrating patient's spiritual or religious perspectives in optimising treatment impact

recalibration when a treatment fails and a new one is initiated. Continued belief in spiritual support will give a patient hope and peace of mind, which will reduce stress levels and thus have health benefits [8, 59].

Only if health-care workers acknowledge and respect religious beliefs and spiritual perspectives of patients can we ensure that these beliefs provide optimal support for them in coping with the health issues they are facing (see Fig. 2.1). Coyle suggests that health-care workers need to show respect but also familiarise themselves with the spirituality of the people in their care [27]. Often transcendent or religious beliefs can be aligned effectively with perceived medical and/or psychological mechanisms, but sometimes such beliefs may interfere. The understanding of HIV-AIDS internationally is a good example of where spiritual and medical explanations of the illness sometimes clash, with devastating effect for the trust in medical treatment and the motivation to refrain from unprotected sex. Consideration of matters of trust is crucial, because psychological research has demonstrated convincingly that trust is easily broken and hard to re-establish [60]. As a health-care worker, it is essential to pay attention to this process.

> **Implications for Health-Care Practice I**
> It is essential that medical and psychological factors in health, illness and health care are well enough understood by patients but also that patients are supported in activating their own positive beliefs, including religious or spiritual ones, in relation to healing and recovery (see Fig. 2.1). While specific transcendent beliefs that health-care workers have themselves should be subordinate to the patient's beliefs, understanding core spiritual principles may help in understanding how these can benefit patients, even if their specific beliefs are different. Question: Which core spiritual principles might help us to make this link?

2.5.2 The Health Benefit of a Meaningful Life

Both the search for and an achieved sense of meaning in one's life is part of an overall motivational mechanism. We are 'driven' to look for and find meaning in life in work, love, raising children, making a difference in other people's lives, etc. Many psychologists consider this an essential function, and some don't shy away from advocating that a spiritual approach to the meaning of life is essential to an overarching motivational theory [61]. Meaning in life has been associated with higher levels of mental health and well-being [62], a buffer against stress [63] and as a mediator between religiousness and psychological health [64].

There is evidence to suggest that significant health scares lead people to reconsider their perspectives on the meaning of life or may add or emphasise a more spiritual or religious aspect to it [65]. What gives meaning to life differs for each individual and often changes throughout the lifespan. Younger adults tend to 'search' for meaning, while older adults more often identify a 'presence' of meaning.

Implications for health care II: What gives meaning to our life?		
If we want to identify a person's answer to this question, it may be useful to ask about all three aspects. We may want to start with ourselves		
Individual or self-related	Family, community, society related	Spiritual or religious aspect

Fig. 2.2 Three domains of meaning in life

Meaning in life tends to be associated with higher well-being [66], but more prominently in older adults [67]. Ageing itself may also play an important role in this, but since many life-threatening illnesses are most likely to affect us later in life, these tendencies may well amplify each other.

The great advantage of a spiritual or religious perspective on the meaning of life is that it can be maintained even when social, individual or occupational circumstances which give meaning are diminished. In particular when people end up in hospital for a considerable period of time, the emerging crisis [68, 69] is likely to be exacerbated because all sorts of meaning-giving activities fall by the way side. Achievement through work, being part of a community and excelling in sport or other activities will be out of the question, and thus life ceases to provide the same sense of meaning, once in a hospital bed (see Fig. 2.2). It should not surprise us that people become more spiritual or religious under those circumstances. In this sense it can be a compensatory mechanism.

2.5.3 Reduction of Human Suffering and Fear of Death

As there is evidence for higher quality of life in those engaging in spirituality or religion when affected by chronic illness, such as cancer [5], there is also the suggestion that those engaging in spirituality may be more effective at coping with human suffering [70]. The calming and balancing effect of being connected to transcendental elements is one factor. The other is that acts of meditation or prayer may reduce fear, stress, anxiety and pain and increase wellness [71]. People engaged with spirituality have lower risk of suicidality [72].

A strong appeal of most religions is that they include elements that reduce suffering or perceived levels of suffering. Jesus's intense suffering is an essential aspect of Christianity and emphasises that most of our own suffering is insignificant in comparison. This may help in pain management. Any form of sanctification or transcendental experience of childbirth might also have such an impact [73]. Spiritual aspects of relaxation exercises and meditation are bound to add to the impact of such techniques to reduce stress and cope effectively with pain and discomfort.

Belief in an afterlife is most helpful when death approaches. This is why spirituality is often so central in palliative care [9].

Much of our suffering is of a mental nature. Specifically inner conflict about important self-related matters can make us feel bad about ourselves [74]. When being made to think one is wrong, immoral, bad, stupid, hypocritical, etc., this is bound to affect us most. Spiritual or religious inner conflicts may be involved in this. It disrupts our peace of mind and sometimes generates a degree of heartache more intense than physical pain. It expresses itself in guilt, shame, embarrassment, regret, remorse or self-directed anger and motivates efforts to continue looking for a resolution, until solace has been found. And while values, beliefs or faith may be part of the inner conflict, spiritual or religious answers can also be helpful to reduce the inner turmoil.

> **Implications for Health-Care Practice III: Spiritual responses to reduce Inner Conflict**
>
> How we experience and respond to inner conflicts is best explained by cognitive dissonance theory [74–76] which suggests that we are motivated to seek and maintain internal consistency in our thinking and behaviour and find inconsistency or 'dissonance' uncomfortable. Dissonance between our behaviour and important standards we hold ourselves to can be the source of intense discomfort. Ideally we bring our behaviour back in line with these standards. However, sometimes actions lead to damage to self or other that cannot be reversed. Consequently the person may be unable to resolve the related dissonance and may experience prolonged mental anguish. It is in these cases that a spiritual or religious approach may provide solace. Let us consider the following scenarios:
>
> Matt [23] is in hospital with several non-life-threatening injuries following a traffic accident in which he was the driver. His girlfriend died in the accident. He had been drinking. As his physical state improves, his mental state deteriorates. He says that he wished he was dead.
>
> Fatima [57] is overweight and suffering from diabetes. She has come to the realisation that her illness is the result of long-term lack of physical activity and an unhealthy diet. She is ashamed and does not want to see her family.
>
> Jane [77] is on life support and reflecting on her life. She is talking about an abortion she had a long time ago and how subsequently she could not conceive and remained childless. She says that she still regrets this and does not know how to make peace with herself.
>
> **Question:** Can you think of a spiritual approach to assist Matt, Fatima and Jane in coming to terms with what happened and alleviate the mental pain they are experiencing? (Consider first how you would find out what their spiritual beliefs are. Then reflect on how meditation, prayer, confession, seeking forgiveness, establishing transcendent meaning or other aspects might benefit them).

2.5.4 Health Benefits of Spiritual and Religious Social Support

We are social animals [78]. This is reflected also in how transcendent beliefs are experienced and the strength of the community bond these shared beliefs may generate. While the survival and reproductive advantages have already been outlined in the above, the direct health benefits of social and spiritual support still require some comment. Perhaps most obviously, church membership tends to imply support from the church community whenever a member is unwell. This support has been shown to be beneficial in a variety of contexts [79]. This makes sense, because it is well documented that social support in general has many physiological benefits [80] especially for the endocrine, cardiovascular and immune system [81] with many studies indicating that social support and inclusion moderate a negative impact of stress on health [82] and mental health [83].

Churches and spiritual organisations also engage actively in providing health care and support. This relationship may have its origin in shamanistic health-care duties in hunter-gatherer societies [84] and is evidently still playing a dominant role in health care today. Think of all the hospitals run by religious orders and organisations like the Red Cross or Red Crescent. While the times of specific hospitals for specific religious grouping has gone, a religious ethos often still shines through underneath a secular veneer. At the same time, the growing ethnic and religious diversity within the patient populations in most hospitals in Europe and the USA have led to individualised spiritual support. One can request a visit from clergy of a variety of backgrounds, according to one's expressed preference. This practice is particularly prevalent around life-threatening operations and in end-of-life care. While the impacts of such supports are notoriously difficult to establish, the evidence is not overly favourable [85]. The fit between the person and the preferred spiritual support may be crucial in this respect. Research on music as a preoperative or pain reduction intervention showed that self-selected music was most effective [86]. It may well be the same for spiritual support. This is an argument to suggest that health-care workers may need to become more familiar with the different kinds of spiritual perspectives generally encountered in practice, in order to provide optimal support [27].

The combined impact of social and spiritual support is most evident where organisations with a faith-based foundation have set up patient or peer support groups for specific conditions. A review of the literature shows that such programmes tend to be aimed at primary prevention, general health, cardiovascular health or cancer and may lead to significant reductions in blood pressure, cholesterol, weight and illness symptoms [77]. In addition widespread initiatives such as Alcoholics Anonymous, which incorporate a spiritual aspect, have been demonstrated to be effective [87]. Even web-based spiritual supports for patient groups are potentially helpful [88]. Some religious and spiritual organisations use their health and mental support efforts to recruit people. The Scientology Church is an example of this. Other organisations tend to pre-empt this ethical issue, by being as all-inclusive as possible and avoiding proselytising as part of their health-care activities. As a result, the religious or spiritual identity of their support activities may remain implicit.

2.6 Conclusion

After a brief introduction to the psychology of spirituality, this chapter has aimed to provide an understanding of the possible development of religiosity and spirituality rooted in evolutionary psychology. A novel model has been proposed which suggests that 'believing' in information that could not be verified was an essential adaptation for our hunter-gatherer ancestors. It had benefits for the transfer of information and added 'drive' or motivation to activities. Moreover, shared beliefs would have facilitated social bonding. Transcendent beliefs may have been particularly attractive as they added meaning to life, reduced suffering and often provided a way of reducing fear of death. Strong transcendental beliefs may have superseded kinship as a binding factor and will have promoted social interaction beyond the family. This may have reduced the risk of inbreeding, potentially a very important adaptation. The core factors mentioned here also play a role in how psychological mechanisms mediate between religion/spirituality and health benefits. This has significant implications for health care. Health-care workers might consider reminding patients of how they see meaning in life, how to integrate their transcendent perceptions in the understanding of treatment, and how to assist patients in using a spiritual perspective to reduce mental distress.

References

1. Chiu L, Emblen JD, Van Hofwegen L, Sawatzky R, Meyerhoff H. An integrative review of the concept of spirituality in the health sciences. West J Nurs Res. 2004;26(4):405–28.
2. Hill PC, Pargament KI. Advances in the conceptualization and measurement of religion and spirituality: implications for physical and mental health research. Psychol Relig Spiritual. 2008;S(1):3–17.
3. Paloutzian RF, Park CL. Handbook of the psychology of religion and spirituality. New York: Guilford; 2014.
4. Van Cappellen P, Toth-Gauthier M, Saroglou V, Fredrickson BL. Religion and well-being: the mediating role of positive emotions. J Happiness Stud. 2016;17(2):485–505.
5. Visser A, Garssen B, Vingerhoets A. Spirituality and well-being in cancer patients: a review. Psycho-Oncology. 2010;19(6):565–72.
6. Clayton-Jones D, Haglund K. The role of spirituality and religiosity in persons living with sickle cell disease: a review of the literature. J Holist Nurs. 2016;34(4):351–60.
7. Unterrainer H-F, Lewis AJ, Fink A. Religious/spiritual well-being, personality and mental health: a review of results and conceptual issues. J Relig Health. 2014;53(2):382–92.
8. Koenig HG. Religion, spirituality, and health: a review and update. Adv Mind Body Med. 2015;29(3):19–26.
9. Sinclair S, Pereira J, Raffin S. A thematic review of the spirituality literature within palliative care. J Palliat Med. 2006;9(2):464–79.
10. Ogden J. Health psychology. London: McGraw-Hill Education; 2012.
11. Kumar V, Kumar S. Workplace spirituality as a moderator in relation between stress and health: an exploratory empirical assessment. Int Rev Psychiatry. 2014;26(3):344–51.
12. Martin RV. Spirituality in law enforcement: an exploration of possible correlations of spirituality to burnout and job satisfaction for police officers. Regent University; 2016.
13. Cladder JM. Past-life therapy with difficult phobics. J Regres Ther. 1986;I(2):81–5.
14. Miner M, Dowson M. Spirituality: perspectives from psychology. In: Spirituality across disciplines: research and practice. Basel: Springer; 2016. p. 165–78.

15. Rogers CR. The place of the person in the new world of the behavioral sciences. J Couns Dev. 1961;39(6):442–51.
16. Maslow AH, Frager R, Fadiman J, McReynolds C, Cox R. Motivation and personality. New York: Harper & Row; 1970.
17. Vitz PC. Psychology as religion: the cult of self worship. Grand Rapids: William b. Eerdmans Publishing Co.; 1977. p. 144.
18. Rhine J. The relation between parapsychology and general psychology. J Parapsychol. 1949;13:215–24.
19. Tenhaeff W. Some aspects of parapsychological research in the Netherlands. Int J Neuropsychiatry. 1966;2(5):408.
20. Boerenkamp HC. Helderziendheid Bekeken. Haarlem: De Toorts; 1988.
21. Seligman ME, Csikszentmihalyi M. Positive psychology: an introduction. Washington, DC: American Psychological Association; 2000.
22. Langer EJ, Moldoveanu M. The construct of mindfulness. J Soc Issues. 2000;56(1):1–9.
23. Reuder ME. A history of Division 36 (psychology of religion). In: Unification through division: histories of the divisions of the American Psychological Association, vol. 4. Washington, DC: American Psychological Association; 1999. p. 91–108.
24. Zinnbauer BJ, Pargament KI, Cole B, Rye MS, Butter EM, Belavich TG, et al. Religion and spirituality: unfuzzying the fuzzy. J Sci Study Relig. 1997;36(4):549–64.
25. Hill PC, Pargament KI, Hood RW, Mccullough ME, Swyers JP, Larson DB, et al. Conceptualizing religion and spirituality: points of commonality, points of departure. J Theory Soc Behav. 2000;30(1):27.
26. Falb MD, Pargament KI. Religion, spirituality, and positive psychology: strengthening well-being. In: Teramoto Pedrotti J, Edwards L, editors. Perspectives on the intersection of multi-culturalism and positive psychology. Dordrecht: Springer; 2014. p. 143–57.
27. Coyle J. Spirituality and health: towards a framework for exploring the relationship between spirituality and health. J Adv Nurs. 2002;37(6):589–97.
28. Tarakeshwar N, Stanton J, Pargament KI. Religion: an overlooked dimension in cross-cultural psychology. J Cross-Cult Psychol. 2003;34(4):377–94.
29. Heine SJ. Cultural psychology: third international student edition. New York: WW Norton & Company; 2015.
30. Allport GW. The individual and his religion: a psychological interpretation. Oxford: Macmillan; 1950.
31. Fowler JW, Levin RW. Stages of faith the psychology of human development and the quest for meaning. Int J Philos Relig. 1984;15(1):89–92.
32. Fallot RD. Spirituality and religion in psychiatric rehabilitation and recovery from mental illness. Int Rev Psychiatry. 2001;13(2):110–6.
33. Spilka B, Hood RW, Hunsberger B, Gorsuch R. The psychology of religion: an empirical approach. 3rd ed. New York: Guilford; 2003.
34. Galen L. Overlapping mental magisteria: implications of experimental psychology for a theory of religious belief as misattribution. Method Theory Study Relig. 2017;29(3):221–67.
35. Spilka BE, McIntosh DN. The psychology of religion: theoretical approaches. Boulder: Westview Press; 1997.
36. McNamara P. The neuroscience of religious experience. New York: Cambridge University Press; 2009.
37. Fingelkurts AA, Fingelkurts AA. Is our brain hardwired to produce God, or is our brain hardwired to perceive God? A systematic review on the role of the brain in mediating religious experience. Cogn Process. 2009;10(4):293–326.
38. van Elk M, Zwaan R. Predictive processing and situation models: constructing and reconstructing religious experience. Relig Brain Behav. 2017;7(1):85–7.
39. Gaulin SJ, McBurney DH. Psychology: an evolutionary approach. Upper Saddle River: Prentice Hall; 2001.
40. Buss DM. Evolutionary psychology: the new science of the mind. Boston: Allyn & Bacon; 1999.

41. Tooby J, Cosmides L. The past explains the present: emotional adaptations and the structure of ancestral environments. Ethol Sociobiol. 1990;11(4):375–424.
42. Buss DM, editor. The handbook of evolutionary psychology, volume 1: foundation. Hoboken: Wiley; 2015.
43. Kirkpatrick LA. Attachment, evolution, and the psychology of religion. New York: Guilford; 2005.
44. Kirkpatrick LA. Religion is not an adaptation. In: McNamara P, editor. Where men and god meet: how brain and evolutionary studies alter our understanding of religion, vol. 1. Santa Barbara: Praeger; 2006. p. 159–79.
45. Flannelly KJ. Belief in god as an attachment figure and mental health. In: Religious beliefs, evolutionary psychiatry, and mental health in America. Cham: Springer; 2017. p. 211–23.
46. Sosis R. The adaptationist-byproduct debate on the evolution of religion: five misunderstandings of the adaptationist program. J Cogn Cult. 2009;9(3):315–32.
47. Sosis R, Alcorta C. Signaling, solidarity, and the sacred: the evolution of religious behavior. Evol Anthropol Issues News Rev. 2003;12(6):264–74.
48. Baddeley A. The magical number seven: still magic after all these years? Psychol Rev. 1994;101(2):353–6.
49. Fiske ST. Stereotyping, prejudice, and discrimination at the seam between the centuries: evolution, culture, mind, and brain. Eur J Soc Psychol. 2000;30(3):299–322.
50. Bering J. The belief instinct: the psychology of souls, destiny, and the meaning of life. New York: Norton & Company; 2012.
51. Mogenson GJ, Jones DL, Yim CY. From motivation to action: functional interface between the limbic system and the motor system. Prog Neurobiol. 1980;14(2):69–97.
52. Jones WE. The goods and the motivation of believing. Epistemic Value. 2009;10:139–62.
53. Bulbulia J. The cognitive and evolutionary psychology of religion. Biol Philos. 2004;19(5):655–86.
54. Beauregard M. Mind does really matter: evidence from neuroimaging studies of emotional self-regulation, psychotherapy, and placebo effect. Prog Neurobiol. 2007;81(4):218–36.
55. Bensing JM, Verheul W. The silent healer: the role of communication in placebo effects. Patient Educ Couns. 2010;80(3):293–9.
56. Boozang KM. The therapeutic placebo: the case for patient deception. Fla Law Rev. 2002;54:687.
57. Enck P, Benedetti F, Schedlowski M. New insights into the placebo and nocebo responses. Neuron. 2008;59(2):195–206.
58. Wager TD, Atlas LY. The neuroscience of placebo effects: connecting context, learning and health. Nat Rev Neurosci. 2015;16(7):403–18.
59. Koenig HG. Religion, spirituality, and health: the research and clinical implications. ISRN Psychiatry. 2012;2012:278730.
60. Kosfeld M. Trust in the brain. EMBO Rep. 2007;8(1S):S44–S7.
61. Emmons RA. The psychology of ultimate concerns: motivation and spirituality in personality. New York: Guilford; 1999.
62. Zika S, Chamberlain K. On the relation between meaning in life and psychological well-being. Br J Psychol. 1992;83(1):133–45.
63. Park J, Baumeister RF. Meaning in life and adjustment to daily stressors. J Posit Psychol. 2017;12(4):333–41.
64. Steger MF, Frazier P. Meaning in life: one link in the chain from religiousness to well-being. J Couns Psychol. 2005;52(4):574.
65. Phelps AC, Maciejewski PK, Nilsson M, et al. Religious coping and use of intensive life-prolonging care near death in patients with advanced cancer. JAMA. 2009;301(11):1140–7.
66. Krause N. Longitudinal study of social support and meaning in life. Psychol Aging. 2007;22(3):456.
67. Steger MF, Oishi S, Kashdan TB. Meaning in life across the life span: levels and correlates of meaning in life from emerging adulthood to older adulthood. J Posit Psychol. 2009;4(1):43–52.

68. Moos RH, Schaefer JA. The crisis of physical illness. In: Coping with physical illness. Boston: Springer; 1984. p. 3–25.
69. de Vries J, Timmins F. Understanding psychology for nursing students. London: Sage; 2017.
70. Karekla M, Constantinou M. Religious coping and cancer: proposing an acceptance and commitment therapy approach. Cogn Behav Pract. 2010;17(4):371–81.
71. Goyal M, Singh S, Sibinga EM, Gould NF, Rowland-Seymour A, Sharma R, et al. Meditation programs for psychological stress and well-being: a systematic review and meta-analysis. JAMA Intern Med. 2014;174(3):357–68.
72. Edwards MJ, Holden RR. Coping, meaning in life, and suicidal manifestations: examining gender differences. J Clin Psychol. 2001;57(12):1517–34.
73. Hall J, Taylor M. Birth and spirituality. In: Normal childbirth: evidence and debate. New York: Elsevier; 2004. p. 41–56.
74. Aronson E. The theory of cognitive dissonance: a current perspective. Adv Exp Soc Psychol. 1969;4:1–34.
75. Cooper J. Cognitive dissonance: 50 years of a classic theory. London: Sage; 2007.
76. Festinger L. A theory of cognitive dissonance. Stanford: Stanford university press; 1957.
77. DeHaven MJ, Hunter IB, Wilder L, Walton JW, Berry J. Health programs in faith-based organizations: are they effective? Am J Public Health. 2004;94(6):1030–6.
78. Aronson E. The social animal. 9th ed. New York: Worth; 2004.
79. Nooney J, Woodrum E. Religious coping and church-based social support as predictors of mental health outcomes: testing a conceptual model. J Sci Study Relig. 2002;41(2):359–68.
80. Cooper CL, Quick JC. The handbook of stress and health: a guide to research and practice. Hoboken: Wiley; 2017.
81. Uchino BN, Cacioppo JT, Kiecolt-Glaser JK. The relationship between social support and physiological processes: a review with emphasis on underlying mechanisms and implications for health. Psychol Bull. 1996;119(3):488.
82. Thoits PA. Stress and health: major findings and policy implications. J Health Soc Behav. 2010;51(1_suppl):S41–53.
83. Wang X, Cai L, Qian J, Peng J. Social support moderates stress effects on depression. Int J Ment Heal Syst. 2014;8(1):41.
84. Winkelman M. Shamanism. In: Encyclopedia of medical anthropology. New York: Springer; 2004. p. 145–54.
85. Candy B, Jones L, Varagunam M, Speck P, Tookman A, King M. Spiritual and religious interventions for well-being of adults in the terminal phase of disease. Cochrane Database Syst Rev. 2012;5:CD007544.
86. Nilsson U. The anxiety-and pain-reducing effects of music interventions: a systematic review. AORN J. 2008;87(4):780–807.
87. Humphreys K, Blodgett JC, Wagner TH. Estimating the efficacy of alcoholics anonymous without self-selection bias: an instrumental variables re-analysis of randomized clinical trials. Alcohol Clin Exp Res. 2014;38(11):2688–94.
88. Pierce LL, Steiner V, Havens H, Tormoehlen K. Spirituality expressed by caregivers of stroke survivors. West J Nurs Res. 2008;30(5):606–19.

Spiritual Assessment in Healthcare: An Overview of Comprehensive, Sensitive Approaches to Spiritual Assessment for Use Within the Interdisciplinary Healthcare Team

3

Wilfred McSherry, Linda Ross, Karnsunaphat Balthip, Natasha Ross, and Sadie Young

Abstract

The provision of healthcare involves dialogue and interaction between those receiving and those providing care. These interactions incorporate the need for building relationships based upon mutual trust and respect. The delivery of healthcare across all professions necessitates the need to conduct some form of assessment to identify an individual's healthcare needs. This assessment should be holistic in nature addressing all aspects of the person including physical, psychological, social and spiritual domains. However, because of the misconceptions and assumptions associated with the concept of spirituality, spiritual needs of the person are often overlooked and neglected in the delivery of healthcare. Therefore, this chapter provides a brief overview of some of the key features of spiritual assessment offering a new pragmatic two-question model for spiritual

W. McSherry (✉)
Department of Nursing, School of Health and Social Care, Staffordshire University, Stafford, UK

The University Hospitals of North Midlands, NHS Trust, Stoke-on-Trent, UK

VID Specialized University (Haraldsplass Campus), Stavanger, Norway
e-mail: w.mcsherry@staffs.ac.uk

L. Ross · S. Young
Faculty of Life Sciences and Education, School of Care Sciences, University of South Wales, Pontypridd, UK

K. Balthip
Public Health Nursing Department, Faculty of Nursing, Prince of Songkla University, Hatyai, Songkhla, Thailand

N. Ross
Faculty of Life Sciences and Education, School of Psychology and Therapeutic Studies, University of South Wales, City Campus, Newport, UK

assessment and goes on to explore how the model may be useful in addressing spiritual needs in a range of different settings.

3.1 Introduction

The information used in most patient care plans, whether written or electronic, is primarily derived from and based upon some form of standard assessment tool. Spiritual assessment is '…an attempt to enquire positively and unobtrusively with a patient/client or their carers into areas of life that are associated with their health and well-being. It is more than just an enquiry into physical health' ([1], p. 61). Spiritual assessment involves action and the process of enquiry combined with information gathering and interpretation [2]. Patient care plans should therefore be rooted in a variety of diverse assessments that cover the multiplicity of patient care [3, 4]. Whether or not the evaluation of a person's spiritual needs is called 'screening' or 'assessment', for healthcare professionals, this type of activity ought to be encompassed within standardised approaches to assessment. An 'appropriate spiritual assessment' allows the healthcare professional to identify the personal, religious and spiritual needs, resources and coping mechanisms of a patient.

There is recognition across healthcare practice and education that a more open qualitative approach to spiritual assessment is most appropriate, despite a growing focus and desire for more quantitative methods and scientific evidence [5]. As such, any form of spiritual assessment ought to be based upon local needs and agreements and not simply a 'tick box' exercise. The style and language should be practical, clear and simple and ideally developed with staff and patients to ensure fitness for purpose and to maximise utility [1]. It is important to note that the tool has no magic formula in itself. Its usefulness in addressing spiritual need will be entirely reliant on the discernment and sensitivity of the healthcare professional using it [5].

This chapter will briefly explore some key features of spiritual assessment and its implementation and operation across the healthcare team. The chapter offers a new pragmatic two-question model for spiritual assessment and goes on to explore how the model may be useful in addressing spiritual needs in a range of different settings.

3.2 Aims

This chapter will:

1. Explore what is meant by the term spiritual assessment, outlining the different types and approaches.
2. Describe the main features of a spiritual assessment tool giving consideration to how these will influence care.
3. Provide a pragmatic two-question model for undertaking a spiritual assessment within healthcare practice and explore its application in different settings.

3.3 Background

Healthcare is dynamic and constantly changing to meet the diverse needs of individuals and societies. Despite the vast improvements, innovations and technologies that have enhanced available treatments, the delivery of healthcare still involves the recognition and validation of the person, in a caring relationship that is dignified, respectful and compassionate. Healthcare that is devoid of these humanistic and altruistic elements can feel overly scientific and 'heartless' [6].

It is widely accepted that healthcare must attend to the holistic needs of individuals: physical, psychological, social and spiritual [7, 8]. In reality, however, although many healthcare professionals feel comfortable in assessing and supporting individuals with the first three dimensions, they feel less confident and competent with the spiritual dimension of care [9].

In recent years, healthcare provision has been driven by the scientific, medical and curative model of care. The mantra of evidence-based practice has echoed across health and care services shaping practice and the delivery of care. Spiritual aspects of care appear to be being forced or 'shoehorned' down a narrower scientific paradigm. This is evident by the development of a large number of quantitative studies [10] and bespoke indicator-based, and value clarification, spiritual assessment tools [11]. Whilst the rationale may be to gain scientific/academic credibility by producing quantifiable evidence that demonstrates impact and better outcomes, recognition must also be given to the more subjective and qualitative nature of spirituality making it difficult to measure and quantify.

We suggest that the hierarchy of scientific evidence which values meta-analysis and systematic reviews more highly than qualitative evidence may need reconsideration and remodelling when applied to the spiritual dimension. This is important because what constitutes credible and trustworthy scientific evidence is certainly influencing and directing how healthcare professional assess, plan, implement and evaluate care, including spiritual care. Attempts to redress this balance can perhaps be seen in the Patient-Reported Outcomes Measures (PROMs) and Patient-Reported Experience Measures (PREMs) movement in its attempts to capture the patient/client experience, but again PROMs try to capture qualitative accounts using objective measures [12].

3.4 Undertaking a Holistic Patient Assessment

In the United Kingdom, the Nursing and Midwifery Council (NMC), the professional regulatory body for nurses and midwives, states:

> Registered nurses prioritise the needs of people when assessing and reviewing their mental, physical, cognitive, behavioural, social and spiritual needs. They use information obtained during assessments to identify the priorities and requirements for person-centred and evidence based nursing interventions and support. They work in partnership with people to develop person-centred care plans that take into account their circumstances, characteristics and preferences. ([13], p. 13)

This statement affirms it is the responsibility of all nurses to undertake a holistic assessment of their patient's needs in partnership with people important to them and members of the multidisciplinary team. This holistic assessment includes a spiritual assessment, an area that nurses often struggle with [9] and which this chapter seeks to address.

The following exercise (3.1) invites you to consider these different dimensions of care when undertaking a holistic assessment. The case involves admitting a patient into the emergency department. (This exercise was created by Sadie Young based on her presentation 'Incorporating spirituality into holistic patient assessment' at the 8th International Student Conference on Spiritual Care, Copenhagen, Denmark, 20–22 September 2017).

Introductory Exercise 3.1

As the admitting nurse, you have to undertake a holistic assessment of Gerry's needs. These are listed in Table 3.1. What order would you place them in? And why?

Here is some demographic and medical information about Gerry you are admitting:

Setting:	emergency department
Patient:	Gerry, 60-year-old male
Presenting complaint:	ischaemic stroke
Previous medical history:	high blood pressure
Social:	lives at home with his wife
Plan:	thrombolysis, rehabilitation

Linda Ross's group, who undertook this exercise, temporarily put them in the following order (see Table 3.2). 'Informal spiritual assessment', 'social needs' and 'mental capacity' moved around from moment to moment, which is why they are arranged around the outside.

Compare your list and prioritisation with the list presented in Table 3.2, and note the different positioning of the items. There are a number of points that this exercise highlights with regard to undertaking a holistic assessment upon admission to hospital, and these have implications for the delivery of healthcare practice:

Table 3.1 Gerry's needs

Needs/action	Order
Social needs	
Mental capacity	
Mobility	
Formal spiritual assessment, full documented assessment	
Informal spiritual assessment	
Past medical history	
Psychological assessment	
Washing, dressing, continence, eating and drinking	
Neurological assessment; Glasgow Coma Scale	
Blood pressure, pulse, respiration rate, blood glucose, ECG	

Table 3.2 Feedback on activity

	Informal spiritual assessment	
Social needs	Blood pressure, pulse, respiration rate, blood glucose, ECG	Mental capacity
	Neurological assessment, Glasgow coma scale	
	Washing, dressing, continence, eating and drinking	
	Psychological assessment	
	Past medical history	
	Formal spiritual assessment, full documented assessment	
	Mobility	

- Assessment of patient needs is a fluid concept. The nurse can begin their assessment at handover and develop the identification of needs through observing and talking with the patient. There is no hard and fast rule of what is going to be the right procedure for every patient.
- Patient needs and assessments are subjective and individual so the nurse needs to be aware of the risks of following an overly structured and prescriptive approach.
- This task may help to illuminate the nurse's own preconceptions of their patients. Reflecting on how you undertook this exercise may highlight strengths and weaknesses within your skill set.

3.5 Approaches to Spiritual Assessment

There are many approaches to spiritual assessment well documented in the healthcare literature ranging from the informal to the more formal [2, 3, 14]. McSherry and Ross [2, 14] list six categories of approach to spiritual assessment:

Direct methods:	asking direct questions about personal, religious, spiritual needs.
Indicator-based models:	spiritual distress, diagnosis.
Audit tools:	institutional attempts to audit practice in this area.
Value clarification:	Likert-type scales to explore values/perceptions of spirituality and spiritual need.
Indirect methods:	Cues to potential spiritual needs are identified through observation of the environment and/or demeanour/attitudes/behaviours of the individual.
Acronym-based models:	simple models incorporated within the general assessment process, simple to administer and use.

This list shows that spiritual assessment spans a continuum of approaches and that the terminology can be confusing. For example, in some countries (e.g. the United States and Canada), the term 'screening' (direct method) tends to refer to the initial enquiry about a person's personal, religious and spiritual beliefs and can be conducted by any healthcare professional. The outcome of the initial screening may identify the need for a more in-depth spiritual 'history' or 'assessment' which would require referral to the specialist healthcare chaplain.

Informal (indirect) methods necessitate the healthcare practitioner using a range of communication and interpersonal skills (verbal and non-verbal) to observe and assess patient need. This will require establishing rapport and a trusting meaningful relationship with the patient. First impressions are important, so an open, friendly and polite welcoming approach upon admission is vital to enabling the individual to feel comfortable and relaxed within the caring environment.

To launch directly into the admission process with a range of intrusive personal questions such as 'Do you have a religion?' or 'Do you have any personal, religious, spiritual beliefs?', for example, if the patient is in excruciating pain or experiencing severe nausea and vomiting, would certainly be inappropriate. Therefore, it is important for informal spiritual assessment to be continuous in nature and sensitive to the priorities that have resulted in admission.

Once the reasons for admission have been resolved and the patient is comfortable, it may be appropriate to ask a simple screening question to identify any urgent personal, religious and spiritual beliefs but not in any formal or structured manner. This information could be obtained during the admitting conversation or dialogue.

Formal spiritual assessment may involve the use of a structured assessment tool. Examples of acronym-based tools include *P*ermission, *L*imited information, *A*ctivating resources, *N*on-nursing assistance (PLAN) [15] and *F*aith or beliefs, *I*mportance and influence, *C*ommunity and *A*ddress (FICA) [16] and *H*, sources of hope, strength, comfort, meaning, peace, love and connection; *O*, the role of organised religion; *P*, personal spirituality and practices; *E*, effects on medical care and end-of-life decisions (HOPE) ([17], p. 81). These models are primarily used in the initial consultation, or upon first meeting the patient, to obtain information that may be indicative of underlying spiritual needs. Close attention should be given to how these tools are used and introduced within the admission process.

As highlighted above, the NMC calls for nurses to include a spiritual assessment as part of the 'holistic' care they are called to deliver. This makes sense because the nurse is in the unique position of being with the patient 24 h/day, 7 days/week. The nurse also performs advocacy and signposting roles, for example, to specialist spiritual care services. It has been argued that unless nurses identify patients' spiritual concerns, it is very likely that these concerns will go unrecognised and unmet [18].

Spiritual assessment tools have been available in the literature for almost four decades and are mostly American in origin. One of the pioneering tools was developed by Stoll [19] titled 'Guidelines for Spiritual Assessment'. This was a direct method of assessment asking a number of questions focusing upon religious beliefs, practices and sources of support. Many contemporary tools have built upon this original work.

Despite the rhetoric indicating that nurses and healthcare professionals should undertake a spiritual assessment, the evidence suggests that they find this challenging, preferring informal rather than formal approaches. Recent surveys in the United Kingdom and Australia have shown that only 2.2% ($n = 3$ out of 139, [9]) and 26% ([20], $n = 18$ out of 191) of nurses/healthcare professionals, respectively, said they used formal spiritual assessment tools. In both these studies, the most frequent means of identifying patients' spiritual needs was informally by picking up on cues from the patient, by listening and by observation.

3.6 An Integrated Approach

The overriding concern when conducting any form of spiritual assessment is that it is integrated with the entire process of care, rather than being an 'add-on' or 'optional extra'. Clarke [21] captures this when she writes:

> Nurses are in the privileged position of being able to touch and work with people's bodies in a unique way, yet have been seduced into believing that talking was the only way to provide spiritual care. This book has challenged that view and argued that there is another way to provide spiritual care by embedding it into every encounter and relationship and into the physicality of everyday nursing and midwifery care.

This quotation is important and radical in terms of its implication for spiritual assessment because it suggests a new paradigm is required around the way we conceive and undertake it in practice. It implies that spiritual assessment should be integrated within everyday nursing practice and in each patient encounter.

3.7 Introducing an Alternative Pragmatic Model for Spiritual Assessment

So far we have seen that spiritual assessment is expected of nurses as part of the wider holistic assessment they are called to undertake, but that this may not happen, certainly not in any formal way. So, how realistic is it to expect nurses to carry out a spiritual assessment in the current climate with staff shortages, where they are already overstretched and are struggling to meet immediate physical or mental health needs and to provide safe (clinical) care?

3.7.1 A Reflection upon Current Practice: A Colleague's Experience

Let us reflect on a recent example from practice. A colleague, Maggie, has just returned to work following surgery. I (LR) asked her about her experience of the nursing care. She responded by saying:

> The nurses were great but they were so rushed off their feet. They could barely fit in taking a medical history so they certainly didn't have time to ask me about my spiritual needs. But I did have spiritual needs although I might not have recognised them as such at the time.

Maggie was very frightened one night when she felt really poorly after surgery and was worried about dying. When I asked her who she would have liked to have talked to, she said a chaplain or anyone with time to listen, but not family for fear of worrying them. Her spiritual needs were never addressed and highlight Ross's [18] concerns noted above.

In this case Maggie had spiritual needs (to talk about fear of dying), but nurses were too busy to pick up on this. So, how realistic is it to expect nurses to carry out a formal spiritual assessment? Can we really expect them to carry out an additional assessment on top of everything else and to deliver spiritual care as an add-on to the other nursing care? Maybe these expectations are not realistic.

However, what if you could carry out a spiritual assessment without the need for any special assessment tool and without the need for much extra time? What if all that was needed was keeping in mind two simple questions that could be used on admission and at any point during the shift thereafter, ensuring that the care being given at any point is responsive to real and current need?

These two questions are 'What is important to you right now' and 'How can we help?' (see Fig. 3.1).

Let's see how these questions might work in the above situation with Maggie. She may have responded to the first question by saying 'I'm really scared and worried about dying' and to the second question with 'I'd really like to speak to a chaplain'. Her need could have been addressed without involving much 'extra' time, as these questions could have been asked whilst the nurse was giving other care, for example, whilst helping her to turn or go to the bathroom. The only extra time needed would have been in making the phone call to the chaplaincy team. The science (helping Maggie to turn or go to the bathroom) and the art (responding to her fear about dying) of nursing would both have been evident in this example resulting in the best outcome for Maggie at that moment in time. What was important to Maggie (that which gave her meaning and purpose and which is therefore spiritual) at that moment would have been addressed. Fast forward to the morning, asking the same questions again 'what's important to you right now?' and 'how can we help' might elicit a different response such as 'I really need to get to the bathroom' and 'can you please wheel me there'. This time there is a physical need. Later, the same questions might trigger the response 'I'm really worried that my daughter hasn't arrived; she said she was coming' and 'is it possible for me to call her?' This time there is a psychosocial need.

3.7.2 Benefits of This Model

Using the same two questions for each episode of care throughout an entire shift does a number of important things:

– It ensures that *assessment is continuous*, not something that is just done on admission and then is forgotten.
– It deals with the most important (meaningful and therefore it could be argued 'spiritual') issue for the patient at any moment in time.
– The care resulting from that assessment is *dynamic*, *person-centred* and *needs led* providing the potential for the best care outcome to be achieved.
– It provides a model for holistic assessment, with the spiritual at the heart (always focusing on what is meaningful to the patient during any care episode), without the need for a special tool, much extra time or additional documentation. Needs and care can be documented as part of the normal documentation processes so there is no need for additional care plans or reporting sheets.

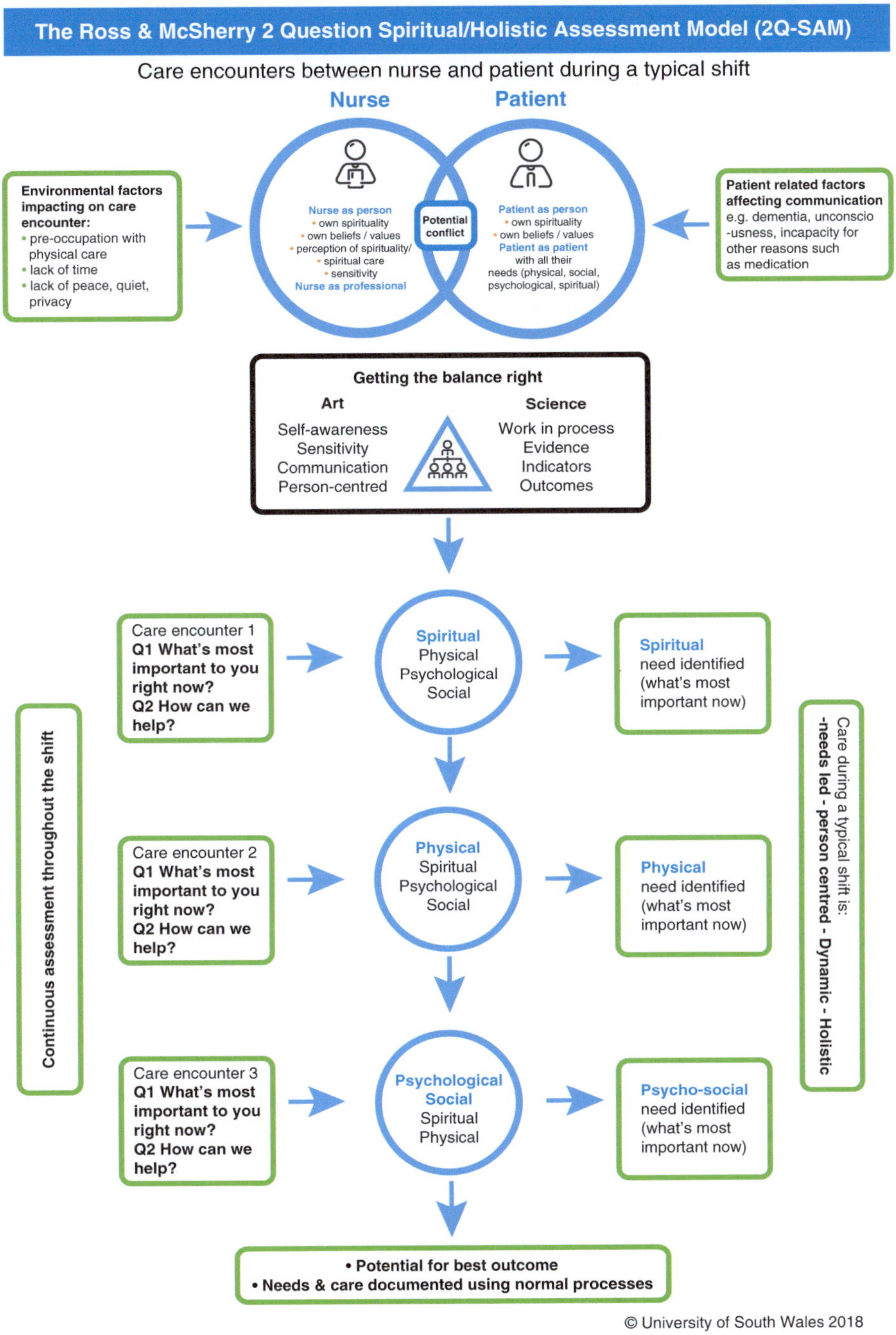

Fig. 3.1 Incorporates aspects of the following models: 'Factors which appeared to influence spiritual care' in Ross [22]. The need for balance in spiritual care in McSherry and Ross [2]. Reproduced by kind permission from M&K Update Ltd, UK from the original image drawn by Mary Blood (2010) ISBN: 9781905539277

3.7.3 Caveats in the Model

3.7.3.1 Self-Awareness

It can be seen that, in the above example, both the *art and the science* of nursing are intermingled and care emanates within the milieu of the nurse-patient relationship. This last point is crucial, because sensitive interpersonal skills, attitude, 'way of being' and personal warmth (*art*) are key to the entire care episodes' success or otherwise. It is here that the nurse's sensitivity and awareness of their own spirituality, beliefs and values is important as evidence shows that these affect the care given [22–26]. So nurses need to be aware of their beliefs/values and their own limitations, knowing when to refer on to another healthcare professional to ensure that what is important to the patient is addressed and not ignored [22].

The Caroline Petrie case (see [27]) highlights the importance of self-awareness and maintaining personal and professional boundaries.

3.7.3.2 The Unconscious Patient

Any factor interfering with the ability of the patient to communicate their need presents a challenge for holistic assessment (Fig. 3.1). So how can what is important to the unconscious patient be elicited? The question is still a valid and important one, but the patient cannot be asked. Perhaps it is down to the nurse asking the 'importance' question of friends and family combined with what information she/he can glean from the notes about what seems to have been important to the person before they became ill. Critical care diaries might be useful here as a means of identifying what is important and keeping a record of that to enable the patient to 'fill in the gaps' of that lost time after recovery [28].

3.7.3.3 The Person Who Is Conscious But has Difficulty in Articulating Their Spiritual Needs

This might apply to people with learning disabilities, dementia, or people, such as Maggie, who had difficulty in expressing how she felt about what was important to her due to the effect of strong analgesia post-surgery (PCA). In these circumstances, is the 'importance' question still useful and who is the best person to ask it? This will very much depend on the person, but someone with learning disabilities might still be able to say 'what's important' to them or to answer a variant of that, such as 'what's on your mind?' or 'what's worrying you?', which may allow them to articulate their spiritual needs. Their key worker might be the best person placed to facilitate this discussion. For the person with dementia, the care co-ordinator may be best placed to ask this question in conjunction with the family and with information obtained from the 'this is me' document and other documentation about their past life before dementia took hold. Variants of that question might include 'what gave your life meaning?', or 'what once gave you hope?'

In the case of Maggie, where powerful medication masked her ability to communicate her spiritual needs, there are perhaps two stages in this process. In response to being asked 'what's important to you right now', she may have said that she felt very unwell and was concerned about having a temperature and infection (physical health) to which the nurse may have provided reassurance. The follow-on question here might have been 'so as well as your concerns about your temperature, is there anything else on your mind that you are concerned about right now?' This follow-on question would have given Maggie permission to raise the more difficult subject about being afraid of dying. This is important in an environment which focuses predominantly on physical aspects of care (see top left box in Fig. 3.1). This question of 'being able to speak about what's on my mind' has been identified as an important question in hospital chaplaincy [29].

3.8 Application of the Model in Different Settings

Let's see how these two questions and this proposed model might work in other situations involving other disciplines.

Example from nursing/medicine: Resuscitation in the emergency department. Sam and the medical model. The following is taken from Piles ([30], pp. 36–37):

> About 12 years again, a code [resuscitation] was called in a critical care unit while I was the faculty member for students practising in this area. ... The resuscitation team rushed in because Sam was in ventricular fibrillation. One member pounded his chest and started sticking needles in him to open a central line. Sam asked, "Am I going to die?" No one acknowledged his existence except to say "Breathe Sam!" Everyone was busy doing all the things they had been trained to do to restore a heartbeat. Sam asked once again, "Am I going to die?" No response except another harsh, "Breathe Sam!" More people entered the room to observe the [resuscitation] team in action but no one spoke to Sam. All Sam finally said was "I am going to die!!" Within 15 min, Sam was pronounced dead. The renunciation team left the room convinced they had done everything possible but the patient died anyway.
>
> My reaction was one of horror. There were 20 people in Sam's room but he died alone. Why didn't someone speak to that man, comfort that man, hold that man's hand, pray with that man? Had the science of nursing overshadowed the art of nursing?

So, in this scenario, had the nurse asked Sam 'What is most important to you right now?' he might have answered 'For someone to answer my question "Am I going to die?"'.

What is important to Sam (acknowledging his urgent existential question about death) seems to be in direct conflict with the healthcare team's perception of what is most important (the preservation of life).

In this situation, the nurse's role is to advocate on the patient's behalf, ensuring that what's important to the patient is acknowledged (the art) but also ensuring that the staff's concern to preserve life (science) is addressed. So there is another caveat in the model, that of conflicting priorities and how to manage that.

Example from psychology (provided by Natasha Ross, based on her presentation 'Students' perceptions of spirituality/religion and spiritual coping' at the 8th International Student Conference on Spiritual Care, Copenhagen, Denmark, 20–22 September 2017).

The two questions can equally apply in non-clinical settings, such as in psychology. As part of a university dissertation eight university students (both religious and non-religious) were interviewed about their perceptions of spirituality and the role of spiritual coping in helping them deal with student life [31]. Although the question 'what is most important to you' was not asked in that way during the interviews, students in effect answered that question by saying that a number of things were important to them as follows (from thematic analysis of the eight interviews).

Meaning and purpose: e.g. '…being a Christian kinda gives me meaning and purpose in life…and gives me energy, gives me hope all of those kind of things'. Pt. 4

Morals and values: e.g. '…I always relate back to those like core values and those basic ways of acting with people and I mean, everyone gets into conflict with people…and I suppose spirituality and religion have sort of helped me bite my tongue a bit more'. Pt 3

Connection with the self: e.g. '…I think that you realise who you are and it (spirituality), helps you to become the person you wana be, not so materialistic, not so judgemental you know being the better version of you'. Pt 7

Connection with others: e.g. '…I think because I feel spiritually connected to people um and their personalities obviously that spiritual connection gives my life meaning and purpose as well'. Pt 3

Connection with the transcendent: e.g. '…I understand other people you know, they look at it (spirituality) as being close to God which is in my opinion, I don't see it as a difference to me seeking to be close to my soul…'. Pt 5

They also said that what helped them to cope with university life ('how can we help' question) included:

Religious and non-religious coping: e.g. '…meditation is a big one that helps me to cope massively…if I'm just feeling stressed I'll do it because…it just helps me to calm down it just, makes my mind a lot clearer…'. Pt 8

Comfort—in an afterlife: e.g. 'I think the greatest way it helps me to cope is…hope that there's a better world and um, yeah hope that this isn't it uh a hope that suffering is not the be all and end all…'. Pt 4

Comfort—journey in this life: e.g. '...I suppose God does have his best interest for you you've just got to be able to, see the good in the situation...when bad things come they're not easy but it sort of helps you to get through it a lot better'. Pt 6

So these two questions could potentially be helpful to universities in planning how they may more effectively support their students throughout their studies. For example, staying connected (to self, others, transcendent) was important and was an issue raised for discussion by the participants attending the workshop at the Student Conference. Discussion centred on the loneliness and isolation felt by students even although they were very well connected by social media. So universities might foster a sense of connection by providing 'social spaces' for students to meet face to face and by including, for example, meditation/mindfulness events within wellbeing initatives which would facilitate time for self. The latter was suggested by interviewees as a tool which would ease stress and anxiety.

Interestingly the themes identified in this small study endorse some of the key attributes of spirituality outlined in recent definitions [32, 33].

Example from Thailand: Adolescent living with HIV/AIDS.

In Thailand it is normal practice for young people diagnosed with HIV/AIDS to visit the hospital HIV clinic (located in the outpatient department) following referral by their doctor. The HIV clinic administers antiretroviral therapy as part of the patient treatment and care package.

The primary focus of Thai nurses in the HIV clinic is on assessing the physical health status (science) of the young person to receive antiretroviral therapy, maximise adherence and minimise side effects. Due to workload demands, holistic assessments (art), which include a spiritual assessment, are not always undertaken.

Although the spiritual part of life is widely accepted as important by Thai scholars, the Thai academic community and the Thai government and lay Thai people including Thai adolescents do not have an expectation that their spiritual needs (which are important to them) will be addressed as part of healthcare [34–36]. Moreover, as Thailand transitions from a traditional to a modern society, a study has found that, despite Thai adolescents still continuing to pray or worship, a decreasing percentage of them believe in the law of karma as part of their Buddhist philosophy [37]. So, in the more modern Thai society, it may be more appropriate to enquire about young people's spiritual needs by asking the more generally phrased questions 'What is important to you right now' and 'How can we help?' However, the model may require to be adapted for the Thai culture by including some preliminary stages as follows.

Before asking these two questions, it would be customary to say 'Sawasdee ka or Sawasdee krub'. This greeting is about acknowledging and recognising the person. The nurse may then begin the dialogue by asking 'how are you feeling today?' whilst making eye contact and physical contact with the patient (e.g. holding the patient's hand or touching the shoulder). This shows genuine concern and compassion and establishes trust paving the way for the young person to express any deeper fears or concerns they may have. The two questions from the model can now be asked. The following is an actual response from a young person:

> I take the ARV drugs on time because I want to be healthy. I don't want to die before my grandparents who take care of me… My grandmother has lost her daughter (my mother)… I have to live to be the representative of my mum. … I should have good behaviour. I want to continue my life [35, 36].

This young person was able to articulate his psychosocial and spiritual needs in response to those two questions. He had a strong bond with his grandparents and wanted to continue to live with them and do his best for them. Being able to do this was what was most important to him giving 'meaning and purpose' to his life, a term which may be more culturally meaningful than 'spirituality'. Follow-up questions could be phrased 'You said, you want to live with your grandparent, why is this?' and 'What is the main purpose in your life?' and 'How can we help you achieve your purpose in life?' These questions are more culturally appropriate variants of 'What is important to you right now' and 'How can we help?'.

3.9 Conclusion

This chapter provides a brief overview of the different approaches to spiritual assessment. It highlights the importance of ensuring that such assessments are conducted in a respectful, sensitive manner enabling the patient to express what is most important to them at any point in time. The new 'two-question model for holistic/spiritual assessment' suggested in this chapter provides a practical and flexible means of undertaking a holistic patient-centred assessment without the need for a special tool or extra time or paperwork. As such, it is responsive to patient need and healthcare provider need for 'prudent healthcare'. The practice examples provided show that the model is relevant and adaptable to a wide range of clinical contexts and social settings ensuring that care is truly person-centred and needs led.

3.10 Summary Points

- Careful consideration must be given to the design, development and use of spiritual assessment tools within healthcare practice.
- Spiritual assessment may be conducted along a continuum involving a range of approaches and strategies; it must always be person-centred and conducted sensitively and in a nonintrusive manner.
- Conducting a spiritual assessment must never interfere with the delivery of dignified, humanistic and compassionate care.
- Spiritual assessment tools have the potential to make a significant contribution to the delivery of holistic care.

Acknowledgement We would like to thank Professor Maggie Kirk for sharing her experience of being a patient. Maggie was Professor of Genetics Education, School of Care Sciences, Faculty of Life Sciences and Education, University of South Wales, before she retired.

References

1. McSherry W. Spiritual assessment: definition, categorisation and features. In: McSherry W, Ross L, editors. Spiritual assessment in healthcare practice. 1st ed. Keswick: M&K Publishing; 2010.
2. McSherry W, Ross L, editors. Spiritual assessment in healthcare practice. 1st ed. Keswick: M&K Publishing; 2010.
3. Draper P. An integrative review of spiritual assessment: implications for nursing management. J Nurs Manag. 2012;20:970–80.
4. Pierce B. The introduction and evaluation of a spiritual assessment tool in a palliative care unit. Scott J Healthcare Chaplaincy. 2004;7(2):39–43.
5. Gordon T, Mitchell D. A competency model for the assessment and delivery of spiritual care. Palliat Med. 2004;18:646–51.
6. The Mid Staffordshire NHS Foundation Trust Public Inquiry. Report of the Mid Staffordshire NHS Foundation Trust public inquiry: executive summary. 2013. Available from http://webarchive.nationalarchives.gov.uk/20150407084003/http://www.midstaffspublicinquiry.com/. Accessed 28 Nov 2017.
7. NHS England. NHS Chaplaincy guidelines 2015. Promoting excellence in pastoral, spiritual & religious care. London: NHS England; 2015.
8. NICE. Care of dying adults in the last days of life. 2015. Available at https://www.nice.org.uk/guidance/ng31. Accessed 28 Nov 2017.
9. Royal College of Nursing. Spirituality survey 2010. 2010. Available at https://www.rcn.org.uk/professional-development/publications/pub-003861. Accessed 28 Nov 2017.
10. Koenig H, King D, Carson VB. Handbook of religion and health. 2nd ed. Oxford: Oxford University Press; 2012.
11. Baldacchino D. Indicator-based and value clarification tools. In: McSherry W, Ross L, editors. Spiritual assessment in healthcare practice. 1st ed. Keswick: M&K Publishing; 2010.
12. Nelson EC, Eftimovska E, Lind C, Hager A, Wasson JH, Lindblad S. Patient reported outcome measures in practice. BMJ. 2015;350:g7818. https://doi.org/10.1136/bmj.g7818.
13. Nursing and Midwifery Council. Future nurse: standards of proficiency for registered nurses. 2018. Available from https://www.nmc.org.uk/globalassets/sitedocuments/education-standards/future-nurse-proficiencies.pdf. Accessed 12 Nov 2018.
14. McSherry W, Ross L. Dilemmas of spiritual assessment: considerations for nursing practice. J Adv Nurs. 2002;38(5):479–88.
15. Highfield MF. PLAN: a spiritual care model for every nurse. Qual Life. 1993;2(3):80–4.
16. Puchalski C, Romer AL. Taking a spiritual history allows clinicians to understand patients more fully. J Palliat Med. 2000;3(1):129–37.
17. Anandarajah G, Hight E. Spirituality and medical practice: using the HOPE questions as a practical tool for spiritual assessment. Am Fam Physician. 2001;63(1):81–8.
18. Ross L. Nurses' perceptions of spiritual care. Aldershot: Avebury; 1997.
19. Stoll R. Guidelines for spiritual assessment. Am J Nurs. 1979;1:1572–7.
20. Austin P, MacLeod R, Siddall P, McSherry W, Egan R. Spiritual care training is needed for clinical and non-clinical staff to manage patients' spiritual needs. J Study Spirituality. 2017;7(1):50–3. https://doi.org/10.1080/20440243.2017.1290031.
21. Clarke J. Spiritual care in everyday nursing practice a new approach. London: Palgrave Macmillan; 2013.

22. Ross LA. Spiritual aspects of nursing. J Adv Nurs. 1994;19:439–47.
23. van Leeuwen R, Tiesinga LJ, Middel B, Post D, Jochemsen H. The effectiveness of an educational programme for nursing students on developing competence in the provision of spiritual care. J Clin Nurs. 2008;17(20):2768–81.
24. Cone P, Giske T. Nurses' comfort level with spiritual care concerns. A mixed method study among working nurses. J Clin Nurs. 2017;26:3125–36. https://doi.org/10.1111/jocn.13660.
25. Ross L, van Leeuwen R, Baldacchino D, Giske T, McSherry W, Narayanasamy A, Downes C, Jarvis P, Schep-Akkerman A. Student nurses perceptions of spirituality and competence in delivering spiritual care: A European pilot study. Nurse Educ Today. 2014;34:697–702.
26. Ross L, van Leeuwen R, Baldacchino D, Giske T, McSherry W, Narayanasamy A, Downes C, Jarvis P, Schep-Akkerman A. Factors contributing to student nurses'/midwives' perceived competency in spiritual care. Nurse Educ Today. 2016;36:445–51.
27. Alderson A. Nurse suspended for offering to pray for elderly patient's recovery. 2009. Available from http://www.telegraph.co.uk/news/health/news/4409168/Nurse-suspended-for-offering-to-pray-for-patients-recovery.html. Accessed 27 Nov 2017.
28. Egerod I, Christensen D, Schwartz-Nielsen KH, Ågård AS. Constructing the illness narrative: a grounded theory exploring patients' and relatives' use of intensive care diaries. Crit Care Med. 2013;39(9):1–7.
29. Snowden A, Telfer IJM, Kelly EK, Bunniss S, Mowat H. I was able to talk about what was on my mind'. The operationalisation of person centred care. Scott J Healthcare Chaplaincy. 2013;16:14–24.
30. Piles C. Providing spiritual care. Nurse Educ. 1990;15(1):36–41.
31. Ross N. Exploring students' perceptions of their spirituality and the role of this in coping. Unpublished BSc Psychology and Counselling dissertation: The University of Northampton; 2017.
32. Puchalski CM, Vitillo R, Hull SK, Reller N. Improving the spiritual dimension of whole person care: reaching national and international consensus. J Palliat Med. 2014;17(6):642–56.
33. Weathers E, McCarthy G, Coffey A. Concept analysis of spirituality: an evolutionary approach. Nurs Forum. 2016;51(2):79–96.
34. Balthip Q. Achieving harmony of mind: a grounded theory study of people living with HIV/AIDS in the Thai context. Unpublished doctoral dissertation, Massey University, Palmerston North, New Zealand; 2010.
35. Balthip K, McSherry W, Nilmanat K. Spirituality and dignity of thai adolescents living with HIV. Religion. 2017;8:257.
36. Balthip K, McSherry K, Petchruschatachart U, Piriyakoontorn S, Liamputtong P. Enhancing life purpose amongst Thai adolescents. J Moral Educ. 2017;46(3):295–307. https://doi.org/10.1080/03057240.2017.1347089.
37. Ramajitti Institute. Child watch during 2011–2012. 2012. http://www.teenpath.net/data/r-research/00011/tpfile/00001.pdf. Accessed 2 June 2017.

Suggested Reading

McSherry W, Ross L, editors. Spiritual assessment in healthcare practice. 1st ed. Keswick: M&K Publishing; 2010.
Puchalski C, Romer AL. Taking a spiritual history allows clinicians to understand patients more fully. J Palliat Med. 2000;3(1):129–37.
Stoll R. Guidelines for spiritual assessment. Am J Nurs. 1979;1:1572–7.

Spirituality as a Public Health Issue: The Potential Role of Spirituality in Promoting Health

Richard Egan and Fiona Timmins

Abstract

The public health mandate is to improve, promote and protect human health and well-being: arguably, spirituality is both a dimension and a determinant of both. Although there is growing support for a more holistic public health approach, spirituality itself is not often deemed a public health priority. This chapter aims to highlight the potential for further integration of spirituality within the realm of public health research and practice. Overall, the published spirituality in healthcare research has an almost exclusively 'downstream' focus, meaning that the research focuses on patients, families and disease states. An 'upstream' focus would focus on policy factors. Despite there being abundant clinically focused evidence, spirituality still remains a forgotten element in much of the public health research to date. Furthermore, spirituality is virtually absent from the public health research agenda. Spirituality in public health must be encouraged via a new and improved research agenda. Importantly, the inclusion of spirituality within national public health remit may provide a new lens through which to examine fundamental questions about our collective values, principles, purpose and meaning.

R. Egan (✉)
Cancer Society Social and Behavioural Research Unit,
Department of Preventive and Social Medicine
Dunedin School of Medicine, University of Otago
Dunedin, New Zealand
e-mail: richard.egan@otago.ac.nz

F. Timmins
School of Nursing and Midwifery, Trinity College Dublin
Dublin, Ireland

Abbreviations

EPICC   Enhancing Nurses and Midwives' Competence in Providing Spiritual Care through Innovation Education and Compassionate Care
NZ   New Zealand
RWJF   Robert Wood Johnson Foundation
UK   United Kingdom
UN   United Nations
WHO   World Health Organization

4.1 Introduction

The public health mandate is to improve, promote and protect human health and well-being: arguably, spirituality is both a dimension and a determinant of both. Unfortunately, although there is growing support for a more holistic public health approach, spirituality itself is not often deemed a public health priority. This chapter aims to highlight the potential for further integration of spirituality within the realm of public health research and practice. Overall, the published spirituality in healthcare research has an almost exclusively 'downstream' focus, meaning that the research focuses on patients, families and disease states. An 'upstream' focus would focus on policy factors. Despite there being abundant clinically focused evidence, spirituality still remains a forgotten element in much of the public health research to date. Furthermore, spirituality is virtually absent from the public health research agenda. Spirituality in public health must be encouraged via a new and improved research agenda. Importantly, the inclusion of spirituality within national public health remit may provide a new lens through which to examine fundamental questions about our collective values, principles, purpose and meaning.

4.2 Background

Public health is often described as "the science and art of preventing disease, prolonging life and promoting health through the organised efforts of society" [1]. Public health, as opposed to the publicly funded health system, is a discipline that aims to prevent illness and protect and promote population health and well-being. The task of 'keeping people healthy' focuses not on individuals, but rather on communities and other populations. Public health efforts have largely centred on the understanding, tracking and prevention of diseases. However, there is growing support for a 'new public health' approach, which takes a holistic view, encompassing four key dimensions of health: physical, mental, social and spiritual. Spirituality and faith-based health are becoming of increasing importance in the contemporary international healthcare context. Globally healthcare providers recognise the need to address spirituality or faith in the context of hospitalised healthcare, although there is minimal attention paid to the role of these concepts in the support and provision of public health. Additionally there are inherent challenges to addressing spirituality and faith needs of populations due to lack of knowledge and understanding, lack of perceived need, inherent bias and population diversity. Spirituality, like public health, is often narrowly understood and not usefully defined. Public health is often understood to include the publicly funded health system, while spirituality may be interpreted merely as religion. In both cases, these interpretations are wrong. There are, in fact, numerous definitions of spirituality, with Unruh et al. claiming as many as 92 within the published literature [2]. From an international perspective, Puchalski et al. have published this widely used definition:

> Spirituality is a dynamic and intrinsic aspect of humanity through which persons seek ultimate meaning, purpose, and transcendence, and experience relationship to self, family, others, community, society, nature, and the significant or sacred. Spirituality is expressed through beliefs, values, traditions, and practices. [3]

What are your views on this definition?
Pause for a moment and consider how this definition links to public health?
Consider whether you agree that spirituality is a public health issue rather than a personal one?

This summative description of spirituality may include religion, but is also inclusive of humanist or existential approaches, and allows for spirituality to be broadly understood and defined by the user. Most authors agree that spirituality and religion are different, albeit connected, concepts [4]. It is useful to think of spirituality as a continuum of beliefs. Globally, healthcare providers recognise the need to address spirituality or faith in the context of hospitalised healthcare; however there is minimal attention paid to the role of these concepts in the support and provision of public health.

The growing attention that is being paid to the importance of spirituality in healthcare arises particularly from within the nursing profession, where there is increasing attention to the requirement to identify and address the spiritual needs of people receiving healthcare. An important step in this is the determination of core competencies for spiritual care that are now well underway in a European context through the recent acquisition of *Erasmus Plus* funding to support this innovation [5]. This aforementioned project—Enhancing Nurses and Midwives' Competence in Providing Spiritual Care through Innovation, Education and Compassionate Care (EPICC)—will be crucial to the support of spiritual care in healthcare for the future by building a European network of nursing and midwifery educators, supported by other key stakeholders in order to share knowledge and skills in spiritual care. From December 2016 to August 2019, this network will review good practice and develop new resources that can be applied to nursing and midwifery education in higher education institutions across Europe. The project is informed by the views of patients, students and the public and led by nurse educators from six universities in Malta, the Netherlands, Norway and the UK and will pave the way for optimal, informed spiritual care delivery in European healthcare. Building on this the next phase of work in this area needs to consider the evidence for, importance of and ways to develop and support workplace spirituality in healthcare. From a public health point of view, we hope this project will have an impact at an institutional policy level.

Within medicine less attention is paid to the topic. However testament to the growing importance of spirituality as a global concern and public health issue is the 2015 Lancet series on faith-based healthcare drew some attention to the importance of addressing patients' faith-related needs in the healthcare context [6–8]. The authors suggested that "…the present, all too common, practice of berating or ignoring faith groups, often on the basis of hearsay, is totally unacceptable" [8]; they further called for urgent action in relation to policy and practice in the field and urged those from various disciplines (e.g. health professionals, faith leaders, policymakers) to "…work together for improving health care" [8]. An overall lack of knowledge with regard to faith as a predictor of health, and the potential importance of faith in supporting global healthcare concerns, emerged as a key message, which was welcomed and supported by an international audience [9–11]. This discussion and debate is encouraging insofar as it opens up the discussion that spirituality or faith may serve to empower public health practices. Indeed it is also encouraging that there is growing support for an emerging approach, which takes a more holistic view and encompasses four key dimensions of health: physical, mental, social and spiritual [12]. Indeed, in *The New Public Health*, Baum insists that "…public health is nothing if not multidisciplinary and holistic" [13]. While traditionally, however, public health efforts have centred largely on the understanding, tracking and prevention of diseases among communities and other populations—an approach that does not adequately address the determinants of health across economic, environmental, social and cultural spheres [14].

The need for a holistic approach to health promotion has been acknowledged, for instance, in policy and approaches aimed at addressing the health of New Zealand (NZ) Māori (the indigenous population of NZ), for instance, in the Māori health model, Te Whare Tapa Wha [15] (Fig. 4.1). New Zealand is, in fact, leading the world in this respect. Public health approaches in this country theoretically incorporate Māori perspectives, which highlight the interdependence of Te Taha Wairua (spirituality), Te Taha Hinengaro (emotional and psychological health), Te Taha Tinana (physical health) and Te Taha Whānau (social wellbeing) [16]. This model of health is taught in all NZ state schools and in both medical and nursing pre-service education. Spirituality is considered to be central to Māori health, but this is yet to be acknowledged or addressed by mainstream health provision, let alone public health.

There are, of course, other examples related primarily to indigenous populations internationally [18]. Nonetheless, in both NZ and abroad, public health engagement with the spiritual dimension remains largely theoretical, and consideration of this concept is notably absent from most public health endeavours in NZ, with the exception of some work involving Māori [19] and Pacific peoples [20]. In the UK, the health service appears to be more accepting of a patient's expression of their spiritual needs, and there is growing impetus for progress internationally as well [9, 21, 22, 55]. The Robert Wood Johnson Foundation (RWJF), the largest public health-focussed private institution in the USA, suggests that public health is becoming peripheral and potentially "redundant" [23]. The foundation, which is known for promoting a "culture of health", insists that "a new perspective on health", which includes spiritual well-being, is required [24]. At a global level, the World Health Organization [25] and the United Nations (UN) [26] have both held formal discussions about the place of spirituality in people's lives. Importantly, a report from the UN Round Table during the 2005 World Health Assembly noted that "the spiritual dimension is common to all faiths, cultures and traditions; the spiritual dimension is universal in nature and can support to transcend boundaries of religion and of nationality" [26]. The ways in which public health entities might choose to respond to this acknowledgement are of prime importance.

If you are a nurse or nursing student, you may have said from a nursing perspective, and taking into account the four aspects of Māori health as outlined in Fig. 4.1, that it would be important to address Anna's physical but also

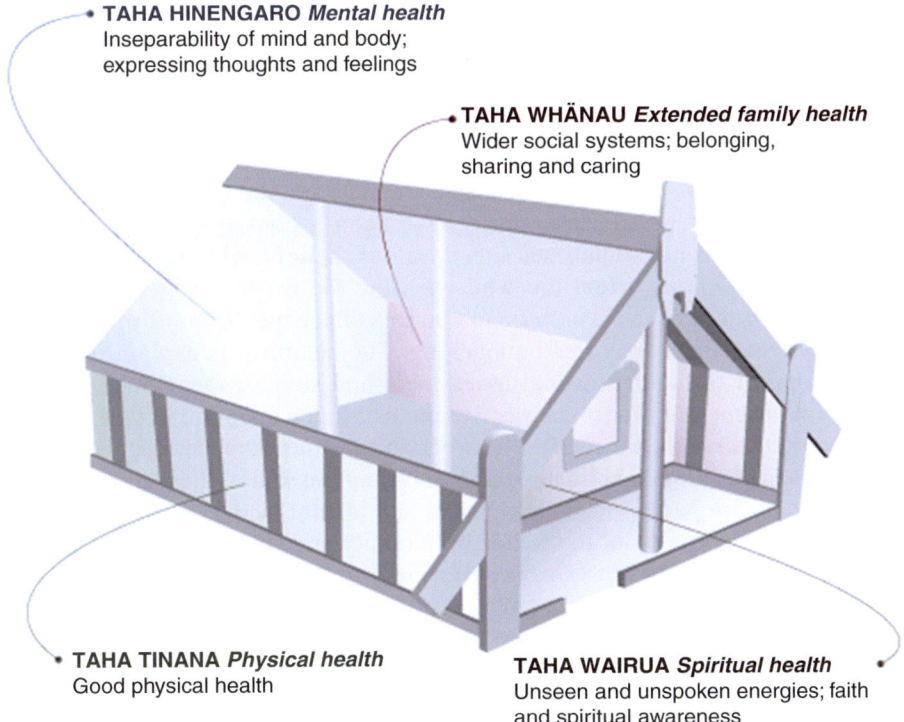

Fig. 4.1 Māori health model: te whare tapa whā [17]

> **Case Study Activity**
> Anna Harp is a 64-year-old woman receiving hospice care for advanced stages of breast cancer. Consider your encounter with Anna firstly from your distinct role perspective but also from the wider public health/health promotion perspective.
> You find Anna to be breathless, and although she is receiving pain medication, she still reports pain. She is in a single-bedded room, with a view of an opposite wall, and although her two daughters and husband visit regularly, she is reported as having lost interest in visitors, activities and eating over the past few days. Anna was diagnosed in very advanced stages of the disease, and her eldest daughter reports that she is very worried now about the daughter's developing breast cancer and she also feels guilty for having the disease and believes that she has done something wrong to deserve this.

psychosocial spiritual needs. As a first step, having first secured her physical comfort by assessing her pain/breathlessness and providing medication and comfort, it might be useful to address the source of her lack of interest by referring her to the hospice counsellor. Not only will this assist with exploring emotional reactions to this illness, it may uncover deeply health beliefs (see Chap. 2) that could either be having a negative affect or could potentially influence Anna's outlook in a positive way. As many chapters of this book have outlined, addressing Anna's spiritual beliefs could form an important element of improving her current condition. This would centre on a brief or detailed spiritual assessment (see Chaps. 1 and 2) and the recognition that her own beliefs about her disease could have been a consequence of her own actions. These strong, sometimes subconscious, beliefs, which may have religious influences, can affect the way we view the world. Regardless of the authenticity or not of these beliefs, to aim to address the discomfort that Anna currently feels, these may need unpacking. The healthcare chaplain is a very useful support for such spiritual assessment and support (see Chap. 7), and taking into account a Māori perspective on health, the chaplain in this circumstance might serve as the conduit between the various perspectives. By working as a member of the healthcare team, the chaplain will witness the attention that the team are paying to both physical and mental health, and in their role as chaplain, they can work to include both family and spiritual aspects of care. Finding out whether or not Anna is suffering from spiritual distress (see Chap. 8) is important. This may explain her loss of interest. A plan of care that would address all four aspects of health (family, spiritual, physical and mental) would likely entail a family-based approach that would address current healthcare needs. Examples of interventions, which could be planned with the family, would be the creation of a life diary, termed 'spiritual legacy' [27]. Simple interventions may have a positive impact on Anna's well-being, such as exploring the possibility of moving to a room with a view of nature or displaying appropriate artwork in the room.

Now that you have considered the impact of a holistic view of promoting health, which includes the spiritual, at a downstream individual and family level, let's now consider a public health approach to this case.

> Consider Anna Harp's late presentation with breast cancer. Is there anything that can be done to improve women's early access to healthcare, and encourage them to attend for or practice breast cancer screening initiatives, that draws on the model outlined in Fig. 4.1? Screening usually involves breast self-examination and/or mammography, and some female populations [28] are known to present late despite national encouragement of these preventions.

You might have suggested that approaches to screening for breast cancer could be carried out at local, family and community level. This would work well with this model. From a spiritual perspective, faith communities and other community groups could be useful in promoting healthcare screening interventions. Community-based innovations are likely to be less daunting and perhaps less costly than hospital-based interventions. For example, women could be encouraged to carry out breast self-examination by targeting local community with flyers, Facebook and WhatsApp notices. Mobile breast mammography units could be mobilised to work directly with community figures, as intermediaries for the women, and would work well to encourage attendees from within the community rather than without. The mobility of such units would also address the issue of rural dwelling of many of these women, thus overcoming access issues. Finally national campaigns targeting health promotion would need to be mindful to reflect the worldviews and beliefs of people and their commitment to the four cornerstones of health (Fig. 4.1) by reflecting appropriate imagery and targeted messages for communities. Any such campaign needs to also take account of potentially low literacy levels among some populations, ensuring that its message is clear and simple.

However while it is notable that NZ approaches to public health incorporate the concept of spirituality, despite the recognition within the social determinants of health [13, 29], as enshrined in the Ottawa Charter [30] at the first World Health Organization (WHO) health promotion conference in 1986, where arguably spirituality is both a dimension [31] and a "key determinant of health" [32], and despite abundant clinically focused evidence, spirituality still remains a forgotten element in much of the public health research to date. Furthermore, spirituality is virtually absent from the public health research agenda, and yet in the case of Anna Harp above, clearly person-centred care warrants attention to the spiritual, particularly in minority groups where health disparities exist but who also have a strong cultural tradition of spirituality and/or community.

4.3 Research to Date

Since the turn of the millennium, the study of spirituality in healthcare has grown almost exponentially [33]. Review articles [34–36], meta-analysis [37] and seminal texts [38] have drawn together a growing body of evidence, which now underpins the discourse on spirituality in healthcare. Combining much of the research to date, Cobb et al. published the ground-breaking *Oxford Textbook of Spirituality in Healthcare* [38], which points out just how mainstream the topic of spirituality has become. Perhaps unsurprisingly, there are disputes within the published literature with regard to definitions of spirituality [37, 39, 40], the current state of the science [41, 42] as well as inappropriate cultural generalisations [43].

Few published health promotion interventions or analyses include spirituality amongst other factors [44, 45], while some focus on religious spirituality [46, 47]. Some studies have considered spirituality and health-related attitudes and behaviours [48, 49]: Rew et al., in a recent review, concluded that religiosity and spirituality may be important to adolescent health [50]. Mental health promotion is one of the few areas that consistently includes spirituality in both definitions [51] and policy efforts [52–54].

Overall, the published research has an almost exclusively 'downstream' focus. The areas of palliative care [55, 56], cancer [57, 58], nursing [59, 60], ageing [61, 62], mental health [63, 64], social work [65, 66] and general medicine ([3, 67]: Koenig, 2014 #5053) as well as some indigenous work [18, 68–70] tend to dominate the published literature on spirituality. Although clinically oriented, this research has led to certain policy and practice developments: healthcare professional training, for instance, is now beginning to include courses on spirituality [71]. This body of evidence has impacted policy to a certain extent as well: the Scottish National Health Service has, for instance, produced a spirituality resource for all staff members [72]; in the USA, the Joint Commission on Accreditation of Healthcare Associations now assesses how spiritual care is delivered in hospitals [73].

Despite there being abundant clinically focused evidence, spirituality still remains a forgotten element in much of the public health research to date [74]. Furthermore, spirituality is virtually absent from the public health research agenda. This is despite an international mandate that health promotion be centred around an "inclusive concept of health…, encompassing spiritual well-being" [12].

Examining spirituality both independently and as a component of broader research priorities would help to identify barriers to, and enablers of, spiritual care in the UK, the USA, NZ and elsewhere. Spirituality, it may be argued, is theoretically part of the "new public health" but has yet to truly find its place in research, policy and practice. There is certainly a need to further investigate the relationship between spirituality and public health, so as to continue to develop this important field. Classic epidemiological approaches and tools that are commonly used in public health domains may be used, for instance, to better understand spirituality at a population level.

Regarding the field of health promotion, as directed by the Ottawa Charter [30], spirituality could be effectively integrated into existing systems and services, further lending to the creation of supportive environments [75]. Spirituality in public health must be encouraged via a new and improved research agenda. Questions remain with regard to measurement [76–78], culturally appropriate and responsive approaches, spiritual literacy and building systemic approaches to spirituality within the public health system. High-quality research and practice (from needs analysis through to evaluation of interventions) that is based on public health values and ethics must take the spiritual dimension into account. As asked by Professor Ursula King, "what kind of spirituality can truly meet the urgent needs and new opportunities of a global world?" [79]

4.4 Conclusion

We currently live in multi-cultural and multifaith societies with growing secular populations. It is of profound importance that we identify ways in which to foster spiritual harmony, and public health has an important role to play in this work. Importantly, the study of spirituality in public health may provide a new lens through which to examine fundamental questions about our collective values, principles, purpose and meaning [80]. Such a lens may provide a means of increasing our capacity to influence public policy, which ultimately has important impacts on equity, mental health and social norms.

> **Key Messages**
> - There is increased interest internationally in the role of spirituality in healthcare.
> - While there is some agreement internationally that supporting patients' spiritual needs is important, limited attention is given to the potential contribution of spirituality to public health.
> - Public health without spirituality is not truly holistic and risks omitting an important determinant and dimension of human health and well-being.

Acknowledgements We acknowledge Anna de Mello for her comments and edits on the final draft of this chapter.

References

1. Acheson D. Public health in England. Report of the Committee of Inquiry into the future development of the public health function. London: Her Majesty's Stationery Office; 1988.
2. Unruh AM, Versnel J, Kerr N. Spirituality unplugged: a review of commonalities and contentions, and a resolution. Can J Occup Ther. 2002;69(1):5–19.
3. Puchalski CM, Vitillo R, Hull SK, Reller N. Improving the spiritual dimension of whole person care: reaching national and international consensus. J Palliat Med. 2014;17(6):642–56.
4. Weaver AJ, Pargament KI, Flannelly KJ, Oppenheimer JE. Trends in the Scientific Study of Religion, Spirituality, and Health: 1965–2000. J Relig Health. 2006;45(2):208–14.

5. McSherry W. EU project champions the 'spiritual' care of patients: Staffordshire University; 2018. Available from http://www.staffs.ac.uk/news/eu-project-champions-the-spiritual-care-of-patients-tcm4293731.jsp.
6. Olivier J, Tsimpo C, Gemignani R, Shojo M, Coulombe H, Dimmock F, et al. Understanding the roles of faith-based health-care providers in Africa: review of the evidence with a focus on magnitude, reach, cost, and satisfaction. Lancet. 2015;386(10005):1765–75.
7. Karam A, Clague J, Marshall K, Olivier J. The view from above: faith and health. Lancet. 2015;386(10005):e22–e4.
8. Tomkins A, Duff J, Fitzgibbon A, Karam A, Mills EJ, Munnings K, et al. Controversies in faith and health care. Lancet. 2015;386(10005):1776–85.
9. Barmania S, Aljunid SM. Faith-based health care. Lancet. 2016;387(10017):429.
10. Messinger R. Faith-based organisations and health care: invest, don't proselytise. Lancet. 2015;386(10005):1733.
11. Summerskill W, Horton R. Faith-based delivery of science-based care. Lancet. 2015;386(10005):1709–10.
12. WHO. The Bangkok charter for health promotion in a globalized world. Geneva: World Health Organisation; 2005.
13. Baum F. The new public health. 4th ed. Oxford: Oxford University Press; 2015.
14. Dahlgren G, Whitehead M. Policies and strategies to promote social equity in health. Stockholm: Institute for Future Studies; 1991.
15. Durie MA. Maori perspective of health. Soc Sci Med. 1985;20(5):483–6.
16. Ministry of Health. Te pai me te oranga o ngā iwi. Health for all people: an overview of public health. Wellington: Ministry of Health; 2002.
17. Durie M. Māori health: te whare tapa whā model The Encyclopedia of New Zealand: The Encyclopedia of New Zealand; 1998. Available from https://teara.govt.nz/en/diagram/31387/maori-health-te-whare-tapa-wha-model.
18. Capstick S, Norris P, Sopoaga F, Tobata W. Relationships between health and culture in Polynesia - a review. Soc Sci Med. 2009;68(7):1341–8.
19. Rochford T. Whare Tapa Wha: a Māori model of a unified theory of health. J Prim Prev. 2004;25(1):41–57.
20. Counties Manukau District Health Board. Lotu Moui: mind body spirit. Auckland: Counties Manukau District Health Board; 2005.
21. Swift C. Hospital chaplaincy in the twenty-first century; 2009.
22. Koenig HG. Religion, spirituality, and health: a review and update. Adv Mind Body Med. 2014;29(3):19–26.
23. Kuehnert P, Palacio H. Transforming public health in the United States. Perspect Public Health. 2014;134(5):251–2.
24. Plough A, Chandra A. From vision to action: a framework and measures to mobilize a culture of health. 2015. Available from http://www.rwjf.org/content/dam/files/rwjf-web-files/Research/2015/RWJF_From_Vision_to_Action_2015-FullReport.pdf. Accessed 13 Sept 2016.
25. Khayat MH (Deputy Regional Director WHO's Office for the Eastern Mediterranean). Spirituality in the Definition of Health The World Health Organization's Point of View. 1996. Available from http://www.medizin-ethik.ch/publik/spirituality_definition_health.htm. Accessed 19 Sept 2016.
26. Luedemann WP. Spirituality, religion & social health: panel report. Geneva: United Nations; 2005.
27. Piderman KM, Radecki Breitkopf C, Jenkins SM, Lapid MI, Kwete GM, Sytsma TT, et al. The impact of a spiritual legacy intervention in patients with brain cancers and other neurologic illnesses and their support persons. Psychooncology. 2015;26:346–53.
28. Lawrenson R, Seneviratne S, Scott N, Peni T, Brown C, Campbell I. Breast cancer inequities between Māori and non-Māori women in Aotearoa/New Zealand. Eur J Cancer Care. 2016;25(2):225–30.
29. Office of Disease Prevention and Health Promotion. Healthy people 2020 framework. Washington, DC: Office of Disease Prevention and Health Promotion; 2010. Available from https://www.healthypeople.gov/sites/default/files/HP2020Framework.pdf.

30. World Health Organisation. Ottawa Charter for health promotion. First International Conference on Health Promotion; 17–21 November; Ottawa. Copenhagen: World Health Organisation Regional Office for Europe; 1986.
31. Durie M. An Indigenous model of health promotion. Health Promot J Austr. 2004;15(3):181–5.
32. Fleming S, Evans DS. The concept of spirituality: its role within health promotion practice in the Republic of Ireland. Spiritual Health Int. 2008;9(2):79–89.
33. Kharitonov SA. Religious and spiritual biomarkers in both health and disease. Religion. 2012;3(2):467.
34. Chiu L, Emblen JD, Van Hofwegen L, Sawatzky R, Meyerhoff H. An integrative review of the concept of spirituality in the health sciences. West J Nurs Res. 2004;26(4):405–28.
35. Cotton S, Zebracki K, Rosenthal S, Tsevat J, Drotar D. Spirituality and adolescent health outcomes: a systematic review. J Adolesc Health. 2005;36(2):119.
36. Gijsberts M-JHE, Echteld MA, van der Steen JT, Muller MT, Otten RHJ, Ribbe MW, et al. Spirituality at the end of life: conceptualization of measurable aspects—a systematic review. J Palliat Med. 2011;14(7):852–63.
37. Salsman JM, Fitchett G, Merluzzi TV, Sherman AC, Park CL. Religion, spirituality, and health outcomes in cancer: a case for a meta-analytic investigation. Cancer. 2015;121(21):3754–9.
38. Cobb M, Puchalski C, Rumbold B, editors. The oxford textbook of spirituality in healthcare. Oxford: Oxford University Press; 2012.
39. Salander P. Whether "spirituality" can be a meaningful concept is still open to question. Palliat Support Care. 2014;13:101–2.
40. Swinton J, Pattison S. Moving beyond clarity: towards a thin, vague, and useful understanding of spirituality in nursing care. Nurs Philos. 2010;11(4):226–37.
41. Sloan R, Bagiella E, VandeCreek L, Hover M, Casalone C, Hirsch TJ, et al. Should physicians prescribe religious activities? N Engl J Med. 2000;342(25):1913–6.
42. Stefanek M, Green MP, Hess SA. Religion, spirituality and cancer: Current status and methodological challenges. Psychooncology. 2005;14(6):450–63.
43. la Cour P, Hvidt NC. Research on meaning-making and health in secular society: secular, spiritual and religious existential orientations. Soc Sci Med. 2010;71(7):1292–9.
44. Lee RLT, Loke AJTY. Health-promoting behaviors and psychosocial well-being of university students in Hong Kong. Public Health Nurs. 2005;22(3):209–20.
45. Tol A, Tavassoli E, Shariferad GR, Shojaeezadeh D. Health-promoting lifestyle and quality of life among undergraduate students at school of health, Isfahan university of medical sciences. J Educ Health Promot. 2013;2(1):11.
46. Marshall J, Archibald C. The influence of spirituality on health behaviors in an Afro-Caribbean population. ABNF J. 2015;26(3):57–62.
47. Michael WP, Jeffrey MB, Phillip B, Mary H, et al. A multidisciplinary model of health promotion incorporating spirituality into a successful aging intervention with African-American and white elderly groups. The Gerontologist. 2002;42(3):406.
48. Tan M-M, Chan CKY, Reidpath DD. Religiosity and spirituality and the intake of fruit, vegetable, and fat: a systematic review. Evid Based Complement Alternat Med. 2013;2013:18.
49. Waite PJ, Hawks SR, Gast JA. The correlation between spiritual well-being and health behaviors. Am J Health Promot. 1999;13(3):159–62.
50. Rew L, Wong YJ. A systematic review of associations among religiosity/spirituality and adolescent health attitudes and behaviors. J Adolesc Health. 2006;38(4):433–42.
51. Leibrich J. Heart and soul matters: a guide to providing spiritual care in mental health settings. 2016. Available from: http://www.spiritualhealthvictoria.org.au/our-publications. Accessed 22 Sept 2016.
52. Mental Health Foundation. Making Space for Spirituality. How to support services users. London: Mental Health Foundation; 2007.
53. Kobau R, Seligman MEP, Peterson C, Diener E, Zack MM, Chapman D, et al. Mental health promotion in public health: perspectives and strategies from positive psychology. Am J Public Health. 2011;101(8):e1–9.
54. 5th World Conference on the Promotion of Mental Health and the Prevention of Mental and Behavioural Disorders. The Melbourne Charter for Promoting Mental Health and Preventing

Mental and Behavioural Disorders. 2008. Available from https://www.vichealth.vic.gov.au/media-and-resources/publications/melbourne-charter. Accessed 22 Sept 2016.
55. Puchalski CM, editor. A time for listening and caring: spirituality and the care of the chronically ill and dying. New York: Oxford University Press; 2006.
56. Grant L, Murray SA, Sheikh A. Spiritual dimensions of dying in pluralist societies. BMJ. 2010;341:c4859.
57. Puchalski CM. Spirituality in the cancer trajectory. Ann Oncol. 2012;23(suppl 3):49–55.
58. Holloway M, Adamson S, McSherry W, Swinton J. Spiritual care at the end of life: a systematic review of the literature. London: Department of Health; 2011.
59. Baldacchino DR. Teaching on the spiritual dimension in care to undergraduate nursing students: the content and teaching methods. Nurse Educ Today. 2008;28(5):550–62.
60. Creedy D, Tiew L. Integration of spirituality in nursing practice: a literature review. Singapore Nurs J. 2010;37(1):15–21.
61. MacKinlay E. Palliative care, ageing and spirituality: a guide for older people, carers and families. London: Jessica Kingsley Publishers; 2012.
62. Jackson D, Doyle C, Capon H, Pringle E. Spirituality, spiritual need, and spiritual care in aged care: what the literature says. J Relig Spiritual Aging. 2016;28:281–95.
63. Swinton J. Spirituality and mental health care: rediscovering a 'forgotten' dimension. London: Jessica Kingsley Publishers; 2001.
64. Colucci E. Recognizing spirituality in the assessment and prevention of suicidal behaviour. World Cult Psychiatry Res Rev. 2008;3(1):77–95.
65. Crisp BR. Social work and spirituality in a secular society. J Soc Work. 2008;8(4):363–75.
66. Duncan-Daston R, Foster S, Bowden H. A look into spirituality in social work practice within the hospice setting. J Relig Spiritual Soc Work Soc Thought. 2016;2016:1–22.
67. Koenig H. The spiritual history. South Med J. 2006;99(10):1159–60.
68. Tse S, Lloyd C, Petchkovsky L, Manaia W. Exploration of Australian and New Zealand indigenous people's spirituality and mental health. Aust Occup Ther J. 2005;52(3):181–7.
69. Durie M. Whaiora: Māori health development. 2nd ed. Auckland: Oxford University Press; 1998.
70. Fleming J, Ledogar RJ. Resilience and indigenous spirituality: a literature review. Pimatisiwin. 2008;6(2):47.
71. Lambie D, Egan R, Walker S, Macleod R. How spirituality is understood and taught in New Zealand medical schools. Palliat Support Care. 2013;13:1–6.
72. NHS Education Scotland. Spiritual care matters: an introductory resource for all NHS Scotland staff. Edinburgh: NHS Education for Scotland; 2009.
73. Joint Commission on Accreditation of Healthcare Associations. The source: evaluating your spiritual assessment process. Washington: Joint Commission on Accreditation of Healthcare Organisations; 2005. Contract No.: 2.
74. Vader JP. Spiritual health: the next frontier. Eur J Pub Health. 2006;16(5):457.
75. Egan R. Health Promotion and spirituality: making the implicit explicit. Keeping up to date [Internet]. 2010. 22 Sept 2016.; 34:[1–4 pp.]. Available from http://www.hauora.co.nz/keeping-up-to-date.html.
76. Kapuscinski AN, Masters KS. The current status of measures of spirituality: a critical review of scale development. Psychol Relig Spiritual. 2010;2(4):191.
77. Rumbold B. Assessing Assessments in Spiritual Care. First National Conference on Spirituality & Health, University of Adelaide South Australia; 29 July 2005; University of Adelaide South Australia. University of Adelaide South Australia; 2005.
78. Rumbold B. A review of spiritual assessment in health care practice. Med J Aust. 2007;186(10 Suppl):S60–S2.
79. King U. Can Spirituality transform our world? J Study Spirituality. 2011;1(1):17–34.
80. González G. Towards an existential archeology of capitalist spirituality. Religion. 2016;7(7):85.

Health Outcomes of Religious and Spiritual Belief, Behavior, and Belonging: Implications for Healthcare Professionals

Elizabeth Johnston Taylor

Abstract

Thousands of empirical studies now document that aspects of religion or spirituality are linked with desirable health outcomes. This chapter provides an overview of how religious or spiritual (R/S) beliefs, behaviors, and belonging to a faith community contribute to health outcomes. When living with a health challenge, individuals often use R/S beliefs to cope with their circumstances. These beliefs can be positive or negative; they also impact healthcare decision-making. R/S behaviors observed to be associated with health outcomes include attendance at religious services and various practices such as prayer and meditation. For those who belong within a faith community, that community may provide social support and informal caregiving. This evidence ought to prompt healthcare professionals to plan and implement care that supports R/S in an ethical manner. Indeed, there is evidence that indicates when healthcare professionals support patient R/S, it is associated with various positive outcomes.

A mother refuses vaccinations for her child because of her Christian Science convictions. A Sikh gentleman who was shaved in preparation for surgery latter takes his life because of the significance his religion places on hair as a body organ. A Christian with fundamentalist leanings insists on intubating her brain-dead husband, because "God can still perform a miracle." These diverse real cases illustrate the powerful role that religion can contribute to how a person addresses a health-related situation. Not all religious influences, however, are so dramatic.

E. J. Taylor (✉)
School of Nursing, Loma Linda University, Loma Linda, CA, USA
e-mail: ejtaylor@llu.edu

© Springer Nature Switzerland AG 2019
F. Timmins, S. Caldeira (eds.), *Spirituality in Healthcare: Perspectives for Innovative Practice*, https://doi.org/10.1007/978-3-030-04420-6_5

Consider the following: A patient newly diagnosed with a chronic illness wonders if it is because God is punishing him for something he did in his youth. Another patient prays for guidance prior to making a treatment decision. Another reads scripture and meditates to cope with anxiety and discomfort. For these patients, a clinician may never objectively observe these religious beliefs or behaviors, yet they significantly affect how the patient adapts to the illness.

Whether these beliefs, behaviors, and belonging are invisible or openly expressed by a patient, they have a significant impact on physical, psychosocial, and, of course, spiritual health-related outcomes. Indeed, Koenig and colleagues [1, 2] identified over 3300 studies which investigated this linkage between R/S and health and observed that most researchers found R/S to be associated with or contributed to health outcomes significantly and positively. Koenig et al.'s massive review identified that about 80% of these studies examined R/S in relation to psychological factors. Table 5.1 provides a summary of this review of the health-related R/S research published in peer-reviewed publications. Whereas this review focused on mental and physical health outcomes, others have found evidence which indicates that R/S contributes to overall quality of life and life satisfaction among persons with cancer and various other chronic illnesses [3–7].

Furthermore, there is a growing body of evidence that indicates when healthcare professionals support patient R/S, it is associated with various positive outcomes. For example, in studies of American hospitalized patients, those who received spiritual support from chaplains and/or from members of the healthcare team were found to have greater patient satisfaction with healthcare than those who did not receive such support [8–10]. Findings from a study of 343 patients with late-staged cancer found that when spiritual needs are addressed, healthcare costs are lessened, quality of life is improved, and patients are more receptive to hospice [11]. Spiritual therapeutics (e.g., dignity therapy—a manualized reminiscence therapy, meditation or mindfulness training, meaning-centered group therapy) delivered by healthcare professionals likewise have been observed to contribute to various positive outcomes [12–16]. Together, this evidence suggests not just that R/S is linked with health but that healthcare professionals are careless if they do not provide R/S support when caring.

Thus, this chapter will provide an overview about how religious or spiritual (R/S) beliefs, behaviors, and belonging (to a R/S community) contribute to health outcomes. Implications of caring for a patient in a religiously/spiritually sensitive manner will be offered. To provide a foundation first, a theoretical framing for this is reviewed.

5.1 How Faith Affects Health: Levin's Model

The findings presented in Table 5.1 provide overwhelming evidence that R/S, in general, is positively associated with numerous psychological and physical health outcomes. Why is this? What is it about the R/S in people that makes them less anxious, depressed, and obese? Why is R/S higher in people who live longer? Why do people with higher R/S tend to have better immune function and less disease?

Table 5.1 Religiosity/spirituality (R/S) and health-related outcomes: Koenig's [1, 2] synthesis of evidence

Health-related outcome	Number of quantitative, peer-reviewed studies (prior to mid-2010)	Percentage of studies finding positive/beneficial association with R/S[a]	Percentage of studies finding a negative/harmful association with R/S[a]
Coping with adversity (in a wide variety of illnesses and circumstances)	344	"Overwhelming majority"	Not provided
Well-being/happiness	326	79%	<1%
Hope	40	73%	0
Optimism	32	81%	0
Meaning and purpose	45	93%	Not provided
Self-esteem	69	61%	3%
Sense of control in difficult life circumstances	21	61%	14%
Depression	444	61%	6%
Suicide variables	141	75%	3%
Anxiety	299	49%	11%
Mental health illnesses/diagnoses (bipolar, psychotic disorders, substance abuse)	325	79%	5%
Social support	74	82%	0
Cigarette smoking	137	90% (0%)	0
Exercise	37	68%	16%
Healthful diet	21	62%	5%
Weight/body mass index	36	39%	19%
Risky sexual activity	95	86%	1%
Heart disease	19	63%	5%
Hypertension	63	57%	11%
Cerebral vascular disease (risk for stroke)	9	44%	11%
Dementia	21	48%	14%
Immune function	27	56%	4%
Endocrine function	31	74%	0
Cancer onset or mortality	29	55%	7%
Physical function (activities of daily living)	61	36%	23%
Self-rated health	50	58%	10%
Physical pain	56	39%	25%
Longevity	121	68%	5%

[a]Percentages do not add up to 100 because some studies had mixed or inconclusive evidence

Jeffrey Levin, who describes himself as an epidemiologist of religion and one of the earliest to conduct a comprehensive review of research about religion and its association with health, offered a theoretical model to explain religion's salutatory effects [17, 18]. Levin provides a taxonomy where he identifies five mechanisms whereby religion affects human health. He labels these mechanisms as behavioral/conative, interpersonal, cognitive, affective, and psychophysiological. A closer look at each of these mechanisms is in order:

- Behavioral/conative (or motivational) mechanisms refer to health-promoting behaviors that often are prompted by religious prescriptions and proscriptions. These healthful lifestyles and choices have an impact on the immune and endocrine systems in ways that promote health and prevent disease. For example, most religions advise monogamy within a covenantal relationship and consider any breach of a marriage as unethical; thus, those who follow this prescription are at lower risk for genital cancers and sexually transmitted diseases, never mind the psychosocial sequelae associated with an extramarital affair. Likewise, many faith traditions encourage temperance or abstinence from alcohol; others provide advice regarding diet and fasting for which recent research findings provide support.
- Interpersonal mechanisms of faith involve the individual connecting either with others of similar R/S views or with the divine (or divine entities, such as angels or saints). Either provides the individual with companionship—social support—a vital factor known to prevent disease and promote health. Thus, for the R/S person who participates in a faith community of some sort (e.g., engages informally or formally with a community of fellow believers at a church, synagogue, mosque, gurdwara, temple, or devotional meeting), this community can provide friendship and a social safety "net." More accessible, however, is the fellowship with the divine (e.g., God, saint, guardian angel) that can provide one with a sense of comfort and safety. The decreased chance for experiencing isolation, thus, undoubtedly helps people of faith to avert illness and be well.
- Cognitive mechanisms of faith refer to the intellectual schema developed to explain why things happen in life as they do and to the beliefs we hold to make sense of our world. For example, inherently, religions offer myths about how the universe was created and how it will continue or end. For example, many faith traditions (e.g., Christianity and Islam) hold that there will be a judgment at the end of temporal time, and most traditions hold that there will an afterlife (e.g., in a heaven, reincarnated state). Such belief not only motivates a believer to live well in the present life but also provides comfort when considering one's mortality. Religious theologies also provide, to some degree, psychologically comforting explanations for tragedy and suffering. For example, some may view their suffering as a consequence of personal or collective disobedience to God's laws, while others may view it as an invitation to draw closer to a loving God or an opportunity for spiritual transformation. These theological meanings persons ascribe to life and its experiences are thought to have an impact on the psyche and, in turn, be expressed somatically to some degree.

- Affective mechanisms refer to how R/S beliefs and practices can create comforting emotions, the neurochemistry of which may function to buffer and decrease disease processes and/or enhance the immune system and other health-promoting physiology. For example, persons of faith can experience warmth, peace, joy, harmony, perspective, gratitude, and so forth during prayer, chanting, worshipful singing, meditation, communion with fellow believers, and so forth. Such positive emotions are known to be health-promoting.
- Psychophysiological mechanisms refer to those aspects of faith that create hope and optimism, which in turn create a somatic response. Levin acknowledged that all five of these salutatory mechanisms of faith could be classified as psychophysiological but reserved this last category for acknowledging the linkage between the mind and body.
- For example, hope that rests in knowing there is a God who will make all things well will help to ease one's burdens; the comfort of knowing one is not alone also can provide the will to live and endure suffering [17, 18].

Although he did not develop this as a category, Levin did acknowledge that additional mechanisms may exist for the observed faith and health linkage. For example, there may be health that is explained by nonlocal consciousness or unitive experiences with what is transcendent (e.g., "miracles"). Because he delimited his categories of mechanisms to that which can be linked to existing science about mind-body interactions, Levin expressed confidence that this theorizing is plausible.

5.2 Nursing Implications

Given that R/S is significantly associated with health outcomes and we have reviewed several mechanisms likely involved in explaining this faith-health connection, we will explore how all this should impact the care delivered by clinicians. We will merge some of Levin's categories and discuss healthcare implications that emerge from evidence about how a patient's R/S beliefs, behaviors, and belonging do influence healthcare.

5.3 Religious/Spiritual Beliefs

Hebrew scripture posits, "For as he thinketh in his heart, so is he" (Proverbs 23:7; KJV). Indeed, what persons believe is the reason for life and living, for illness, for suffering, for death, and for where people come from and to where they are going—essentially R/S beliefs—certainly will affect how they respond to a health challenge. These S/R beliefs about existence will undoubtedly impact how the health challenge is interpreted, how the treatment decisions are made, as well as how health is defined and pursued in general.

5.4 R/S Beliefs About Living Healthfully

Given R/S beliefs offer a believer existential explanations, it is unsurprising that R/S beliefs permeate how persons define and pursue health in general. R/S beliefs (often intertwined with cultural traditions) can influence what one believes is healthful food, drink, hygiene, and lifestyle, whether and what healers should be sought, and other health behaviors [19]. Consider these examples:

- Christian view their bodies as the temple for God; thus good health habits allow one to more fully experience the indwelling of the divine.
- Jews perceive their bodies as God's property; thus, the body is to be maintained and respected.
- Muslims pursue health by pursuing equilibrium in their lives and making choices for good rather than evil (e.g., balancing work with prayer and sleep, focusing on what is beneficial).
- Sikhs view the human body as the ultimate creation and believe health results when they care for themselves holistically; this is done through adherence to religious principles, service, and daily prayer and showering (to cleanse the mind and body).
- Hindus likewise perceive health as balancing mind, body, and soul (where consciousness resides); health is determined by the law of *karma* (i.e., actions and deeds contribute to good or bad reactions—in this life or then next).
- Christian Scientists explain health as the by-product of spiritual mindedness (e.g., compassion, forgiveness, fearlessness, etc.). Healthy mindedness contributes to physical health.
- Buddhists seek health by recognizing the following insights: All things are impermanent, one is incapable of making true happiness, and one's existence is neither inherent nor eternal [19].

R/S beliefs also shape how persons of faith think about what is illness, suffering, and death. Whereas the Eastern religious traditions (e.g., Buddhism, Sikhism, Hinduism) tend to see illness resulting from an imbalance, disharmony, or lack of moderation in physical, mental, or spiritual pursuits, the Abrahamic faiths (i.e., Judaism, Christianity, and Islam) link illness and death with "sin" and accept Western scientific causal explanations. Although (as the evidence to follows substantiates) many from Christian backgrounds entertain the notion that their illness is punishment, this is not a position most Christian denominations espouse [19].

Empirical evidence linking R/S with various health-related outcomes often intertwines the R/S beliefs with R/S behaviors. Although this chapter will attempt to tease these two aspects of R/S apart in the discussion to follow, one example of this is appropriate here. A number of studies, especially with samples of patients with HIV, have observed some aspect of R/S contributes to medication adherence [4, 20]. Whereas most found a positive relationship, many observed some aspect of religiosity linked with poorer adherence. Indeed, it is easy to surmise that the more religious a patient is (i.e., the more one accepts that his or her body is a temple of God, as most in these studies were from cultures influenced by Christianity), then the more likely the patient will be to take their medication. The implication for clinicians may be obvious: Assess R/S, and when it is present, use it therapeutically to motivate health-promoting behaviors. Conversely, when patients are making poor choices impacting their health, screening for R/S struggle—or negative interpretations of their circumstances—may provide insight.

5.5 Negative vs. Positive Religious Interpretations

Given R/S beliefs about health and illness vary, it is helpful to consider how beliefs impact adjustment to illness. One of most frequently used instruments for measuring how a person interprets and copes with an illness or tragedy is the Brief RCOPE or Religious Coping Questionnaire [21]. This questionnaire includes two scales: one measuring positive religious coping while the other quantifying negative religious coping. Table 5.2 provides the items from this instrument to illustrate what is positive and negative religious coping. To summarize, however, positive religious coping involves a secure attachment to God and a sense of connectedness with a benevolent God and faith community. For persons using negative religious coping, there is a sense of abandonment and punishment by God, isolation from their faith community, doubts about the power of God, and thinking that one's illness is caused by a dark or devilish force. Note: Although atheists/agnostics/humanists, by definition, question or reject there is a divine being, Exline et al. [22] found that some atheists harbor a long-seated anger toward God.

Findings from numerous studies firmly establish negative religious coping as maladaptive and positive religious coping as adaptive among persons with various illnesses [23]. Indeed, negative religious coping, or religious struggle (the term

Table 5.2 Illustrations of positive and negative religious coping: the Brief RCOPE [21]

Positive religious coping items
• Looked for a stronger connection with God
• Sought God's love and care
• Sought help from God in letting go of my anger
• Tried to put my plans into action together with God
• Tried to see how God might be trying to strengthen me in this situation
• Asked forgiveness for my sins
• Focused on religion to stop worrying about my problems
Negative religious coping items
• Wondered whether God had abandoned me
• Felt punished by God for my lack of devotion
• Wondered what I did for God to punish me
• Questioned God's love for me
• Wondered whether my church had abandoned me
• Decided the devil made this happen
• Questioned the power of God

currently used), may be surprisingly frequent among patients with particularly difficult health challenges. For example, findings from a large American study of hematopoietic cell transplant survivors ($N = 1449$) revealed 27% reported some degree of negative religious coping [24]. Although this religious struggle was not associated with how long it was since the transplant, it was directly correlated with depression and quality of life and inversely related to age. Other research results have documented rates of spiritual struggle to be as high as 56% (among hospitalized Swiss patients) [25], 58% (for American patients hospitalized for coronary conditions) [26], and 61% (for Tanzanian women with an obstetric fistula) [27], whereas <13% of a large sample of Danes who had coped with a crisis in their past used negative religious coping [28].

Regardless of prevalence, it is important for clinicians to appreciate that religious struggle is associated with depression, anxiety, and other poor outcomes [25, 27, 29, 30]. Indeed, findings from a well-designed study of 101 Americans with end-stage congestive heart failure found that R/S struggle predicted future hospitalization and physical functioning in [29]. Such evidence should prompt clinicians to assess for spiritual struggle among patients and make referrals to experts who can sensitively address the psychospiritual complexities of spiritual struggle.

5.6 R/S Beliefs Affecting Treatment Decision-Making

R/S beliefs can impact treatment decision-making. The evidence about this primarily involves how patients (or their surrogates) are influenced to some degree by R/S when making decisions related to birthing (e.g., genetic testing, pregnancy termination) or dying (e.g., whether to accept life-sustaining treatment such as a tube feeding or resuscitation) [30–32]. Researchers, however, have also documented how R/S beliefs affect decisions about organ transplantation [33] and cancer treatment [34] and other medical issues [35]. Several themes emerge from this body of evidence.

First, R/S beliefs guide persons as they make healthcare decisions. Although this is typically not described well, it appears that this guidance comes in different ways. R/S provides practices that facilitate decision-making or discernment (to use a religious term); for example, praying about what to do is common [34, 35]. Also, religious traditions typically offer standards or counsels that can explicitly guide a patient to know what is right [19, 33]. For example, a Jehovah's Witness has explicit guidelines on what blood products to accept, and the beliefs espoused by many faith traditions refute abortion and euthanasia.

Second, when persons are making a major decision such as a treatment decision, some variation in the perception of control may be evident. For example, Geros-Willfond et al. [35] observed among 46 family members making decisions about their hospitalized elders that some abdicated the decision-making to God, whereas others used a shared control model and viewed the process as engaging both themselves and God in the decision process. Other researchers found that some of the Israeli women with HIV they interviewed acquiesced their decision-making about whether to have a child, illustrated by statements about how it was God who controls reproduction [36]. A third theme in this literature describing how patients' R/S influences healthcare decision-making identifies how a R/S belief in a miracle can create challenges for healthcare providers. Whereas some R/S beliefs lead some persons to accept that death may be the plan God has for them, others may make healthcare decisions to medically prolong life so that God can perform a "miracle" [35].

Indeed, it is essential for healthcare providers to understand how patients' (or their surrogates') R/S beliefs influence their treatment decision-making. This can easily be asked with a question such as "How might your religious or spiritual beliefs inform the decision you are about to make?" Van Norman [37] observed that typically clinicians fail to make such a query when discussing end-of-life issues. Yet there is evidence that R/S beliefs (partially mediated by decisional conflict) explain regret about treatment decision [38]. In a large sample of mostly white American men with prostate cancer, researchers documented that the stronger the R/S beliefs, the less regret about the cancer treatment decision made [38]. Perhaps knowing that God is guiding one's decisions allows one to later be at peace with whatever it is. Furthermore, results from a longitudinal study of late-stage cancer patients in the USA revealed that those who received spiritual support were 3.5 times more likely to accept hospice care than those whose spiritual needs were unmet; furthermore, those who had high religious coping and spiritual support were nearly five times more likely to receive hospice care [11]. This evidence infers that when R/S beliefs are respected, healthcare outcomes likely improve.

Respecting R/S beliefs, however, can be complicated. Patients and their surrogate decision-makers may hold or interpret their R/S beliefs differently, causing intrafamilial conflict when making healthcare decisions [39]. Patients may also misunderstood or be conflicted about their faith tradition's tenets impacting their decision. Consequently, Messina et al. [33] recommended that amidst such circumstances, clinicians engage the patient's religious leader and facilitate accurate religious information for the patient. Decisional conflict may not only exist between patient and surrogates but also between patients/surrogates and clinicians. Based on findings from a survey of 1156 US physicians, Ayeh et al. [40] documented how they were less likely to accommodate client wishes for life-sustaining treatment if the patient/surrogate presented their desire in the context of wanting a miracle or not wanting to give up than if they presented their desire as a mandate of their religion (e.g., "my faith does not permit" or "my religious community does not accept"). In concert, this evidence indicates that respecting the weight of R/S beliefs in healthcare decision-making may not only be respectful, good care but also contribute to positive outcomes. Negotiating the decisional conflict between the stakeholders, however, may be necessary.

5.7 Religious/Spiritual Behaviors

As mentioned earlier, R/S beliefs are intertwined with R/S behaviors; how a patient believes will affect how they behave. Much evidence, however, does provide support for the health benefits of certain R/S behaviors. Consider these examples:

- Attendance at religious services was the greatest predictor of all-cause mortality among African-American women participating in a large epidemiological study ($N = 36,613$), such that those who attended lived longer [41]. Similarly, church activity (mediated and moderated by various other benefits of R/S) predicted decreased mortality in a large sample of Seventh-day Adventists [42].
- R/S practices (i.e., attending services, prayer, meditation), as well as interpreting their illness positively through a R/S lens, having gratitude, and overcoming guilt, when practiced separately or together, predicted increased survival among 177 persons with AIDS 2–4 times [43].
- Various approaches to meditation, a common spiritual practice originating in eastern faith traditions, have received extraordinary and consistent empirical support from research findings obtained over the past couple of decades. The regular practice of meditation contributes to numerous physiologic and psychological outcomes as well as spiritual transformation. Outcomes observed include decreased hypertension, anxiety, depression, increased attention and emotional regulation, and decreased stress (including lower stress hormones) [44–46].
- Although numerous clinical trials have determined that physically ill patients receiving intercessory prayer are no better off than those not receiving this "intervention," [47] many studies show that positively framed personal prayer is associated with positive psychological outcomes [48].
- Fasting, a spiritual discipline many faith traditions expect or encourage, produces several healthful metabolic outcomes in humans and rats, according to a narrative literature review [49].

Indeed, R/S behaviors do affect health whether they involve religious service attendance or private activities.

What are the resulting implications for healthcare providers? Does this evidence mean they should urge patients to attend services or even encourage them to develop private R/S practices like meditation? These questions beg deeper questions about what is ethical, especially when clinicians have a R/S perspective that they believe will be beneficial to patients [50, 51]. Pujol et al.'s [52] observation from interviews with 20 French cancer patients reminds clinicians that their role is not that of clergy: Patients do not seek care from healthcare professionals for R/S support. In the process of receiving healthcare, however, people do not want to be "just 'patients' but human beings with a precious interior life" [52] (p. 733). The admonitions presented in Table 5.3 are offered to avoid any unethical imposition of R/S in patient care.

Table 5.3 Avoiding unethical religious/spiritual support [19, 53]

• Be aware of clinician-patient relationship dynamics
– The relationship is asymmetric; the clinician is in a more powerful position (empowered by knowledge and skills the patient desires to receive)
– Patients enter healthcare organizations to receive healthcare, perceived by patients as care for physical or mental illness
– Whereas some patients (especially those who are older, religious, female, and facing a life-threatening challenge) do want clinicians to make inquiry about their R/S and provide spiritual care, some do not. Those who do not want spiritual care may equate it with religious support
• Recognize what is within the scope of practice for your discipline within healthcare. While the well-trained chaplain is the spiritual care expert, physicians, nurses, and others are spiritual care generalists with limited skills. Care for patients with serious spiritual issues (e.g., negative religious coping) is best provided by experts; a generalist's attempt to care for such serious concerns is potentially harmful
• Evaluate your motives for recommending a R/S belief or practice: Ask yourself, "Whose needs am I meeting?" If your motive is to persuade the patient to accept your perspective because it will make you more comfortable or advance a personal goal, then do not do it
• Assess patient R/S. What are the patient's R/S beliefs, resources, and preferences? How would they want the healthcare team to respect and support these? Provide R/S care that reflects these wishes. When assessing R/S, delimit it to a screening or spiritual history; keep it focused on that which relates to health and that which is within the scope of your professional practice
• Avoid the appearance of coercion, even when providing R/S support that the patient requests
• When introducing R/S into patient care, offer it in such a way that the patient will be free and comfortable to refuse it. (E.g., Evidence indicates meditation is helpful for people with your condition; would you like to attend a class here at the hospital to learn how to do it? Some people in your situation like to have their nurse pray with them; would that be something you'd like?)

5.8 Religious/Spiritual Belonging

A massive demographic study of global patterns of religious affiliation discovered that 84% of the world's population identified with a faith tradition in 2015 [54]. Gleaning data from 2500 censuses and population registers, demographers not only identified current religious affiliation but also projected these rates for the near and more distant future (i.e., 2060). Key findings are presented in Table 5.4. Belonging to a R/S community often means fellow believers become informal caregivers during times of illness; it also can provide a venue for providing health promotion.

5.9 RS Communities: Informal Caregiving

Although 84% may identify to some degree with a religious tradition, of course, many patients may weakly observe their religious beliefs and practices. Many adherents of a religion may not know or accept all the doctrines, rituals, lifestyle recommendations, and so forth. Furthermore, many are influenced to varying

Table 5.4 Prevalence of religion worldwide: major findings from the Templeton-Pew Changing Global Religious Landscape report [54]

• Religions of global population in 2015
– 31.2% Christian
– 24.1% Muslim
– 16% unaffiliated (e.g., atheists, agnostics)
– 15.1% Hindu
– 6.9% Buddhist
– 5.7% Folk religions
– 0.8% other religions
– 0.2% Jewish
• Although "Unaffiliated" will grow during the next 5 years, they will reduce in numbers (to 13%) by 2060 due to fewer births than deaths among women in this category. The majority of Unaffiliated live in Asia and the Pacific regions, Europe, and North America
• Christians and Muslims have grown in numbers due to birth rates; however, by 2060, there will be nearly the same number of Muslims as Christians due to their higher birth rate (31.1% vs. 31.8%, respectively). Muslims and Christians have higher fertility rates than those of other religions; this is the primary factor explaining growth in these traditions
• Religious switching is projected to be largely observed when Christians leave Christianity and Buddhists to a much smaller extent leave Buddhism. Muslims are expected to gain adherents from switching, as well as folk and other religions and "unaffiliated"

degrees by multiple faith traditions (e.g., the person raised Roman Catholic who uses Buddhist meditational practices and currently self-identifies as a Unitarian Universalist). Also, within one religious tradition, there are a myriad of interpretations of the faith's tenets and practices. Varying degrees of engagement, commitment, and orthodoxy will be found within one denomination—and even within one family belonging to the same denomination. This variation in religiosity underscores the importance of assessing the R/S of each patient; each patient has a unique religion (or a religious spirituality) [19].

For those who are integrated to some degree within a religious community, there often are resources that can support patients and their families during times of illness [19]. Latter-Day Saints (Mormons) may be the most organized at providing support to their parishioners or "ward" members. Lay leaders regularly will visit parishioners, identify who is sick or in need, and organize support; the women of the church constitute the "Relief Society" which regularly meets and is instrumental in providing care for those in need. Anabaptist-descended denominations, Seventh-day Adventists, Pentecostals, Roman Catholics, Presbyterians, Orthodox Christians, and other Christian denominations often appoint and/or train lay leaders (especially women, deacons or deaconesses, or those in Stephen's ministries) to visit and support sick church members. In Judaism, such ministry to the sick is regularly performed by members who are part of a *Bikur holim* group. For Muslims, an Islamic center or association likely will offer services for the sick and elderly in the congregation [19].

Indeed, belonging to a religious group not only provides social support in general (as Koenig's [1, 2] review documented), but it often also provides added support—a safety net—for those who are sick and in need. A national study of African-American churchgoers documented types of instrumental support members provided; the more religious and less-educated members provided the most care, which included transportation, help with chores, and even financial support [55]. Yes, a robust faith community will care for its own as would any caring family. The implications for the healthcare professional may be obvious: If the patient consents, clinicians should inform, mobilize, and/or collaborate with these informal caregivers as appropriate. This is particularly true for when patients are discharged home or institutionalized for an extended time.

5.10 R/S Communities: Venues for Health Promotion

R/S communities have been harnessed by health professionals for delivering various types of healthcare. Most of this work has involved providing health promotion (e.g., education about advanced care plans, lifestyle programs aimed at reducing obesity, improving diet and exercise) and disease prevention (e.g., HIV and cancer screening programs) [56–61]. Typically, these programs are studied using community-based participatory research methods. Much of the research exploring how healthcare can be delivered in a faith community is conducted in urban US American African-American churches or in churches for Latino or Asian immigrants. Indeed, the R/S community is a venue for reaching populations that otherwise might distrust or be unable to access healthcare. Many of the reports about these church-based health promotion programs identify feasibility and sustainability issues encountered [60–62]; characteristically, however, they also conclude the R/S communities hold great potential for improving health within communities.

5.11 Conclusion

Thousands of studies now document that R/S is linked with desirable health outcomes. Whether the association is because of R/S beliefs, behaviors, or belonging—or a mixture of these aspects of R/S—this evidence ought to prompt healthcare professionals to plan and implement care that supports R/S. A commitment to systematic R/S assessment and ethical care that reflects this assessment is essential for effective healthcare.

References

1. Koenig HG, King D, Carson VB. Handbook of religion and health. 2nd ed. New York: Oxford University Press; 2012.
2. Koenig HG. Religion, spirituality, and health: the research and clinical implications. ISRN Psychiatry. 2012;2012:278730.

3. Bai M, Lazenby M. A systematic review of associations between spiritual well-being and quality of life at the scale and factor levels in studies among patients with cancer. J Palliat Med. 2015;18(3):286–98.
4. Lin CY, Saffari M, Koenig HG, Pakpour AH. Effects of religiosity and religious coping on medication adherence and quality of life among people with epilepsy. Epilepsy Behav. 2017;78:45–51.
5. Freitas TH, Hyphantis TN, Andreoulakis E, Quevedo J, Miranda HL, Alves GS, et al. Religious coping and its influence on psychological distress, medication adherence, and quality of life in inflammatory bowel disease. Rev Bras Psiquiatr. 2015;37(3):219–27.
6. Ramirez SP, Macedo DS, Sales PM, Figueiredo SM, Daher EF, Araujo SM, et al. The relationship between religious coping, psychological distress and quality of life in hemodialysis patients. J Psychosom Res. 2012;72(2):129–35.
7. Szaflarski M, Ritchey PN, Leonard AC, Mrus JM, Peterman AH, Ellison CG, et al. Modeling the effects of spirituality/religion on patients' perceptions of living with HIV/AIDS. J Gen Intern Med. 2006;21(Suppl 5):S28–38.
8. Astrow AB, Kwok G, Sharma RK, Fromer N, Sulmasy DP. Spiritual needs and perception of quality of care and satisfaction with care in oncology patients: a multi-cultural assessment. J Pain Symptom Manag. 2018;55:56.
9. Williams JA, Meltzer D, Arora V, Chung G, Curlin FA. Attention to inpatients' religious and spiritual concerns: predictors and association with patient satisfaction. J Gen Intern Med. 2011;26(11):1265–71.
10. Hodge DR, Sun F, Wolosin RJ. Hospitalized Asian patients and their spiritual needs: developing a model of spiritual care. J Aging Health. 2014;26(3):380–400.
11. Balboni T, Balboni M, Paulk ME, Phelps A, Wright A, Peteet J, et al. Support of cancer patients' spiritual needs and associations with medical care costs at the end of life. Cancer. 2011;117(23):5383–91.
12. Breitbart W, Rosenfeld B, Pessin H, Applebaum A, Kulikowski J, Lichtenthal WG. Meaning-centered group psychotherapy: an effective intervention for improving psychological well-being in patients with advanced cancer. J Clin Oncol. 2015;33(7):749–54.
13. Fitchett G, Emanuel L, Handzo G, Boyken L, Wilkie DJ. Care of the human spirit and the role of dignity therapy: a systematic review of dignity therapy research. BMC Palliat Care. 2015;14:8.
14. Charlson ME, Loizzo J, Moadel A, Neale M, Newman C, Olivo E, et al. Contemplative self healing in women breast cancer survivors: a pilot study in underserved minority women shows improvement in quality of life and reduced stress. BMC Complement Altern Med. 2014;14:349.
15. Hulett JM, Armer JM. A systematic review of spiritually based interventions and psychoneuroimmunological outcomes in breast cancer survivorship. Integr Cancer Ther. 2016;15:405.
16. Marchand WR. Mindfulness-based stress reduction, mindfulness-based cognitive therapy, and Zen meditation for depression, anxiety, pain, and psychological distress. J Psychiatr Pract. 2012;18(4):233–52.
17. Levin J. How faith heals: a theoretical model. Explore (NY). 2009;5:77–96.
18. Levin J. God, faith, and health: exploring the spirituality-healing connection. New York: Wiley; 2001.
19. Taylor EJ. Religion: a clinical guide for nurses. New York: Springer; 2012.
20. Medved Kendrick H. Are religion and spirituality barriers or facilitators to treatment for HIV: a systematic review of the literature. AIDS Care. 2017;29(1):1–13.
21. Pargament K, Feuille M, Burdzy D. The brief RCOPE: current psychometric status of a short measure of religious coping. Religions. 2011;2(1):51–76.
22. Exline JJ, Park CL, Smyth JM, Carey MP. Anger toward God: social-cognitive predictors, prevalence, and links with adjustment to bereavement and cancer. J Pers Soc Psychol. 2011;100(1):129–48.
23. Pargament KI, Ano GG. Spiritual resources and struggles in coping with medical illness. South Med J. 2006;99(10):1161–2.

24. King SD, Fitchett G, Murphy PE, Pargament KI, Martin PJ, Johnson RH, et al. Spiritual or religious struggle in hematopoietic cell transplant survivors. Psycho-Oncology. 2017;26(2):270–7.
25. Fitchett G, Winter-Pfandler U, Pargament KI. Struggle with the divine in Swiss patients visited by chaplains: prevalence and correlates. J Health Psychol. 2014;19(8):966–76.
26. Magyar-Russell G, Brown IT, Edara IR, Smith MT, Marine JE, Ziegelstein RC. In search of serenity: religious struggle among patients hospitalized for suspected acute coronary syndrome. J Relig Health. 2014;53(2):562–78.
27. Watt MH, Wilson SM, Joseph M, Masenga G, MacFarlane JC, Oneko O, et al. Religious coping among women with obstetric fistula in Tanzania. Glob Public Health. 2014;9(5):516–27.
28. Hvidtjorn D, Hjelmborg J, Skytthe A, Christensen K, Hvidt NC. Religiousness and religious coping in a secular society: the gender perspective. J Relig Health. 2014;53(5):1329–41.
29. Park CL, Wortmann JH, Edmondson D. Religious struggle as a predictor of subsequent mental and physical well-being in advanced heart failure patients. J Behav Med. 2011;34(6):426–36.
30. Pinter B, Hakim M, Seidman DS, Kubba A, Kishen M, Di Carlo C. Religion and family planning. Eur J Contracept Reprod Health Care. 2016;21(6):486–95.
31. Chakraborty R, El-Jawahri AR, Litzow MR, Syrjala KL, Parnes AD, Hashmi SK. A systematic review of religious beliefs about major end-of-life issues in the five major world religions. Palliat Support Care. 2017;15(5):609–22.
32. Delgado-Guay MO, Chisholm G, Williams J, Bruera E. The association between religiosity and resuscitation status preference among patients with advanced cancer. Palliat Support Care. 2015;13(5):1435–9.
33. Messina E. Beyond the officially sacred, donor and believer: religion and organ transplantation. Transplant Proc. 2015;47(7):2092–6.
34. Lifford KJ, Witt J, Burton M, Collins K, Caldon L, Edwards A, et al. Understanding older women's decision making and coping in the context of breast cancer treatment. BMC Med Inform Decis Mak. 2015;15:45.
35. Geros-Willfond KN, Ivy SS, Montz K, Bohan SE, Torke AM. Religion and spirituality in surrogate decision making for hospitalized older adults. J Relig Health. 2016;55(3):765–77.
36. Leyva B, Nguyen AB, Allen JD, Taplin SH, Moser RP. Is religiosity associated with cancer screening? Results from a national survey. J Relig Health. 2014;54:998.
37. Van Norman GA. Decisions regarding forgoing life-sustaining treatments. Curr Opin Anaesthesiol. 2017;30(2):211–6.
38. Mollica MA, Underwood W 3rd, Homish GG, Homish DL, Orom H. Spirituality is associated with less treatment regret in men with localized prostate cancer. Psycho-Oncology. 2017;26(11):1839–45.
39. Noh H, Kwak J. End-of-life decision making for persons with dementia: proxies' perception of support. Dementia. 2018;17:478.
40. Ayeh DD, Tak HJ, Yoon JD, Curlin FA. U.S. physicians' opinions about accommodating religiously based requests for continued life-sustaining treatment. J Pain Symptom Manag. 2016;51(6):971–8.
41. VanderWeele TJ, Yu J, Cozier YC, Wise L, Argentieri MA, Rosenberg L, et al. Attendance at religious services, prayer, religious coping, and religious/spiritual identity as predictors of all-cause mortality in the Black Women's Health Study. Am J Epidemiol. 2017;185(7):515–22.
42. Morton KR, Lee JW, Martin LR. Pathways from religion to health: mediation by psychosocial and lifestyle mechanisms. Psycholog Relig Spiritual. 2017;9(1):106–17.
43. Ironson G, Kremer H, Lucette A. Relationship between spiritual coping and survival in patients with HIV. J Gen Intern Med. 2016;31(9):1068–76.
44. Buttle H. Measuring a journey without goal: meditation, spirituality, and physiology. Biomed Res Int. 2015;2015:891671.
45. Boccia M, Piccardi L, Guariglia P. The meditative mind: a comprehensive meta-analysis of MRI studies. Biomed Res Int. 2015;2015:419808.
46. Roberts L, Ahmed I, Hall S, Davison A. Intercessory prayer for the alleviation of ill health. Cochrane Database Syst Rev. 2009;(2):Cd000368.

47. Anderson JW, Nunnelley PA. Private prayer associations with depression, anxiety and other health conditions: an analytical review of clinical studies. Postgrad Med. 2016;128(7):635–41.
48. Persynaki A, Karras S, Pichard C. Unraveling the metabolic health benefits of fasting related to religious beliefs: a narrative review. Nutrition. 2017;35:14–20.
49. Pesut B, Thorne S. From private to public: negotiating professional and personal identities in spiritual care. J Adv Nurs. 2007;58(4):396–403.
50. Polzer Casarez RL, Engebretson JC. Ethical issues of incorporating spiritual care into clinical practice. J Clin Nurs. 2012;21(15-16):2099–107.
51. Post SG, Puchalski CM, Larson DB. Physicians and patient spirituality: professional boundaries, competency, and ethics. Ann Intern Med. 2000;132(7):578–83.
52. Pujol N, Jobin G, Beloucif S. 'Spiritual care is not the hospital's business': a qualitative study on the perspectives of patients about the integration of spirituality in healthcare settings. J Med Ethics. 2016;42(11):733–7.
53. Taylor EJ. What do I say? Talking with patients about spirituality. West Conshohocken, PA: Templeton Press; 2007.
54. Center PR. The changing global religious landscape. Pew Research Center; 2017. http://www.pewforum.org/2017/04/05/the-changing-global-religious-landscape/.
55. Taylor RJ, Chatters LM, Lincoln K, Woodward AT. Church-based exchanges of informal social support among African Americans. Race Soc Probl. 2017;9(1):53–62.
56. Sun A, Bui Q, Tsoh JY, Gildengorin G, Chan J, Cheng J, et al. Efficacy of a church-based, culturally tailored program to promote completion of advance directives among Asian Americans. J Immigr Minor Health. 2017;19(2):381–91.
57. Derose KP, Griffin BA, Kanouse DE, Bogart LM, Williams MV, Haas AC, et al. Effects of a pilot church-based intervention to reduce HIV stigma and promote HIV testing among African Americans and Latinos. AIDS Behav. 2016;20(8):1692–705.
58. Moore EW, Berkley-Patton JY, Berman M, Burleson C, Judah A. Physical health screenings among African-American church and community members. J Relig Health. 2016;55(5):1786–99.
59. Powell TW, Herbert A, Ritchwood TD, Latkin CA. "Let me help you help me": church-based HIV prevention for young black men who have sex with men. AIDS Educ Prev. 2016;28(3):202–15.
60. Ralston PA, Young-Clark I, Coccia C. The development of health for hearts united: a longitudinal church-based intervention to reduce cardiovascular risk in mid-life and older African Americans. Ethn Dis. 2017;27(1):21–30.
61. Williams MV, Derose KP, Aunon F, Kanouse DE, Bogart LM, Griffin BA, et al. Church-based HIV screening in racial/ethnic minority communities of California, 2011-2012. Public Health Rep. 2016;131(5):676–84.
62. Beard M, Chuang E, Haughton J, Arredondo EM. Determinants of implementation effectiveness in a physical activity program for church-going Latinas. Fam Community Health. 2016;39(4):225–33.

Spirituality and Childbirth

Colm OBoyle and Vivienne Brady

Abstract

Birth is widely recognised as a spiritual experience. In this chapter, we explore spirituality in pregnancy, birth and early parenthood and the extent that spirituality is supported or enriched by midwifery care. While a precise definition of spirituality remains elusive, there is growing acceptance that spirituality concerns the need for personal connectedness, desire for meaning in life, transformation and transcendence. The ability to ascribe meaning is a human attribute, and in health care, the significance of meaning making in and around the end of life is now widely recognized. The significance of meaning making at the start of life, is not so extensively explored.One reason may be that childbirth, in the Western world at least, is largely hospitalised, where medical intervention, maternity structures, and technology can deter from a personal, and spiritual birth experience. Mothers can struggle to find ways to give meaning to birth events, to connect with others and to recognise the transformative and perhaps even transcendent nature of pregnancy, childbirth and parenthood. Spirituality is not necessarily mediated through religious belief, although for many it is. Many midwives identify the privilege of being with woman and witnessing human creation as particularly meaningful and worthy of metaphors, such as sacred or divine. Birth brings new life and is, or should be, a joyful and empowering experience. In the following pages, we consider some of the ways that science and medicine, faith and religion, and feminist discourse contribute to discussion about spirituality and spiritual care in childbirth.

C. OBoyle · V. Brady (✉)
Trinity College, Dublin, Ireland
e-mail: coboyle@tcd.ie; bradyvi@tcd.ie

6.1 Introduction

The aim of this chapter is to explore spirituality in pregnancy, birth and early parenthood. While our discussion is predominantly concerned with women's experiences, we recognise the experiences of the family and birth attendant also. An examination of the spirituality of the baby, in utero and at birth, as part of the total well-being of the family is acknowledged, but is beyond the scope of this chapter.

The rationale for this work is to give attention to spirituality during the pregnancy, birth and motherhood continuum. The first step is to acknowledge and value spiritual aspects of birth and then to offer the reader some language with which to communicate about spirituality in childbirth.

The chapter is divided into the following sections: a consideration of spirituality in pregnancy, birth and new parenthood; the influence of religious, medical and feminist discourses; the importance of relationship in meaning making; and, finally, the transformative and potentially transcendent nature of childbirth. Reflective exercises will prompt readers to explore their own concepts of spirituality, and beliefs about spirituality and childbirth, and spiritual care in midwifery practice.

6.2 Spirituality

Spirituality has been referred to as finding meaning and purpose in life events, as connectedness to others and/or a higher power, as holism and as self-transcendence [1]. Spiritual experience is so exceptional from our ordinary physical and rational experience that we humans use metaphors to try to describe the concept; terms such as 'the divine', 'the sacred', 'spirit', 'God', 'transcendence' or 'higher power'. Some may consider existential matters, such as life's meaning and purpose without reference to the word 'spirit' or the concept of 'spirit'. Many, however, identify spiritual concepts to be significant sources of life meaning.

The lack of a precise definition of spirituality makes discussion about spirituality in health care challenging. We, like Moloney [2] and Sellers and Haag [3], for example, take the ontological position that spirituality is implicit to humanity. We believe that the human search for the meaning and purpose of existence includes a spiritual dimension, in whatever way one tries to define 'spiritual'.

6.3 Spirituality in Pregnancy, Birth and New Parenthood

Childbirth is meaningful to women, to families and to humanity. The existential experiences of pregnancy, labour, childbirth and new parenthood are so personally and socially transformative that the meaning given to these experiences is very often described as deeply spiritual.

This is consistent with Klassen's [4] exploration of spirituality in birth as encompassing reverence for nature, transcending the physical and trusting in a higher power [4]. Birth has been described as miraculous, mysterious and transformational [5], but exceeding religion [4]. Many other authors confirm that spirituality is central to women's and midwives' experience of reproduction and birth [4, 6–17]. Since first published in 1975, Ina May Gaskin's [12] *Spiritual Midwifery* has enduring popularity among birthing mothers and midwives and demonstrates spirituality has long been a concern, however muted, in birth discourse. Most recently, Crowther and Hall [18] have edited a book with contributions from midwives and obstetricians who are engaged in exploring spirituality in maternity care. Parratt [19] in the same book describes couples' spiritual experiences at birth and cites many more academic papers in the field.

Consideration and celebration of birth and birth attendance, as spiritual, is inhibited by the intersection of several strongly held and potentially counter discourses. These are a reductionist view of health and humanity by science and medicine that suggests wariness of faith and religion, and a feminist critique of religious and medical rhetoric, that is believed to perpetuate biological essentialism and patriarchal hegemony in human reproductive and health-care practices. In the following pages, we will, consider some of the ways these discourses can complicate discussion of spirituality and spiritual care in childbirth.

6.4 Religion

An enormous body of academic writing and debate about human understanding of spirituality exists in the fields of philosophy, theology and religious studies. Religious and theological discourses already describe spiritual concepts in subtle detail, which can be very useful to explore the subject of spirituality[1]. Spirituality, for some, overlaps with religion and trust in a higher power [4, 20].

> For most of these women, Christians, Jews, spiritual feminists, new agers and even some "non-religious" women, spirituality was an evocative and useful term to describe their births, generally meaning a personal and embodied connection with a supernatural power that anyone who made the effort could access. ([4], p. 73)

Religion, therefore, can provide a language and metaphor with which to speak of the immanent (real, here and now, embodied) and transcendent (supernatural, infinite) conceptions of spiritual aspects of human and birth experience. Women may draw upon spiritual language and symbolism in childbirth, without considering themselves to be religious or practising religious beliefs [1].

As Klassen [4] points out, patriarchal religions of Judaism and Christianity (and Islam) have not traditionally celebrated the spiritual or sacred nature of birth. A growing secularism in Ireland and elsewhere, however, reveals some antagonism to the dominance and perceived ownership of spiritual discourse by religious authorities. Christian interpretation of Genesis 3:16 'in sorrow thou shalt bring forth

---

[1] We have not sourced Islamic tradition related texts published in English.

children', for instance, has held that suffering in childbirth is punishment and atonement for the sins of Eve [21]. This clearly misogynistic religious perspective is unlikely to be a useful opening to a discussion on the spirituality of birth. Thus, religious expression of spiritual experience may be problematic. Integrating secular meaning making in health care in Northern Europe is not adequately addressed in language that is exclusively spiritual or religious. La Cour and Hvidt [22] therefore, incorporate psychological and social dimensions in meaning making. Cognition (knowing/asking), practice (doing/acting) and importance (being/feeling) are useful dimensions for considering existential issues, whatever a person's secular, spiritual and/or religious viewpoints.

The midwife/birth attendant needs to be familiar with, and balance, their own and women's varied approaches to spirituality. Where religious expression enhances the woman's spiritual experiences and expectations of pregnancy, birth and new motherhood, the midwife should endeavour to understand and welcome this expression as an essential aspect of care. Where the woman's perception is that religious interpretations detract from her experience,[2] the midwife should also identify this and explore with the woman how spirituality in birth, if relevant, may manifest in other ways.

Midwives need to be open to discuss the meaning (-fulness) of pregnancy, birth and motherhood/parenthood. This openness includes the possibility of ambivalence about spirituality within ourselves, in other birth attendants and in women/mothers themselves. Unconditional positive regard is necessary for a therapeutic mother–midwife relationship, and so we should not impose our views [24] but rather enhance the coherence or harmony of the woman's experience and world view [25].

6.4.1 Exercise

Do you consider yourself to be spiritual? If so, how does this shape your perspectives on midwifery care and childbirth?

Can and/or must your personal views (e.g., on religion or politics) be held only outside of your professional practice?

6.5 Medicine

Marjorie Tew [26] dispelled the myth that medical advances in surgery, antibiotic therapy and hospitalisation of birth led to improved birth outcomes in the twentieth century. As important as these advances were, social factors, such as sanitation, housing and women's reproductive control, and their consequent effects on living standards accounted for the most significant improvements in maternal and perinatal mortality and morbidity in the developed world.

---

[2] See Pargament et al. [23] for positive and negative religious coping.

In a similar vein, taking mortality and morbidity as the best or only measures of quality in maternity care is too simplistic a view of human experience [27]. Birth is complex and multidimensional and midwives must identify and value (count or account for) the 'subjective, personal and particular' of women's childbirth experiences ([28], p. 53).

Contemporary medicine's tendency to compartmentalise the human body into ever more specialised biological systems, to the near exclusion of extra-corporal dimensions [29] has been captured in a relatively recent call to holism. The spiritual dimension of human existence and health, however, remains under-explored. Midwives who recognise the relational aspects of humanity and birth are somewhat closer to acknowledging spirituality as essential to birth attendance [30]. In Ireland at least, but perhaps almost everywhere, the relatively low status of midwifery in social, medical and hospital hierarchies, and the need for midwives to operate within the medical hegemony, has inhibited expression of spiritual midwifery. The pervasive rhetoric of the multidisciplinary team (MDT) quietly ignores the reality of medical power and dominance in contemporary health policy, health-care settings and risk discourse.

Scientific reductionism within medicine and obstetrics has and continues to inhibit both the exploration and integration of spiritual care into contemporary maternity care services [31].

The dominant model of birth in contemporary industrialised countries is consultant-led, hospitalised birth, which anticipates risk and danger, diminishes relationship and privileges surveillance and intervention [32]. The scientific rationality of contemporary Western (allopathic) medicine cannot easily accommodate highly variable subjective human experience, let alone the metaphysical or spiritual. In contrast, midwifery constitutes that women are their own 'deliverers' ([33], p. 298) and emphasises the pursuit of natural and physiological childbirth [34].

6.6 Feminist Discourse

Feminist critique of patriarchy and masculinist thinking in society generally, in law and governance but also in science, medicine and religion, has opened new ways of seeing and being in the world.

Essentialist or reductionist views of women's reproductive capabilities have been subject to feminist critique; one example is Adrienne Rich's [21] analysis of the regulation and control of women's bodies and psyche by the medical institution. There is rejection of the long-standing reduction of gender differences to biological function and capacity for sexual reproduction, to justify highly gendered social role expectations. The highly gendered split between the paid public professional spheres and the unpaid private domestic spheres, has been recognised as arising from gendered social norms and rightly challenged as unequal by feminist thinkers. The danger in attempts to celebrate and give meaning to birth is that even positive attributions may easily become, or be seen to be, justifications for limiting women's role to their reproductive function or diminishing women who cannot, or choose not to, become mothers [21, 35].

As one might expect, there are many feminist perspectives on spirituality, some critiques embody rejection of God and religion as perpetuations of masculinist, patriarchal structures [36]. Others seek to provide an array of positive female metaphors for God and may use female pronouns or the term 'Goddess'. Some women may be familiar with these and consider them useful approaches to talking about spirituality around birth.

Our purpose is to encourage birth attendants to remain open to spiritual expression in whatever way the woman chooses to convey this in pregnancy and childbirth. Midwives could explore the Goddess as metaphor, which could help birthing women access their own meaning in their becoming mother.

If a 'Goddess' does not appeal as an alternative to patriarchal religion and its metaphors, the work of Grace Jantzen [37] might offer an alternative approach. Jantzen proposes that in a feminist philosophy based upon the fact of our birth, our human 'natality' enables a creative and nurturing approach that might be useful in discussing human meaning. Jantzen, in her book, *Becoming Divine* (1999) offers a cogent critique of the dominant focus on human 'mortality' and death, which pervades Judeo-Christo-Islamic religious traditions. Taking human 'natality' as the foundation of human being and becoming (ontology) has obvious resonance in the search for a spirituality of midwifery.

With every birth, hope is reborn, as 'it is in birth, in natality, that newness enters the world, and it is in the fact of new life that every other form of freedom and creativity is grounded...' ([38], p. 6).

6.6.1 Exercise

How do you feel about the representation of 'Goddess' as a means of expressing your own spirituality or relationship with the divine?

What, if anything, blocks your ability to bring such a perspective to women in your care?

Does Jantzen's focus on human embodied 'natality' as a basis for creativity and growth sit well with your view of birth?

Might Jantzen's positive philosophy of natality offer a useful alternative to contemporary focus on risk, danger and mortality in maternity care?

6.7 Meaning Making

Returning to our conception of spirituality as being a central aspect of human meaning making, we will explore the recurring themes of relationship, transformation and transcendence in women's experience of birth as spiritual, and spirituality as giving meaning in childbirth. While any schema is likely to be inadequate for a field that so often references the 'infinite', these themes, for us, capture enough of the meaning of spirituality in childbirth to enable fruitful discussion.

The concept of relationship is central to women's birth experience, and therefore, a midwife should be able to relate, communicate and support the woman's spiritual needs, as part of the central philosophical tenet of midwifery of 'being with'. Pregnancy, labour, birth and new parenthood are undeniably transformative on all levels, physical, emotional, psychological, social and spiritual. A holistic approach to birth cannot deny its spiritual nature and the potential for spiritual growth, enlightenment and transformation in birth. The concept and language of transcendence as an aspect of spirituality and of transformation needs also to be explored. Concepts such as the 'divine' and the 'sacred' are commonly, though not universally, expressed in women's and midwives' birth experiences [4, 39] and discourses, and so, these and related ideas should be incorporated into the midwife's discursive repertoire.

6.8 Relationship in Spiritual Midwifery

Relationship is central to reproduction, pregnancy, birth and parenthood. Each step presupposes a degree of relationship: sexual intimacy between mother and partner; the mother–baby dyad; the development of a new life and body within the living body of another; the dependent nature of a baby, predominantly upon the mother, but to society more broadly; and finally the developing personhood, self-awareness and meaning making of the child. It is only in the context of relationship to others that childbirth can occur and can be understood or given meaning. Our definition of spirituality as a basis for meaning making fits coherently within this framework. Relationship between each of the actors in childbirth will be explored in the following section. For our purposes, most central is the relationship between the woman and her birth companion, the midwife.

The physiology of birth, labour onset and progress depend upon a complex interplay of endocrine and neurological signals that have been shown to be sensitive to the emotional and psychological well-being of the woman, the social setting and the physical and relational context in which she is to birth [40, 41].

Relationships are developed and connections made through negotiating trust and reciprocity [42]. Comfort in 'letting go' in birth is complex and multifaceted and appears to be concomitant with the woman anticipating birth 'not simply a bodily process to undergo, but an experience to be chosen' ([4], p. 63). Human relationships are central to this experience. Fahy and Hastie [43] analyse relational power in psychotherapeutic terms and describe midwifery guardianship as facilitating the mother's letting go of the ego. This is to permit access to the usually repressed unconscious (non-ordinary consciousness) or inner self and to love. According to Fahy and Hastie [43], the ethical accountability of midwife to woman is also a loving act, one that requires the midwife to explore her own unconscious as potentially damaging to the birthing woman's flourishing. This psychoanalytical approach to relationship acknowledges and enables access to human experiences not readily accessed by the rational mind or ego. As has been recognised above, techno-rationality dominates contemporary maternity care, and this concept of midwifery guardianship is a means to move beyond such a limited and limiting perspective.

Reference to empathy and kindness is very easily incorporated in a discussion about love. The centrality of relational concepts of empathy and kindness in midwifery to enhancing a woman's birth, expression of a positive spiritual experience, and resulting confidence in becoming a mother, is illustrated in the findings of Organic Inquiry research by Moloney and Gair [44] with 48 women, including mothers, midwives and counsellors:

> The stories presented above include some shining examples of empathy, kindness and spiritual presence and care, the beauty, awesome power and energy of birth, and the intimate relation-ships between birthing women and midwives. The latter stories appear to exemplify an absence of empathic regard or kindness, a lack of respect for the sacredness of birth, and experiences of enduring disempowerment and trauma for birthing mothers. ([44], p. 327)

These findings echo the work of Jeanne Siddiqui [45] and Marie Berg et al. [46], which suggest that the potential relationship between the woman and her midwife is the very core of human connection and caring. All relationships are context-bound [47], and a positive midwife–mother relationship enhances the experience of birth and safety of mother and her baby [48]. Conversely, negative relationships, or the absence of support, inhibit birth in myriad ways [49]. Schneider's [16] research exploring the significance of childbirth to women moves our conversation to spiritual aspects of relationship. Women's narratives reveal that birth can be:

> A rich source of connection to self, other, community, and the divine, spiritual aspects in one's life serve to inspire, support, and transform'. ([16], p. 212)

Schneider's work resonates with similar themes in midwifery narratives of childbirth as spiritual [12, 44]. Midwives, with a philosophical commitment to relationship, to 'being with' woman during the childbirth experience, are perhaps understandably in tune with a holistic model of birth that incorporates a spiritual dimension. Lundgren and Berg [50] developed the earlier work of Berg et al. [46] and Lundgren [51] and determined the central concepts in the midwife–woman relationship, by secondary analysis of eight Swedish research studies. Pairs of concepts underpinning the larger theme of relationship were identified, each pair describes one aspect from the woman's perspective and, with it, her midwife's response. These are 'surrender–availability', 'trust–mediation of trust', 'participation–mutuality', 'loneliness–confirmation', 'differences–support uniqueness' and 'creation of meaning–support meaningfulness' [50]. While all are essential to the midwife as facilitator of the powerful birth experience, of specific interest to our discussion is explication of the midwife's role in meaning making.

Pembroke and Pembroke [30] integrate women's and midwives' discussion of relationship in childbirth and align the idea of relationship with Martin Buber's [52] concept of human 'responsibility' and Gabriel Marcel's [53] concept of 'availability' to the other. The concept of 'presence' in midwifery care relating to spirituality in midwifery has been identified by Hunter [54], Moloney and Gair [44] and Crowther and Hall [9].

Pembroke and Pembroke [30] describe midwifery 'presence' as a spiritual relationship:

The [ ] central metaphor in our discussion was 'calm presence'. In the midst of the emotional and physical frenzy, the midwife offers calm reassurance.

A spirituality of presence in midwifery requires a commitment to an ongoing movement towards higher levels of responsibility and personal availability. This involves a commitment to self-transcendence. Self-transcendence in the context of midwifery is expressed through a desire to go out of self in order to respond sensitively, respectfully and generously to the values and needs of labouring women. ([30], p. 326)

The idea of transcendence will be revisited later in this chapter. Before that however the idea of transformation will be explored.

6.8.1 Exercise

Walsh [24] observed that the characteristics of childbearing women in labour and birth—'loving, gentle, hopeful, energetic, courageous, grateful, connected, accepting, broad outlook, detached' ([24], p. 484)—were the traits that Beck [55] identified in those who are spiritually aware.

How important do you think these attributes are in the practice of spiritual midwifery?

6.9 Transformation

Transformation, like relationship, is self-evidently a concept central to understanding the meaning of childbirth. A woman is physically and socially transformed by pregnancy, by birth and by motherhood. The transformation is not just physical, nor is it immediate or final but, rather, developmental and set within a series of other physical and social reproductive developments and transformations.

Many social meanings are attached to female personhood and reproduction: menarche (the onset of menstruation), sexual maturity and autonomy, (in)fertility, control (or not) of the reproductive self, (un)planned pregnancy, abortion, motherhood, mothering roles and menopause.

These transformations could be considered purely social, except that in women's explanations of birth as spiritual, the connection with others appears universal and, for some, expands to connection with the divine, as illustrated in Schneider's [16] analysis of spiritual transformation in birth.

Birth is described as miraculous, transformational and mysterious [5]. Moloney [2], from the testimony of women speaking of their experience of pregnancy, birth and motherhood considers that:

The discovery of pregnancy is a life-changing event; it initiates an ontological process of transformation, which, all being well, culminates in the birth of a child, a mother, a family... to be pregnant is to be touched by the creative power of something infinitely greater than self and such proximity with the divine is transformational. ([2], p. 122)

Midwives need awareness, openness, language and ability to support the existentially transformative nature of birth.

6.9.1 Exercise

Which physical and social transformations in childbirth strike you as opportunities to open up discussion with pregnant women/mothers about meaning making or the 'meaning' of their experience?

What transformations, reproductive or otherwise, in your own life can be drawn upon in understanding and facilitating meaning making as birth companions?

Is self-awareness a prerequisite for nurturing self-awareness in others? Discuss.

6.10 Transcendence

Again, like relationship and transformation, the concept of transcendence has a very broad application beyond the childbirth context. Unlike relationship and transformation, however, transcendence is not so obviously or necessarily inherent within childbirth. We wish to explore, not because we are already convinced, but rather explicitly because of how childbirth is related to concepts of transcendence. Self-transcendence beyond the individual self, to awareness of connection to others, expands beyond the purely social to an experience that could be described as meta-social and metaphysical.

The term transcendence, in particular self-transcendence, echoes an awareness of, and transformation from, a purely individualistic conception of the self. The reality of a distinct and separate life within, the duality, two within one of pregnancy or one becoming two of birth is transformative for mother and baby, but for the mother, perhaps necessarily, it is the transcendence of individualistic notions of the self. The desire for, the necessity of, or the recognition of relationship to others beyond the mother–baby dyad, also forms a significant part of the language of birth.

Self-transcendence through duress has been theorised by Reed [56]. Reed's model, though drawn from end-of-life experiences, enables the measurement of transcendence and exploration of concepts related to it. Her sub-themes, generativity, introjectivity, temporal integration and body transcendence, can be utilised to understand the language used by women to describe their experience of spirituality in childbirth [6, 14]. Generativity, the power to reproduce, temporal integration (in the liminal spaces of pregnancy and labour) and body transcendence—perhaps most crucially in labour—all seem appropriate. Introjectivity, the incorporation of others' world view into one's own, is perhaps less clear, but may be relevent in as far as relationships support, enhance and develop one's sense of self, and can be applied to the childbirth experience as readily as to end-of-life experiences.

Budin [6] cites Reed:

6 Spirituality and Childbirth

Reed [56] defines self-transcendence as the experience of extending self-boundaries inwardly, outwardly, and temporally to take on broader life perspectives, activities, and purposes. Although giving birth in modern times is rarely considered a life-threatening illness, I believe that for some women the experience of giving birth can also provide an opportunity for self-transcendence. ([6], p. 39)

Budin considers that the experience of the pain and joy of birth, along with the trust in one's own ability to birth, may lead to an incredible sense of accomplishment in which the woman experiences self-transcendence, as she realises her strength and power. Such experiences of self-transcendence, 'the ability to move beyond one's personal boundaries to gain a wider perspective', can contribute to enhanced meaning and understanding from life events and contribute to overall well-being [57]. Lydon-Lam [58] captures transcendence as an aspect or continuation of personal transformation:

> Transcendence suggests expansion of self-boundaries (a) inward through self-acceptance, with acceptance of what is and can be and (b) an openness to that which is not of the self (others, the divine, nature). This personal growth suggests knowing one-self, in an integrated way of past, present, and future, while living fully in the present moment. ([58], p. 21)

Similarly,

> Spirituality has both an immanent and a transcendental form. An immanent spirituality refers to an orientation in which people believe that all the resources they need to find meaning and value can be found within the self. ([30], p. 322)

Pembroke and Pembroke [30] go on to make explicit the link between relationship and transcendence (personal and/or spiritual) and say:

> Self-transcendence in the context of midwifery is expressed through a desire to go out of self in order to respond sensitively, respectfully and generously to the values and needs of labouring women. ([30], p. 326)

Spiritual transformation, therefore, can be understood as a natural part of the relational and human transformation that happens in birth. Spiritual transcendence becomes available to give further meaning to the very significant life change and transformation that is inevitable at every stage of pregnancy, labour, birth and new parenthood.

6.10.1 Exercise

Is your sense of spirituality immanent (real, here and now, embodied) or transcendent (supernatural, infinite) or some/any combination of these ideas?

What if any of the metaphors around spirituality might be useful or challenging for you?

Examples could include God, sacred, holy, creation, divine and love.

6.11 Conclusion

In this chapter, we have explored spirituality in pregnancy, birth and early parenthood, with reference to women's experiences. We have emphasised the spiritual aspects of birth and have suggested ways to communicate about and respond to spirituality in childbirth. We have aligned spirituality in pregnancy, birth and motherhood with the concept of human meaning making and have considered this briefly in the socio-biomedical context, with reference to religion, medicine and feminist discourse.

Birth is socially embedded, and so the context of the woman's relationship, particularly the relationship between the woman and midwife, is a central concern. Meaning making about birth is also social and relational. The mother–midwife relationship enables exploration of spirituality as an aspect of the birth experience. A spiritual interpretation of the birth experience can offer a means to integrate the transformations involved into the woman's developing self-concept and world view.

Consideration of the physical transformations inherent in childbirth led to an exploration of spiritual transformation and transcendence in birth. Expansion beyond ones previous self and limitations, is to transcend them. Transcendence is a theme that recurs in childbirth stories and is a concept that sits well within a spiritual framework for human meaning making. Throughout the chapter, we have prompted readers to explore their own relationship to concepts of spirituality, spirituality and childbirth and spiritual care in midwifery practice.

References

1. Callister LC, Khalaf I. Spirituality in childbearing women. J Perinat Educ. 2010;19(2):16–24.
2. Moloney S. Dancing with the wind: a methodological approach to researching women's spirituality around menstruation and birth. Int J Qual Methods. 2007;6(1):114–25.
3. Sellers SC, Haag BA. Spiritual nursing interventions. J Holist Nurs. 1998;16(3):338–54.
4. Klassen PE. Blessed events: religion and home birth in America. Princeton: Princeton University Press; 2001.
5. Moore H. Birth and death: a doula's role in sacred moments. Midwifery Today Int Midwife. 2001;58:21.
6. Budin WC. Birth and death: opportunities for self-transcendence. J Perinat Educ. 2001;10(2):38.
7. Carver N, Ward B. Spirituality in pregnancy: a diversity of experiences and needs. Br J Midwifery. 2007;15(5):294–6.
8. Chester DH. Mother. Unmother: a storied look at infertility, identity, and transformation. Qual Inq. 2003;9(5):774–84.
9. Crowther S, Hall J. Spirituality and spiritual care in and around childbirth. Women Birth. 2015;28(2):173–8.
10. Doherty ME. Voices of midwives: a tapestry of challenges and blessings. MCN Am J Matern Child Nurs. 2010;35(2):96–101.
11. Dwinell J. Birth stories: mystery, power, and creation. Santa Barbara: Greenwood Publishing Group; 1992.
12. Gaskin IM. Spiritual midwifery. Summertown: Book Publishing Company; 2010.
13. Linhares C. The lived experience of midwives with spirituality in childbirth: mana from heaven. J Midwifery Womens Health. 2012;57:165–71.

14. McHugh N. Midwives of the soul: the spirituality of birth. Midwifery Matters. 2003;97:4–5.
15. Miller L. Spiritual awareness in life and psychotherapy. In: Rayburn CA, Comas-Dias L, editors. Woman soul: the inner life of women's spirituality. Westport, CT: Praeger; 2010. p. 221–36.
16. Schneider DA. The miracle bearers: narratives of birthing women and implications for spiritually informed social work practice. J Soc Serv Res. 2012;38(2):212–30.
17. Vincent P. Baby catcher: chronicles of a modern midwife. New York: Scribner; 2002.
18. Crowther S, Hall J. Spirituality and childbirth: meaning and care at the start of life. London: Routledge; 2018.
19. Parratt J. Couples' spiritual experiences at birth. In: Crowther S, Hall J, editors. Spirituality and childbirth: meaning and care at the start of life. London: Routledge; 2018.
20. Bélanger-Lévesque MN, Dumas M, Blouin S, Pasquier JC. "That was intense!" Spirituality during childbirth: a mixed-method comparative study of mothers' and fathers' experiences in a public hospital. BMC Pregnancy Childbirth. 2016;16(1):294.
21. Rich A. Of woman born: motherhood as experience and institution. New York: W. W. Norton; 1995.
22. La Cour P, Hvidt NC. Research on meaning-making and health in secular society: secular, spiritual and religious existential orientations. Soc Sci Med. 2010;71(7):1292–9.
23. Pargament KI, Smith BW, Koenig HG, Perez L. Patterns of positive and negative religious coping with major life stressors. J Sci Study Relig. 1998;374:710–24.
24. Walsh D. How's you spiritual life going? Br J Midwifery. 2002;10(8):484.
25. Rumbold BD. A review of spiritual assessment in health care practice. Med J Aust. 2007;186(10):S60–2.
26. Tew M. Safer childbirth? A critical history of maternity care. London: Springer; 1995.
27. Larkin P, Begley C, Devane D. Not enough people to look after you-an exploration of women's experiences of childbirth in the republic of Ireland. Midwifery. 2012;28(1):98–105.
28. Larkin P, Begley C, Devane D. Women's experiences of labour and birth: an evolutionary concept analysis. Midwifery. 2009;25:49–59.
29. Wagner M. Pursuing the birth machine: the search for appropriate birth technology. Sevenoaks: ACE Graphics; 1994.
30. Pembroke NF, Pembroke J. The spirituality of presence in midwifery care. Midwifery. 2008;24:321–7.
31. Barrett A. Spiritual obstetrics. In: Crowther S, Hall J, editors. Spirituality and childbirth: meaning and care at the start of life. London: Routledge; 2018.
32. Murphy-Lawless J. Reading birth and death: a history of obstetric thinking. Cork: Cork University Press; 1998.
33. Oakley A. Women confined: towards a sociology of childbirth. New York: Schocken Books; 1980. p. 10.
34. Kitzinger S. The new experience of childbirth. London: Hachette UK; 2012.
35. Martin E. The woman in the body: a cultural analysis of reproduction. Boston: Beacon Press; 2001.
36. Byrne P. Omnipotence, feminism and god. Int J Philos Relig. 1995;37:145–65.
37. Jantzen G. Becoming divine: towards a feminist philosophy of religion. Bloomington: Indiana University Press; 1999.
38. Jantzen GM. Foundations of violence. London: Routledge; 2004.
39. Crowther S. Sacred space at the moment of birth. Pract Midwife. 2013;16(11):21–3.
40. Gaskin IM. Ina May's guide to childbirth. New York: Bantam Dell, Random House; 2003.
41. Hammond A, Foureur M, Homer C, Davis D. Space, place and the midwife: exploring the relationship between the birth environment, neurobiology and midwifery practice. Women Birth. 2013;26(4):277–81.
42. Hunter B, Berg M, Lundgren I, Olafsdóttir O, Kirkham M. Relationships: the hidden threads in the tapestry of maternity care. Midwifery. 2008;24:132–7.
43. Fahy K, Hastie C. Midwifery guardianship: reclaiming the sacred in birth. In: Fahy K, Foureur M, Hastie C, editors. Birth territory and midwifery guardianship: theory for practice, education and research. Edinburgh: Books for Midwives; 2008. p. 21–37.

44. Moloney S, Gair S. Empathy and spiritual care in midwifery practice: contributing to women's enhanced birth experiences. Women Birth. 2015;28(4):323–8.
45. Siddiqui J. The therapeutic relationship in midwifery. Br J Midwifery. 1999;7(2):111–4.
46. Berg M, Lundgren I, Hermansson E, Wahlberg V. Women's experience of the encounter with the midwife during childbirth. Midwifery. 1996;12:11–5.
47. Kirkham M. The maternity services context. In: Kirkham M, editor. The midwife mother relationship. 2nd ed. Houndmills: Palgrave Macmillan; 2010. p. 1–16.
48. Leap N. The less we do the more we give. In: Kirkham M, editor. The midwife mother relationship. 2nd ed. Houndmills: Palgrave Macmillan; 2010. p. 1–16.
49. Coates R, Ayers S, de Visser R. Women's experiences of postnatal distress: a qualitative study. BMC Pregnancy Childbirth. 2014;14:359.
50. Lundgren I, Berg M. Central concepts in the midwife-woman relationship. Scand J Caring Sci. 2007;21:220–8.
51. Lundgren I. Releasing and relieving encounters: experiences of pregnancy and childbirth. Scand J Caring Sci. 2004;18:368–75.
52. Buber M. Between man and man. Translated by Gregor Smith R. London: Routledge & Kegan Paul; 1947.
53. Marcel G. The mystery of being, vol. I. London: The Harvill Press; 1950.
54. Hunter L. Spirituality and midwifery care. In: Introducing the social sciences for midwifery practices birthing in a contemporary society. New York: Routledge; 2016. p. 87–102.
55. Beck C. Better Schools: A Values Perspective. Faliner Press, London; 1990.
56. Reed PG. Toward a theory of self-transcendence: deductive reformulation using developmental theories. Adv Nurs Sci. 1991;13(4):64–77.
57. Coward DD, Reed PG. Self-transcendence: a resource for healing at the end of life. Issues Ment Health Nurs. 1996;17(3):275–88.
58. Lydon-Lam J. Models of spirituality and consideration of spiritual assessment. Int J Childbirth Educ. 2012;27(1):18.

7. Providing Spiritual Care: An Exploration of Required Spiritual Care Competencies in Healthcare and Their Impact on Healthcare Provision

René van Leeuwen

Abstract

Healthcare workers deliver holistic patient-centred care. Spiritual care is part of that. To deliver spiritual care, the healthcare worker should be competent for that. These competencies could be divided in three domains, namely:

- Awareness and use of self: this domain is about the healthcare workers' intra- and interpersonal communications and attitudes in spiritual care delivery.
- Spiritual dimensions of the nursing process: this domain is about the role of the healthcare worker in spiritual assessment, planning, interventions and evaluation of spiritual care within the integral nursing process.
- Assurance of quality and expertise: this domain of competence is about the healthcare workers' professional development regarding spiritual care.

In this chapter these competencies will be further theoretically clarified and applied in specific exercise that enables the reader to work on his/her spiritual care competence.

R. van Leeuwen (✉)
Viaa Christian University of Applied Sciences, Zwolle, The Netherlands
e-mail: r.vanleeuwen@viaa.nl

7.1 Introduction

> **Box 7.1: An Impression from Healthcare Practice**
> Since 1 year Joan (22) works as a mental health nurse on a critical care ward of a mental health hospital. Joan finds herself spiritual, but not in a religious sense. At the moment Joan cares for Jim (29) who is treated for a depression. Jim was admitted to the hospital because of a suicide attempt. He is deeply depressed and feels guilty to himself, to his family and also to God. Most of the day he lies on his bed, and he is praying all day and reads a lot in Scripture. 'Leave me alone', he said to the nurses. Joan finds it difficult to understand Jim's situation and to cope with it in a professional way. 'Faith can do a lot of harm, why does he still rely on it', she considers for herself. She asks her colleagues for their experiences, but most of them find it also a difficult situation. '"The spiritual" is not really an integrated part of our work, I guess', they say. One of the colleagues says 'we have to take his belief seriously'.

In order to provide holistic care, as a healthcare worker you must be competent to intervene on a physical, mental, social and spiritual level. The situation of Jim described in Box 7.1 makes clear that interventions might be relevant for all of these dimensions of holistic care. For example, what does it mean for his physical condition when he does not leave his bed for a long time? How suicidal is he still at the moment and what actions are required for that? How can you help him from his social isolation? And, what is the relationship between his faith and the mental and social problems he is facing? This last question is focusing on the spiritual dimension of Jim's functioning. This dimension should also be part of the process of clinical reasoning which can lead to specific interventions in this area.

The situation is also pointing on the person of the healthcare worker. It touches also her personal beliefs and views. Is her interpretation of the situation correct as she says that religion has harmed Jim? What does it mean that she wonders that Jim still can rely on his belief? How will she connect with Jim from that perspective? And why is one of her colleagues saying that the patient's belief should be taken seriously? Is she saying that from a professional point of view, or is she reacting in this way because she is religious herself? This situation makes clear that personal convictions and opinions regarding spirituality and spiritual care might be of influence on how you will act in such a situation as a healthcare professional. It is important to be aware of that and reflect on that.

The situation also says something about the way spiritual care might be well integrated within the healthcare policy of a healthcare institution. According to this situation, that can be questioned. It seems every healthcare worker has his/her own vision and a common policy is lacking. It might also be expected from healthcare professionals that they are able to influence the spiritual care policy of the healthcare team they are acting in and play their part in enhancing the quality of spiritual care in healthcare practice.

The above-mentioned three perspectives of spiritual care (the healthcare process, personal attitude and the healthcare policy) cover the three domains of spiritual care competencies of healthcare professionals. The notion of 'competencies' denotes sets of knowledge, skills and attitudes used in a professional context, i.e. the clinical nursing process. Being competent depends on correct assessment of a clinical situation and on the ability to implement knowledge and skills in the right way at the right moment.

According to the findings of a literature review and research in practice, a nursing competency profile for spiritual care was formulated that consisted of three domains and six competencies [1, 2]. Box 7.2 gives an overview of these competencies. In this chapter these six competencies will be worked out in a way that it will help you as a healthcare professional to develop those competencies and apply them in your own healthcare practice.

Box 7.2: Profile of Spiritual Care Competencies

Domain	Competence
Awareness and use of self	1. Attitude towards the patient's spirituality: handling their own values, convictions and feelings in their professional relationships with patients of different beliefs and religions
	2. Communication: addressing the subject of spirituality with patients from different cultures in a caring manner
Spiritual dimensions of the nursing process	3. Assessment and implementation of spiritual care: the nurse collects information about the patient's spirituality and identifies the patient's need
	4. Personal support and patient counselling: discussing with the patient and team members how spiritual care is planned, provided and evaluated
	5. Referral to professionals
Assurance of quality and expertise	6. Contributing to quality assurance and improving expertise in spiritual care in the organisation

---

Exercise 1 'What Is My Starting Point?'

Before studying this chapter, make this exercise in which you assess your own level of competence. For this purpose you can use the Spiritual Care Competence Scale that is added in the Appendix of this book.

Score yourself on the 27 items of this questionnaire, and mark those competencies you personally find you have to/want to develop further.

Discuss the outcome of this exercise with a fellow student or colleague.

7.2 Attitude Towards the Patient's Spirituality

> *Nurse:* 'She has children. She knew she had to leave them. That's what broke her. I thought that was really difficult, because she didn't let anyone near. That gets me thinking. What would I have done? What would help me? It's so difficult. I feel so helpless. I see her struggling. She had philosophical questions, but the spiral was hard to break out of'.
>
> *Social worker:* 'I'm not a religious person, and I can sense a kind of inner friction. For example, when a client tells me about the abuse and what it did to her. How can such a person still believe? Where was that God when things went wrong? I really have difficulty with that'.
>
> *Care provider:* 'Sometimes I can't take it anymore. I feel like crying. That won't happen in front of a patient, but I'll go to my colleagues. I'm able to share my story with them and that's important. It's difficult to cross my own boundaries and to let my own emotions interfere too much. I wonder if I did right, if I didn't go too far'.

Maybe one way or another, these brief descriptions are recognisable from your personal experiences in patient care. These situations make clear that your personal thoughts and feelings are at stake when spirituality and spiritual needs come forward in healthcare. Are you conscious of those situations, thoughts and feelings, and can you imagine what impact they can have on the care you give to a patient? The competence of 'attitude towards the patients' spirituality' is about handling your own values, convictions and feelings regarding spirituality and spiritual care in professional relationships with patients of different beliefs and religions. A healthcare profession is in essence a relational profession. It asks primarily for an open, respectful, emphatic and reflective attitude. As a healthcare worker, you need to be open-minded to spirituality in general, to the individual patient's spirituality and to the impact of your own (spiritual) beliefs and convictions in the caring relationship. How will you react when you see a patient spiritually struggling? How do you respond to a religious patient, when you struggle with that belief yourself? How do you deal with your own emotions? Is showing your own 'weakness' allowed?

Healthcare professionals are often practical-minded. There is a problem that needs to be solved. After all, that is why you are a healthcare professional. However, spiritual issues often cannot be solved easily or solved at all. Within this context, we can refer to the so-called active and the passive side of a caring relationship [3]. The active component is expressed by words such as helping, providing care and assistance, wanting to be of significance to a client, showing you are there, holding a patient's hand, listening to a patient's story and so on. Healthcare professionals often are focussed (too much) on this component. After all, she is a 'doer'. The passive component of care provision is reflected in having to sit by and watch, encountering limitations, being faced with questions that you have no answer to, being affected by a patient's suffering, having to face death and being exposed to feelings of fear, indignation, helplessness and uncertainty. In situations like these, you are thrown upon your own resources or on your team's, and you can only be there for a client, without doing anything to solve it. In these situations, 'being' is equally important as 'doing' [4]. This passive component is essential to the caring relationship with the patient. Delivering spiritual care means that you must allow both the active and the passive aspect of the relationship. It is interesting to explore the balance between that active and passive component of the care you deliver.

> **Box 7.3: Exercise: Explore the Active and Passive Side of Your Caring Relationship**
> The quotes at the start of this section give an impression of the passive component of the care relation. Read the quotes again.
>
> (a) Describe a situation with a client in which you are/were involved and which entails the passive component of care, according to you.
> (b) Indicate on the continuum below where you would position yourself, when it comes to the relation between active and passive action in a care relationship.
>   Active   (doing)   --Passive
>   (being)
>   Give a concise motivation.
> (c) Discuss a and b with fellow students/colleagues.
> (d) Reflect on how you can/want to develop the passive role.

Your attitude towards spirituality and spiritual care asks for an open attitude towards the patients' spirituality. Such an attitude can be defined as 'inner space' [5]. Inner space is a metaphor. It is an inner attitude of rest and relaxation which opens you to learn new things, be patient and do not give way to mood swings or emotions. To define what inner space is not can easily be explained by means of some examples. In your work you can be fully occupied by organising and administrating your work which makes that you cannot pay any attention to patients' questions or you don't even hear the patient asking for help or attention. You do not experience any inner space to be present and attentive for the patient. Another example is about someone who is not open for the subject of spirituality at all, because he or she does not feel spiritual at all. A healthcare professional who is lacking the experience or feeling of any personal spirituality might have a less open space for the spiritual needs of patients. Spiritual needs can be ignored because you do not recognise them or find them not important to address.

> **Box 7.4: Exercise for Self-Reflection: 'How Is Your Inner Space?'**
> Reflect with a fellow student or colleague on the concept of inner space with the help of the following questions:
>
> 1. Do you find yourself a spiritual human being? Explain. What impact does this have on your openness to spirituality in your work?
> 2. Give an example when you had less/much inner space in connection with patients from your own healthcare practice. What factors were of influence?
> 3. What conditions do you need to have inner space for the spirituality and spiritual needs of patients? Give an example!
> 4. How would you describe 'inner space'?

7.3 Communication

You have probably gone through the following yourself: you told a friend about something you felt really sad about, for instance, when you broke up or when a long-cherished dream vanished. How did your friend respond to your story? Did he give comfort or advice or did he really listen? People are inclined to comfort in a situation like that, for instance: 'Bet you will meet a much nicer man'. Or they will advise you: 'You'd better not keep in touch, the sooner you will get over it'. Sometimes, people will tell their own story: 'Well, I've seen something like that myself …'. All of these responses show good intentions and involvement. People really want you to feel fine again soon. Patients often have to deal with situations when something is broken beyond repair and it cannot be fixed. In moments like these, spiritual questions often arise. A person can ask themselves: 'Why me?!' or 'What's next?' Often there are no concrete answers when these questions arise. The competence of communication is about addressing the subject of spirituality with patients from different cultures in a caring manner.

As a healthcare professional, you learn problem-solving methods. As nice as it can be to be able to do something for someone, so helpless you may feel when you are left empty-handed when there are no real solutions. Earlier in this chapter we talked about the active and passive side of helping. An important point of interest in spiritual communication is discerning which problems can be changed and which ones need to be accepted. Questions on spirituality are not always worded as an explicit question. They can be hidden behind the quarrels, irritation and anger. Questions of spirituality are often interwoven with many other questions and issues that patients are struggling with. A simple model can help to bring order in different types of questions [6]. This model assumes you can take a statement literally, but you can also learn to practise 'deep listening', sometimes referred to as 'listening in layers'.

Imagine a patient who is saying to you: 'I often lie awake at night, worrying about my work'. How can you trace the possible spiritual question in this statement? You do this by descending, as it were, from the superficial meaning to deeper layers of meaning by the next four steps:

1. First, you will hear the sentence as a statement about facts. The patient says, in fact, he often lies awake, because he worries about his work. You could fly at it immediately and tell him he should take a sleeping pill or do relaxation exercises. But perhaps that is not what he actually wants to say.
2. The fact that he lies awake means he is concerned about it. In his statement, there is an emotional layer or a perception layer as well. Perhaps he is filled with nostalgia for how he enjoyed his work. Perhaps he thinks now his life is empty and lonely, because he has to end his work which means a lot to him.
3. This emotional layer is connected to his life story. If we let him tell his life story, we will reach the biographical layer of the statement. You will only discover how deep and how important the emotions are when you find out what his work means to him. Maybe it was all the world to him: much more than just a job, a life fulfilment.
4. This brings us to the spiritual layer of the statement. An important source of spirituality comes up for him, something that makes him happy when he thinks about it. It gives him the feeling that his live was meaningful. It is not just something he lies awake about: when he compares his current life with his life in the past, he wonders about the meaning of his present life.

The spiritual layer is often hidden under the other layers. But once you are aware that you can reach spirituality via facts, emotions and biography, it may help you to find out what is of real importance to people. Sometimes, small facts may be of great significance, or things that you assume are important may mean little to your client. You will only find out what is really going on, by listening carefully and by descending in openness the four steps to the deepest layer.

The common goal in communication about spirituality is increasing the inner space of your patient or client, as well as your own inner space. This makes it possible to see things in a new, meaningful light and make changes. Increasing the inner space is realised by appealing to empathy and (self) compassion, tolerating uncertainty and being transparant and self reflective. This allows people to look for meaning together, for a spiritual perspective. This search can be painful and uncertain, because it usually means that people have to accept difficult situations and endure intense feelings. It is a challenge to acknowledge their questions and struggles and to remain empathically present, even when you have no answers yourself. However, you will notice that your urge to look for solutions, even when they do not help at all, can be very strong. This is called 'righting reflex' [7]. This tendency can prevent you from listening openly to people's stories, and it is important to become aware of this tendency. Practical conversational skills and techniques that are helpful are reflecting on feelings, silence, storytelling, metaphors and rituals.

> **Box 7.5: Exercise: Developing Your Spiritual Communication**
> In this box you find some brief communication exercises to enhance your spiritual sensitivity ('inner space'). Consider to study communication skills in depth by using additional literature.
> Reflecting on feelings:
>
> - Exercise your 'deeper listening' in daily life conversations (at home, with colleagues) by asking yourself the following questions: How should this feel for him/her? What does this mean to him/her?
> - What non-verbal behaviour do you observe?
> - Check and discuss your interpretations with the person you are talking with.
>
> Silence:
>
> - Experiment in conversations with patients by being silent. Remark what this silence is doing with you. What do you observe in the client? What is the result of this period of silence?
>
> Storytelling:
>
> - The way patients cope with their illness is also influenced by their life story. Life stories are sources for the way the patient is dealing with spiritual problems and/or needs. Insight in those life stories might be of importance for you as a healthcare professional. So-called ego-document can provide that insight. Ego-documents are published as books, films, letters, etc.
> - Search for an ego-document of a patient, and consider yourself the four steps of finding deeper meaning described earlier in this section of this chapter (facts, emotions, biography, spirituality).
>
> Rituals:
>
> - Think about moments in your life that a ritual is/was apparent. In this case don't think about great life events, but about daily rituals. What does this ritual mean to you?
> - What do you learn from this question about the meaning of rituals for patients?

7.4 Assessment and Implementation of Spiritual Care

Spiritual care is part of the integrated interdisciplinary care process. This integrated approach is recently reflected in the definition of health as formulated by Huber [8]. In this approach health is defined as 'people's ability to adapt and to self-manage, in the face of the life challenges with the objective to make life meaningful'. In this definition health is no longer explicitly focussing on the absence of illness. With the growing amount of patients with chronic diseases, elderly people and the developments in palliative care, this definition becomes more relevant in today's healthcare. In this approach the following six dimensions of health are explicitly distinguished:

- Bodily functions: medical facts and observations, physical functioning, complaints and pain, energy;
- Mental functions and perception: cognitive functioning, emotional state, self-esteem/self-respect, manageability, self-management and experiencing to be in charge, resilience;
- Spiritual/existential dimension: spirituality, striving for aims/ideals, future prospects, acceptance;
- Quality of life: quality of life/well-being, experiencing happiness, enjoyment, zest for life, balance;
- Social and societal participation: social and communicative skills, meaningful relationships, social contacts, experiencing to be accepted, community involvement; meaningful work;
- Daily functioning: activities of daily living, ability to work.

In this approach spirituality is an explicit and essential indicator of health. This dimension is connected with the other dimensions of health. The spiritual dimension can become apparent in all above-mentioned dimensions of human functioning. An example is the relationship with bodily functions. Choices with regard to nutrition may, for instance, be determined by a person's view of life (e.g. veganism). Decisions on quality of life in the case of continuation or ceasing treatment may be determined by someone's (religious) convictions or by the extent to which someone considers their life as meaningful. In the social-societal dimension, the question may arise about what are (still) meaningful relationships for a person. In the care for daily functioning, a Muslim woman may object to showering assistance by a male healthcare professional. This approach makes clear that spirituality can be linked to health and well-being and therefore that it is of relevance for good healthcare. Stating this makes that spirituality should be seen as an integrated part of the caring process. According to that caring process, two approaches can be distinguished: the instrumental approach and the narrative approach [9, 10]. Both approaches are complementary.

The instrumental approach is characterised by its methodical approach. This approach is goal-oriented and systematically worked out in the process stages of assessment, diagnostics, planning, intervention and evaluation. This methodical work is also described as evidence-based practice (EBP). EBP is often reduced to working only based on the latest scientific insights, obtained by research. However, the starting point of EBP is the individual client situation. In a careful process of shared decision-making, care for the patient is planned and executed. EBP is based on three pillars: the experience of the healthcare professional, scientific insights and the values and beliefs of the client. The client perspective is essential in EBP. The spiritual dimension is part of this perspective. Values and beliefs play a defining part in decisions about care. For instance, the personal view on marriage determines one's participation in relationship therapy. Participating in an experimental treatment with new medications is determined by a person's perspective on life. A proper application of the EBP principles in the methodical care process includes spiritual care. The spiritual dimension can play a part in each above-mentioned stage of the healthcare process.

In the assessment phase questions are asked about the patients' spirituality. In Chap. 3 of this book, you find guidelines for this spiritual assessment. The diagnosis phase is about the formulation of spiritual diagnosis if relevant. In the process of clinical reasoning, the healthcare professional can formulate his/her own diagnosis. Besides this, there are evidence-based diagnoses available from different perspectives. Box 7.6 gives an overview of such diagnosis from the perspective of the Omaha System (http://www.omahasystem.org/problemclassificationscheme.html), DSM-5 [11] and NANDA International (http://www.nanda.org/nanda-international-nursing-diagnoses-definitions-and-classification.html).

Box 7.6: Overview: Standard Spiritual Diagnosis
Omaha System for community care

- Expressing spiritual concerns
- Distressed spiritual rituals
- Distressed spiritual trust
- Conflicting spiritual beliefs in relation to treatment and care
- Others

Diagnostic and Statistical Manual of Mental Disorders Fifth Edition (DSM-5)

- Religious or spiritual problem: trauma because of loss of faith or doubt; problems in adapting new faith; doubt about spiritual values

NANDA International

- Spiritual distress: e.g. religious belief is challenged; questioning meaning of life, dying and suffering; questions about sustainability of (religious) convictions
- Risk form spiritual distress: high risk for disturbing values and/or belief
- Limitation in expression of faith: experience of stress as a result of problems in living with religious rules and rituals
- Risk on limitation in expression of faith

Box 7.7: Exercise: Spirituality in the Nursing Process
Discuss the case below with fellow students/colleagues in relation to the six dimensions of health described in the above section of the chapter.

- What explicit spiritual problems and/or needs do you assess, and what are their related factors?

Midland is a district in a medium-sized city. People of various cultural backgrounds live in the district. In due course, the neighbourhood has become impoverished. After their marriage in 1964, Mr. (74) and Mrs. (73) Brook came to live in the district. They have witnessed the change of the district over time. Still they felt at home, all those years. Both of them have participated in community activities for a long time. They were always ready to help anyone. Mrs. Brook had a hair salon at home, until her 68th. Fellow residents called the hair salon 'The Open House'. A lot of people were regular visitors, and they discussed issues at stake in the neighbourhood. Until his retirement, Mr. Brook has worked as an administrator at an insurance company in the city. Until recently, they would go to the bridge club together weekly. Ever since Mrs. Brook is in failing health, she no longer comes along. Now Mr. Brook goes by himself. They still walk the neighbourhood together every week.

The couple has three children. One daughter (50) lives in another part of the country. She only visits them on their birthdays and during some of the public holidays. She is married and has one daughter. Another daughter (41) lives in Midland neighbourhood, like her parents do. She is married and has a busy family with two young children. This daughter stops by weekly for a short visit. Mr. and Mrs. Brook have a son as well, who lives in a city nearby, but they have become estranged. Troubles in the past have led to a rift in their relationship.

Two years ago, Mrs. Brook has had a heart attack, and since then she is experiencing chronic health problems. She becomes increasingly forgetful; she sleeps badly and is restless at night. She has difficulty walking, due to increasing arthritis. Consequently, she has trouble taking care of herself. Six months ago, she has been diagnosed with early dementia, and since then, homecare visits her in the morning, to help her with her physical daily care. Mrs. Brook does not like having to depend on homecare. 'If life has to be like this, then I am not very keen anymore' and 'soon I will only be a burden to you', she occasionally tells her husband. Sometimes, she sits in her chair by the window for hours, staring aimlessly, without saying a word. She seems to brighten up a little when the TV broadcasts choral music. For years, she has sung in a church choir. Mr. Brook helps his wife wherever possible. He hardly dares to leave her alone anymore. She has already left the gas tap on in the kitchen once, and he has found her lying on the bathroom floor one night. He has skipped his weekly bridge party several times already. His daughter has started to buy their weekly groceries. In a conversation with the district nurse, he says he can see his wife's condition failing rapidly. 'Sometimes I do not recognise my wife any longer', he says. Even though he sometimes finds it difficult, he wants to continue caring for his wife. 'I promised to help her for better or for worse', he says. The district nurse notices that Mr. Brook acts curtly lately. He gets angry with municipal institutions, because a request for domestic assistance has been rejected. They believe he is still capable of some housekeeping himself and he should call on his relatives. He argues with his wife more often. It seems like they no longer understand each other. The daily care provided by the district nurse annoys him as well. He thinks they concede too much to his wife's 'fantasy world', as he puts it. He does not approve of the occasional skipping of the showering because his wife is uncooperative. 'She used to be immaculately groomed, she always took good care of herself', Mr. Brook says. The district nurse wishes to coordinate on the situation in the social district team.

In addition to the methodical approach, there is the so-called narrative approach. In the narrative approach, the story of someone's life is expressed. This story provides insight in someone's personal identity, into how someone came to be who she or he is now, into what is important and valued. Each person, however how old or young they are, has a life story. A life story may offer clues for care and guidance and it may also lead to life issues. Life stories play an important role in geriatric care, but it can be employed in any target group. The narrative approach calls for a narrative attitude in caregivers. This involves being sensitive to evoking, listening to and dealing with meaningful information from the stories of patients and clients. This involves also being sensitive to receiving personal signals.

The narrative approach is not opposed to the methodical approach, but it is part of it. An intake or an anamnesis procedure may follow a standardised protocol, but it may imply an open, non-directive approach, based on the narrative approach. In that case, the patient's story is guiding in the assessment, rather than a list of standard intake or anamnesis questions.

Box 7.8: Exercise: Life Story
– Talk with a patient about his or her life story. Prepare yourself by considering what questions you are going to ask.
– Consider during the conversation how the patient reacts. Take note when the patient shows any reluctance to tell further.
– When you have finished the conversation, consider for yourself what you learn from the patient's life story for the care you are giving to that patient

7.5 Personal Support and Patient Counselling

This competence is about the planning and implementation of spiritual care. Personal support and patient counselling in spiritual care by the individual healthcare professional depend most importantly on attitude and communication skills. These aspects were already described earlier in this chapter. Spiritual care is also part of the interdisciplinary caring process. As a healthcare professional, you must be able to discuss the planning and implementation of spiritual care with the patient but also with other healthcare professionals in the multidisciplinary team. The question can be asked what might be expected from every healthcare professional. It is important that every healthcare worker is aware of his/her own possibilities and boundaries. A model that can be helpful to get insight in your role in spiritual care is the so-called Traveller Model [12]. The model shows four stages of spiritual care, and every stage is pointing on the professional responsibility regarding spiritual care. It shows that for every individual healthcare worker, there is a basic responsibility of spiritual awareness and spiritual sensitivity. Every healthcare worker should recognise and assess the significance of spiritual issues of the patient by joining with and listening to the patient. The phases of spiritual empathy and spiritual exploration are reserved for healthcare workers with awareness of their own spirituality and those who have had specific training. They are able to understand the spirituality and/or spiritual need of the patient, and they can interpret that. This model is develop for social work but might be applicable for healthcare in general. The model can surely be discussed, but it shows that spiritual care is bound to specific conditions (Fig. 7.1).

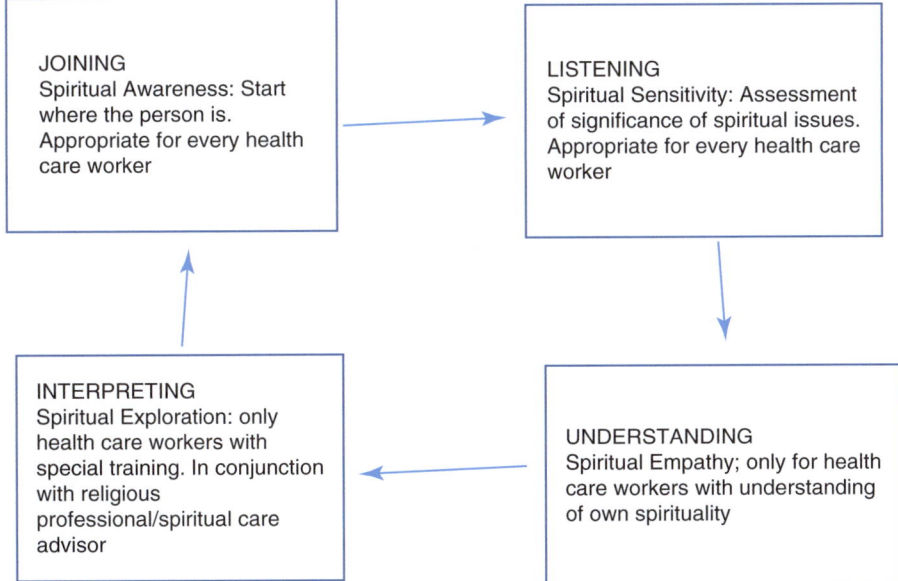

Fig. 7.1 Traveller model

> **Box 7.9: Exercise: What 'Traveller' Are You?**
> - How would you place yourself in the four phases of the above-described Traveller Model?
> - Discuss with a fellow student/colleague the outcome of this question.
> - Discuss the Traveller Model: relevance, applicability, etc.

7.6 Referral

Talking about your professional role in spiritual care in the above exercise makes also clear that there might be boundaries in what you can mean for a patient. Awareness of those boundaries and timely referral are important. Two kinds of boundaries can be distinguished, intrinsic and extrinsic boundaries [13]. Intrinsic barriers are about personal factors in the client or the healthcare professional himself. These are barriers about:

- Communication problems between client and the healthcare worker. There is no relational 'click' between you and the patient or in case of transference and countertransference.
- Lack of awareness of the importance of spirituality in one's personal life or in the working environment
- The subject is too much emotionally burdened

Extrinsic barriers are about organisational factors like lack of privacy, time, personnel, lack of education, etc.

Healthcare workers should be especially aware of the intrinsic (personal) barriers in the delivery of spiritual care. When you feel there is no relational 'click' with the patient, you should refer to another professional. In case of countertransference, you are unconscious of the fact that your reaction to the patient comes from what a patient is expecting from you (transference), but that won't help the patient. These reactions come forward from experiences out of someone's earlier life. You think you are helping a patient but the opposite occurs. The patient might get dependent from you. As a healthcare worker, you can also transfer your feelings to a patient. For example, when you have negative experiences with religion, you can project them on the patient who is struggling with religion, by saying that religion might be no longer important for the patient. Awareness of your personal feelings, opinions and boundaries regarding spirituality is important. You can refer to a colleague or to a spiritual specialist (e.g. a chaplain).

> **Box 7.10: Exercise: Explore Your Barriers**
> Discuss together with fellow students/colleagues your (possible) intrinsic barriers by answering the following questions:

- Mention examples how these barriers can play a role in the patient.
- How do/did you act on these barriers?
- Give an example of a spiritual care situation from you own work in which you faced personal barriers. How did you cope with that situation?
- Discuss together what important rules are for coping with intrinsic barriers regarding spiritual care.

7.7 Contributing to Quality Assurance and Improving Expertise in Spiritual Care in the Organisation

The spiritual care competencies described so far are about the role of the healthcare professional in the caring relationship with the patient and in the methodical caring process. It might also be expected from a healthcare professional that he or she contributes to the improvement of the quality of spiritual care on the personal and team level. On the personal and team level are ongoing education, coaching and training of importance. For example, the development of the professional role in spiritual care can be subject to a process of intervision or supervision on the working place. This can take place by discussing personal cases from your own healthcare practice. Coaching by spiritual specialist (e.g. chaplain) can deepen those learning experiences.

Quality assurance is also about policy development and innovation regarding spiritual care. Possible subjects for this are, for example, developing a spiritual assessment procedure, attention for spiritual care in the multidisciplinary meetings, evaluation regarding patients' spiritual care experiences, etc. The starting point depends on the developmental stage a team is in. It can be helpful to have a team member that has a special responsibility for the quality assurance of spiritual care and that can guide the team in this process.

Box 7.11: Exercise: How Can Spiritual Care Be Developed in Your Working Place?
Organise a team meeting (mono- or multidisciplinary) to discuss about spiritual care in your working place.
Follow the following steps:

1. First answer individually the following question: what subject should be at first picked up to enhance the quality of spiritual care in your team?
2. Present all individual answers (one subject a person)
3. Discuss as a group what subject should be prioritised to take action on at first
4. Discuss how this subject practically will be picked up (objective, actions, planning, responsibilities, evaluation, etc.)

Appendix: Spiritual Care Competency Scale

1 = completely disagree; 2 = disagree; 3 = neither agree or disagree; 4 = agree; 5 = fully agree

Attitude Towards Patient Spirituality

1. I show unprejudiced respect for a patient's spiritual/religious beliefs regardless of his or her spiritual/religious background

1	–	2	–	3	–	4	–	5

2. I am open to a patient's spiritual/religious beliefs, even if they differ from my own

1	–	2	–	3	–	4	–	5

3. I do not try to impose my own spiritual/religious beliefs on a patient

1	–	2	–	3	–	4	–	5

4. I am aware of my personal limitations when dealing with a patient's spiritual/religious beliefs

1	–	2	–	3	–	4	–	5

Communication

5. I can listen actively to a patient's 'life story' in relation to his or her illness/handicap

1	–	2	–	3	–	4	–	5

6. I have an accepting attitude in my dealings with a patient (concerned, sympathetic, inspiring trust and confidence, empathetic, genuine, sensitive, sincere and personal)

1	–	2	–	3	–	4	–	5

Assessment and Implementation of Spiritual Care

7. I can report orally and/or in writing on a patient's spiritual needs

| 1 | – | 2 | – | 3 | – | 4 | – | 5 |

8. I can tailor care to a patient's spiritual needs/problems in consultation with the patient

| 1 | – | 2 | – | 3 | – | 4 | – | 5 |

9. I can tailor care to a patient's spiritual needs/problems through multidisciplinary consultation

| 1 | – | 2 | – | 3 | – | 4 | – | 5 |

10. I can record the nursing component of a patient's spiritual care in the nursing plan.

| 1 | – | 2 | – | 3 | – | 4 | – | 5 |

11. I can report in writing on a patient's spiritual functioning

| 1 | – | 2 | – | 3 | – | 4 | – | 5 |

12. I can report orally on a patient's spiritual functioning

| 1 | – | 2 | – | 3 | – | 4 | – | 5 |

Referral

13. I can effectively assign care for a patient's spiritual needs to another care provider/care worker/care discipline

| 1 | – | 2 | – | 3 | – | 4 | – | 5 |

14. At the request of a patient with spiritual needs, I can in a timely and effective manner refer him or her to another care worker (e.g. a chaplain/the patient's own priest/imam)

| 1 | – | 2 | – | 3 | – | 4 | – | 5 |

15. I know when I should consult a spiritual advisor concerning a patient's spiritual care

| 1 | – | 2 | – | 3 | – | 4 | – | 5 |

Personal Support and Patient Counselling

16. I can provide a patient with spiritual care

| 1 | – | 2 | – | 3 | – | 4 | – | 5 |

17. I can evaluate the spiritual care that I have provided in consultation with the patient and in the disciplinary/multidisciplinary team

| 1 | – | 2 | – | 3 | – | 4 | – | 5 |

18. I can give a patient information about spiritual facilities within the care institution (including spiritual care, meditation centre, religious services)

| 1 | – | 2 | – | 3 | – | 4 | – | 5 |

19. I can help a patient continue his or her daily spiritual practices (including providing opportunities for rituals, prayer, meditation, reading the Bible/Koran, listening to music)

| 1 | – | 2 | – | 3 | – | 4 | – | 5 |

20. I can attend to a patient's spirituality during the daily care (e.g. physical care)

| 1 | – | 2 | – | 3 | – | 4 | – | 5 |

21. I can refer members of a patient's family to a spiritual advisor/pastor, etc. if they ask me and/or if they express spiritual needs

| 1 | – | 2 | – | 3 | – | 4 | – | 5 |

Professionalisation and Improving the Quality of Spiritual Care

22. Within the department, I can contribute to quality assurance in the area of spiritual care

| 1 | – | 2 | – | 3 | – | 4 | – | 5 |

23. Within the department, I can contribute to professional development in the area of spiritual care

1	–	2	–	3	–	4	–	5

24. Within the department, I can identify problems relating to spiritual care in peer discussion sessions

1	–	2	–	3	–	4	–	5

25. I can coach other care workers in the area of spiritual care delivery to patients

1	–	2	–	3	–	4	–	5

26. I can make policy recommendations on aspects of spiritual care to the management of the nursing ward

1	–	2	–	3	–	4	–	5

27. I can implement a spiritual care improvement project in the nursing ward

1	–	2	–	3	–	4	–	5

References

1. van Leeuwen R, Cusveller B. Nursing competencies for spiritual care. J Adv Nurs. 2004;48(3):234–46.
2. Leeuwen van R, Tiesinga LJ, Middel B, Post D, Jochemsen H. The validity and reliability of an instrument to assess nursing competencies in spiritual care. J Clin Nurs. 2009;18:2857–69.
3. van Leeuwen R. Towards nursing competencies in spiritual care. Stud Spiritual. 2009;19:249.
4. Baldacchino D. Spiritual care: being in doing. Floriana: Preca Library; 2009.
5. Leget C. Art of living, art of dying. Spiritual care for a good death. London/Philadelphia: Jessica Kingsley Publishers; 2017.
6. Weiher E. Das Geheimnis des Lebens berühren. Spiritualität bei Krankheit, Sterben, Tod – Eine Grammatik für Helfende (Touching the secret of life. Spirituality of illness, death – a grammar for carers). 2nd ed. Stuttgart: Kohlhammer; 2009.
7. Miller WR, Rollnick S. Motivational interviewing. 3rd ed. New York: Guildford Publications; 2012.
8. Huber M, Kottnerus JA, Green L, Horts van der H, Jadad AR, Kromhout D, Leonard B, Lorig K, Loureiro MI, Meer van der JWM, Schnabel P, Van Wee C, Smid H. How should we define health? Br Med J. 2011;343(4163):235–7.
9. Rumbold B. Models of spiritual care. In: Cobb M, Puchalski CM, Rumbold B, editors. Oxford textbook of spirituality in healthcare. New York: Oxford University Press; 2012. p. 177–84.
10. Kelly E. Competences in spiritual care education and training. In: Cobb M, Puchalski CM, Rumbold B, editors. Oxford textbook of spirituality in healthcare. New York: Oxford University Press; 2012. p. 435–42.

11. American Psychiatric Association. Diagnostic and statistical classification of mental disorders. 5th ed. Arlington: American Psychiatric Association; 2013. www.psychiatry.org.
12. Holloway M. Social work. In: Cobb M, Puchalski CM, Rumbold B, editors. Oxford textbook of spirituality in healthcare. New York: Oxford University Press; 2012. p. 235–42.
13. McSherry W. Making sense of spirituality in nursing and health care practice. An interactive approach. London/Philadelphia: Jessica Kingsley Publishers; 2006.

The Role of the Nurse in Providing Spiritual Care: A Case Study Approach to Exploring Specific Care Provision by Healthcare Workers in the Context of an Interdisciplinary Healthcare Team

Sílvia Caldeira, Joana Romeiro, and Helga Martins

Abstract

The role of nurses within the multidisciplinary healthcare team is to support patients as they navigate health-illness transition. As the discipline has grown, so too has the knowledge that informs nursing practices. Nursing process relates to nursing clinical reasoning when caring for patients as individuals in a holistic paradigm, from assessment to outcomes evaluation, which should include spiritual needs. This chapter will:

1. Explore nursing care, outlining heritage and theories.
2. Describe spiritual care, particularly that provided by nurses.
3. Provide instruments (scales and classifications) for performing nursing process, based on a case.

8.1 Introduction

Nurses are a constant presence in the life experience of individuals, playing an essential role in the promotion (e.g., community nurses), maintenance and recovery of patient health (e.g., in hospitals) [1]. The dichotomist nature of human existence surrounding health-illness exerts the need for nursing diagnosis, planning, intervention and evaluation, which is a process grounded in the assessment of patient needs towards an expected individualized or collective outcome [2].

Evidence reveals the presence of nurses during several transitional phases that patients endure, from the ordinary and expected biological, psychological, mental and spiritual stages of development in a typical life span to those which emerge from an unpredictable health-illness imbalance [3]. At the same time, such changes

S. Caldeira (✉) · J. Romeiro · H. Martins
Institute of Health Sciences, Catholic University of Portugal, Lisbon, Portugal

© Springer Nature Switzerland AG 2019
F. Timmins, S. Caldeira (eds.), *Spirituality in Healthcare: Perspectives for Innovative Practice*, https://doi.org/10.1007/978-3-030-04420-6_8

may raise vulnerability and evoke a sense of a disrupted life followed by diminished well-being and perception of quality of life [3, 4]. A wide spectrum of acute and chronic diseases capable of threatening existence may put individuals not only under physical duress but also put them through an emotionally, psychologically and spiritually demanding journey, challenging coping mechanisms and resilience towards those adverse events [1].

Unlike other members of the multidisciplinary healthcare team, the privileged position of nurses seems to offer an opportunity of becoming close to patients and establishing unique relationships and connections with them, therefore allowing nurses an in-depth, dynamic and contextualized knowledge of a patient's particular needs [1]. This aspect is critical, as nursing interventions are drawn from an accurate diagnoses and, ultimately, from proper identification of patient responses and demands [2]. In addition, theoretical frameworks [4] and internationally accepted nursing classifications and taxonomies intend to guide nursing practice, ensuring a standardized language and common ground for effective application of each step of the nursing process [2]. Nevertheless, nurses' sensitivity and personal skills are recognized as pivotal to adequate care of individuals, couples and communities [5]. A nurse's success lies in his or her ability to assist in different contexts while simultaneously delivering care to patients with distinct health conditions and from diversified cultural and religious backgrounds [3].

Along with technological and medical advances in recent decades, an increased specialization and fragmentation of knowledge throughout areas of professional expertise has emerged [1]. The growing concern over compartmentalized assistance in healthcare and the danger of attention being take off the intricate multidimensionality and wholeness of the patient has raised political and organizational awareness of a holistic view and performance in healthcare [6]. However, such a view is recognized as far from totally and efficiently implemented [6]. In fact, a system that ensures holistic care seems doomed from the start, since the outdated and reductive concept of health assumed by the World Health Organization (WHO) fails to clearly recognize and respect the role of the spiritual dimension [7]. Yet, nursing as a science and a profession goes beyond the former definition, as caring is its core and the embrace of spirituality is a critical component of caring [5]. Researchers have signalled the importance of spirituality and the fundamentals of spiritual care in a vast range of environments and instances. For instance, infertility [8, 9], childbirth and early childhood [10], hospitalization [11] and chronic and life-threatening health conditions [12–14] are events considered to be overflowing with meaning, purpose and suffering; these are some of the underlying characteristics of spirituality, present from the beginning to the end of life [10].

Additionally, spiritual care is positively related to the actual improvement of health-related symptoms [15], and this raises self-awareness in nurses [5] as they help patients in overcoming and recovering the health status or in increasing quality of life, while accepting their new condition or disability [16]. However, a gap in implementing spiritual care is often described based on the following barriers: a subjective definition of spirituality [6]; the vague role each member of the health team in providing spiritual care [6]; the absence in nursing curricula;

inadequate nurse training for properly addressing body-mind-spirit; time constraints; and an adequate hospital environment for patients to express their spirituality [6, 17–19].

In the following sections, the authors acknowledge the heritage of nursing as a science and as a profession, vis-à-vis both theoretical influences and future challenges in the delivery of nursing care.

8.2 Nursing: Heritage and Future Challenges

Nursing is an inevitable result of historical and geographical transitions that took place through time. Furthermore, socio-economic, religious, cultural and technological aspects of each context have inexorably influenced the evolution of nursing as an art and a science, and has evoked changes in the concept and understanding of nursing [1]. Early references place nursing origins in ancient cultures and traditions, such as those of the Greece and Roman eras [20]. However, essential elements of nursing provision can be found as early as the beginning of humankind [20].

The dictionary definition of 'nursing' states it is a profession accountable for the delivery of care to the infirm [21]. Moreover, the word 'infirm' is related to a weak or frail person cared for by nurses, which derives from the Latin expression '*infirmus*,' an aggregation of '*in*' ('*not*') and '*firmus*' ('*firm*') [22]. While previous, related words are only accepted as nouns, 'nurse' is either a noun or a verb [23]. In this case, as a noun, 'nurse' refers to the health professional responsible for taking care of the infirm [23]. Nurse' as a verb denotes not only the act of attending to the needy but also the act of breastfeeding a child [23]. 'Nurse' is considered a variant of '*n(o)urice, norice*' (Old French), '*nūtrīcia*' *(Latin)*, with its feminine '*nūtrīcius*' (nutritious), later '*nursh*' (nourish) [23]. Nurse, therefore, denotes not only a skilled and trained person whose role is of care delivery, it is associated as well with the act of ensuring a child's health by means of woman's exclusive responsibility of breastfeeding [23]. This reflects the closeness of the nursing concept to the unquestionable duty females have owned since the earliest time— looking after children and assisting the weak and the vulnerable [1, 20]. Historically, in Christianity's dissemination era, noble women were presumed to have a charitable duty to serve the infirm [24]. Later, in the early Middle Ages, nuns and monks, following religious precepts, also assumed those tasks [20]. Afterwards, hospitals were raised from these foundations, and supervised care to the unhealthy evolved from the absence of a standardized training in a professional framework capable of educating and molding with growing proficiency nurses' intents and actions [1, 20]. The first proper documentation of nursing practice is widely recognized by researchers to have been made by Florence Nightingale, in 1860, in her published book, *Notes on Nursing: What it is and What it is Not* [25]. The essence of nursing was described in her writings:

> [W]hat nursing has to do … is to put the patient in the best condition for nature to act upon him. Generally the contrary is done. You think fresh air, and quiet and cleanliness extravagant, perhaps dangerous luxuries, which should be given to the patients only when quite

convenient, and medicine the sine qua non, the panacea. If I have succeeded in any measure in dispelling this illusion, and in showing what true nursing is and what it is not, my object will have been answered [25].

The insight given from the care delivered to the war-wounded by Nightingale was of primordial significance to the emergence of foundational theories of nursing as they are known today [1]. Standards for the client-nurse relationship and a holistic attention to the patient were set [1, 4]. In addition, caring was assumed to be a main focus of nursing [26], encompassing subjective and objective aspects along with the multidimensionality of a human being [4]. Since the biological, social, cultural, emotional, psychological and spiritual dimensions of an individual interact, any perceived dysfunction caused in one affects the patient's quality of life and the entire self [3, 4, 16]. These understandings have led to several approaches, since different researchers acknowledge the significance of different theoretical frameworks as structural to the body of knowledge of nursing discipline. Yet, whether one analyses from a holistic point of view embracing individual human needs [4] or from a caring perspective [26], researchers reiterate similar theoretical models, since common aspects can be found. Some authors therefore assume the critical contribution of Nightingale's Environmental Theory (1860), Abdellah's 21 Nursing Problems Theory (1960), Henderson's Nursing Need Theory (1971), Orem's Self Care Theory (1980) and Hall and Watson's Theory of Human Caring (1985), to capture the nursing essence through the patient's human needs [27]. On the other hand, the interactions established in the patient-nursing-environment were considered to be revealed in Peplau's Interpersonal Relations Theory (1952), Orlando's Nursing Process Theory (1961), Wiedenbach's Helping Art of Clinical Nursing Theory (1964), King's Theory of Goal Attainment (1971), Paterson and Zderad's Humanistic Nursing Theory (1988), Erikson, Tomlin and Swain's Modeling and Role-modeling Theory (1983),and Boykin and Schoenhofer's Nursing as Caring Theory (1993) [27]. In addition, systems thinking was uncovered by Johnson's Behavioral Systems Model (1980), Roy's Adaptation Model (1976), Neuman's System Model (1974), Levin's Conservation Theory (1989) and Leininger's Culture Care Theory (1980) [27]. The first attention given to energy fields was in Rogers' Theory of Unitary Human Beings (1980), Parse's Human Becoming Theory (1981) and Newman's Theory of Health as Expanding Consciousness (1983) [27]. Previously mentioned is the significance of theoretical structures to an holistic assessment of nursing care [4]; these include those of the Intersystem Model, Adaptation Model, Integrative process, Theory of Unitary Human Beings, Theory of Health as Expanding Consciousness, and Human Becoming Theory. Further achievements were attained by Abdellah, Roger, Henderson, Leininger, Watson, Neuman and Roy, whose work brought a focus on incorporating spirituality, along with Artinian's Intersystem Model (1997) and Horta's Basic Human Needs Theory (1979) [28].

As they aim to explain and predict events experienced by nurses, theories are considered primordial to the effectiveness of the nursing process, serving as rich guidance in facilitating nursing assessment, promoting an accurate diagnosis, planning interventions, and implementing and evaluating the outcomes. Nursing emerges today in contradiction to the early biomedical paradigm linking it to an occupation whose practitioner assisted the physician in curing the patient [1]. In 1977, Virginia Henderson identified the need to find a common place for and standardized definition of the nursing concept, highlighting its meaning in worldwide recognition of nursing as not only an interdependent but also an independent discipline and profession [1]. Henderson's definition of nursing gave an inside glimpse to the nurse's unique role:

> [To] assist the individual, sick or well, in the performance of those activities contributing to health or its recovery (or to peaceful death) that he would perform unaided if he had the necessary strength, will or knowledge. And to do this in such a way as to help him gain independence as rapidly as possible [29].

On the other hand, the American Nurses Association (ANA) definition states:

> Nursing is the protection, promotion, and optimization of health and abilities; prevention of illness and injury; alleviation of suffering through the diagnosis and treatment of human responses; and advocacy in health care for individuals, families, communities, and populations [30].

The International Council of Nurses (ICN) presents not one but two versions of the nursing concept. The longest description recalls ANA's and Henderson's critical nursing elements, condensed in the following definition:

> Nursing encompasses autonomous and collaborative care of individuals of all ages, families, groups and communities, sick or well and in all settings. Nursing includes the promotion of health, prevention of illness, and the care of ill, disabled and dying people. Advocacy, promotion of a safe environment, research, participation in shaping health policy and in patient and health systems management, and education are also key nursing roles [31].

On the other hand, the Royal College of Nursing (RCN) defines nursing this way:

> The use of clinical judgment in the provision of care to enable people to improve, maintain, or recover health, to cope with health problems, and to achieve the best possible quality of life, whatever their disease or disability, until death [32].

For instance, ANA introduces singular and collective individuals as the target of nursing delivery, ICN adds research to the nurse's role [33] and RCN identifies a holistic view through attention to the quality of patient life.

In spite of Henderson's warnings [1], international nursing organizations present distinct concepts with the inherent risk of perpetuating the blurry boundaries that surround nursing practice, being a reminder of an art and a profession that is still far from being totally apprehended [33]. It is not only important to set and determine the boundaries of nursing practice in order to raise nurses' awareness to the specificities of their particular field of action, it is also necessary to create a wider public acknowledgement of nursing's significance and to increase nursing participation in policy developments [33, 34]. Delineated strategies are therefore placed in interdisciplinary teaching, training and practice [35, 36]. In fact, collaboration is called for, wherein each professional's expertise is respected and each one's work is integrated. At the same time, disciplinary barriers must be eradicated in a way that promotes instead interprofessional action and transdisciplinary action in the future [35, 36].

8.3 The Role of the Nurse in Providing Spiritual Care

Spirituality is regarded as a multidimensional [37], complex and individual experience [38], a reflection of human uniqueness [39], being closely related to personal beliefs [40]. Although difficult to define, the reader can find scattered throughout nursing literature several attempts to apprehend spirituality and its meaning in the pursuit of health [41–48]. The most recent and thorough analysis of the spiritual concept identified connectedness (to self, others, environment and a higher power), transcendence, and meaning in life as spirituality's main attributes [49]. Moreover, researchers have demonstrated the significance of spirituality in patient health, repeatedly identifying it as a resource in the strategies for coping with illness, increasing hope, and reducing suffering [50]. As such, spiritual-based interventions and orientation have shown positive health outcomes that demonstrate spirituality to be a useful therapeutic resource in care provision [51]. It is therefore relevant to explore this dimension of health and the importance of a spiritual role for nurses to play. The following section addresses, firstly, a general approach of spiritual care in nursing. Next, a description of the structural components of the nursing process is addressed, with emphasis placed on the assessment tools available. Then, spiritual care is linked with the nursing process. Finally, nursing care within the healthcare multidisciplinary team is discussed and illustrated by an original case study.

8.3.1 Spiritual Care in Nursing

The spiritual dimension in nursing care has only recently increased in importance and attention compared to how biological and psychosocial dimensions have been traditionally approached and considered more relevant [50]. Nursing is grounded in holism and in consideration of a comprehensive harmony of mind, body, spirit and emotion [52], essential in promoting patient health and wellness [53].

Spirituality is a recognized dimension in nursing, yet spiritual care is often neglected due to nurses' lack of knowledge and understanding [54]. Based on the premise of 'being rather than doing' [55], spiritual care can be defined as the facilitation of the patient's self-identified beliefs, meaning, values, sources of strength and life goals [56].

Historically, nursing has been associated with the personal attention given to a patient's spiritual needs [25], and nursing heritage is deeply linked to religiosity, as stated before. Regardless of the importance of the theme in nursing scientific literature today, spirituality has always been a structural component of nursing [57], but difficulties and barriers continue to be identified and described in daily practice.

According to the International Council of Nurses (ICN), spiritual care is a core element of the code of ethics and a nurse's primary professional responsibility [58]. Therefore, providing spiritual care to patients on a daily basis is an important role of nurses [59] for the integrating not only of direct and objective interventions, such as praying with and listening to patients [60], but also of subjective use of self, as evidenced sensitive and intentional presence [5]. In fact, attributes identified in a previous concept analysis of spiritual care in nursing raised attention to the eight essential factors of nursing's spiritual practice: healing presence, therapeutic use of self, intuitive sense, exploration of the spiritual perspective, patient-centeredness, meaning-centered therapeutic intervention, and creation of nurturing spiritual environment [5]. Still other authors have raised issues of nurse self-awareness, personal beliefs, environment, and their relationships with co-workers as barriers *against* proper spiritual provision [61], a situation that craves a solution in nurse education to overcome perceived difficulties in spiritual approaches to care [61]. As such, the same authors that described the main attributes of spiritual care in nursing also uncovered eight essential, core elements for spiritual care delivery, including spiritual self-care, active learning, professional belonging, personal and professional competencies, gradual evolution under divine guidance, awareness of the spiritual dimension of human beings, occurrence of awakening flashes and incidents during life, and congruence between patient and healthcare provider religious beliefs [62]. Interestingly, personal rather than organizational aspects, even when time-demanding tasks seem to be an issue, have been named to have a more relevant place in the intricate art of caring. In fact, time has been recently identified as an important factor in providing spiritual care—not only as an objective quantitative indicator of care, but as a subjective dimension. Time should be used in a meaningful, intentional and spiritual way, at no cost other than the usual number of minutes spent with the client [63].

8.3.2 Providing Nursing Care: The Nursing Process

Clinical reasoning is an indispensable function in the healthcare setting and in how it plays a vital role in nursing by assuring safe and effective care [64]. Subsequently, the nurse's use of clinical reasoning in providing care allows for effective patient-centered attention, patient empowerment in the decision-making process and accordingly positive healing outcomes. This can only be possible through a continual learning process, a fundamental tool in analysis and reflection skills development [65]. When considering the role of clinical reasoning in spirituality, the nurse anticipates patient needs, especially those patients who experience existential struggling and anxiety [66].

Clinical reasoning is based on the nursing process, which comprises assessment, diagnosis, planning, implementation and outcomes evaluation. Each stage plays an important role performing a logical but dynamic process [67]. The absence of any phase would raise questions with regard to diagnosis accuracy and outcomes [67].

The complexity of the concept spirituality may be challenging within the nursing process [49], as this may require an ontological perspective, but patients' spirituality should be assesse [68]. Additionally, spirituality should be integrated into the assessment performed by nurses with the same investment given to other points of attention [69]. Keeping in mind that assessment is an ongoing process and requires observation, questioning techniques and tools, in order to apprehend patient needs and to allow a proper and individualized implementation of spiritual nursing interventions [66]. So, to conduct an effective assessment it is necessary one take effective time and make information available to all professionals of the multidisciplinary team [70]. The main purpose in assessing spirituality is to identify patient needs and to screen for spiritual distress [68] in order to provide urgent and personalized spiritual interventions [66], helping patients in their self-healing process and in the achievement of a spiritual outcome and well-being. A study conducted on patients undergoing chemotherapy revealed that 40.8% of the participants had spiritual distress [13]. Therefore, it seems relevant to address spiritual needs not only in cancer patients but in other clinical settings where patients have been found to undergo experiences of particular vulnerability. However, nurse unpreparedness whether in the academy or in practice regarding this spiritual domain has been often mentioned [71] and has raised researchers' concerns towards assessment and development of formal and informal frameworks regarding a spiritual approach. On one hand, an informal approach can be done through simple questions and direct observation. On the other hand, a formal assessment can be done though spiritual assessment tools [66]. The myriad of instruments allegedly designed to measure spirituality, however, appear to display several limitations [72], and caution is needed when choosing any of them. In fact, due to the delicate theme, sometimes instruments are not adapted to the characteristics of patients or to settings [55]. For instance, differences can be found in the sensitivity each tool displays to address spirituality in samples of believers and non-believers. In addition, item formulation and the intertwining use of well-being and distress are also features that raise validity doubts and may confuse nurses when selecting instruments [72]. Moreover, the numerous questionnaires that are available enhance that challenge. In 2012, a review identified over 120 instruments to measure spirituality [72]. Although concerns have emerged towards this dimension, its complexity makes measuring a hard and difficult task. In order to improve the use of these tools, below is given a list of some of the most commonly used ones, based on specificity to evaluate general spiritual presence, distress, well-being and spiritual coping (Table 8.1). Nevertheless, further reading is advised of previous researchers' findings and discussions regarding those and other available tools [72–77].

Recalling the aforementioned, nursing practice focus is on a holistic view of patients' human responses and not on illness alone. So, patients having the same pathologic condition (illness) could be diagnosed by nurses with different nursing diagnoses, as these are focused on the answers towards the illness, which are different in each patient [12]. Therefore, assessment is critical in accurately diagnosing and delivering interventions [12] in a culturally competent way [101]. In addition, particular attention should be given not only to patients but also to environment, family communities and even health professionals, since this is the only way to achieve a truly holistic approach [66]. To date, international nursing classifications such as the ones provided by the International Classification of Nursing Practice

Table 8.1 Instruments for assessing spirituality by name, authorship and year, number of included items and country

	Author(s)/Year	Number of items	Country
General spirituality scales			
SAS (spirituality assessment scale) [78]	Howden (1992)	28 items	USA
Ethnic(S) (explanation, treatment, healers, negotiate, intervention, collaborate, spirituality/seniors) [79]	Kobylarz et al. (2002)	7 items	USA
SSCRS (spirituality and spiritual care rating scale) [80]	McSherry (2002)	17 items	UK
The Spirituality Scale [81]	Delaney (2005)	23 items	USA
SHALOM (spiritual health and life-orientation measure) [82]	Fisher (2010)	20 items	Australia
Spiritual distress scales			
Beck Scale of Hopelessness [83]	Beck (1974)	20 items	USA
SPIRIT (spiritual belief system, personal spirituality, integration with a spiritual community, ritualized practice and restrictions, implications for medical care, terminal events planning) [84]	Maugans (1996)	26 items	USA
Existential Loneliness Questionnaire [85]	Mayers et al. (2002)	22 items	Canada
The Meaning in Life Questionnaire [86]	Steger and Frazier (2006)	10 items	USA
Spiritual Distress Scale [87]	Ku et al. (2010)	30 items	Taiwan
VOSS Views of Suffering Scale [88]	Hale-Smith et al. (2012)	30 items	USA
Spiritual well-being scales			
JAREL Spiritual Well-Being Scale [89]	Hungelmann et al. (1996)	21 items	USA
SWB (spiritual Well-being scale) [90]	Ellison (1997)	20 items	USA
FICA spiritual history tool (faith and belief, importance, community, address in care) [91]	Puchalski and Romer (2000)	11 items	USA
			(continued)

Table 8.1 (continued)

	Author(s)/Year	Number of items	Country
HOPE (H– Sources of Hope, strength, comfort, meaning, peace, love and connection; O – The role of organized religion for the patient; P – Personal spirituality and practices; E – Effects on medical care and end-of-life decisions) [92]	Anandarajah and Hight (2001)	18 items	USA
FACIT–Sp (the functional assessment of chronic illness therapy–spiritual Well-being) [93]	Peterman et al. (2002)	12 items	USA
SWBQ (spiritual Well-being questionnaire) [94]	Gomez and Fisher, (2003)	20 items	Australia
WHOQOL SRPB (spirituality, religion and personal beliefs; a cross-cultural study of spirituality, religion, and personal beliefs as components of quality of life) [95]	WHOQOL SRPB Group (2006)	32 items	Switzerland
Spiritual coping scales			
RCOPE scale (the religious coping scale) [96]	Pargament et al. (2000)	87 items	USA
SCS scale (spiritual coping strategies scale) [97]	Baldacchino and Buhagiar (2003)	20 items	Malta
The Spiritual Support Scale [98]	Ai et al. (2005)	12 items	USA
Spiritual and Religious Attitudes in Dealing with Illness [99]	Buessing et al. (2005)	15 items	Germany
The Spiritual Strategies Scale [100]	Nelson-Becker (2005)	18 items	USA

(ICNP), the International Classification of Functioning, Disability and Health (ICF) and the NANDA—International (NANDA-I, previously known as North American Nursing Diagnosis Association) have emerged in an urgent attempt to help nurses in the critical diagnostic phase. These classifications allow the identification of patient health problems and facilitate the planning of adequate nursing interventions [88]. Regardless the incompleteness of spiritual diagnoses [102], the current taxonomy of NANDA-I is claimed to be the most useful due to its ability to conceptually define nursing diagnoses and plan responses to health problems/life processes [103]. Furthermore, NANDA-I features the Nursing Intervention Classification (NIC) and Nursing Outcomes Classification (NOC).

In Table 8.2, the reader can find a concise list of spiritual nursing diagnoses according to each classification, as stated before. In addition, links are provided to easy the access of the content.

8.3.3 Nursing Process and Spiritual Care

In order for nurses to provide spiritual care, specific competencies are required in three different domains such as awareness and use of self, nursing process, and quality of expertise (Fig. 8.1) [104]. Likewise, six core competencies required for the provision of spiritual care have been identified: collection of information, handling one's own beliefs, addressing the subject, collecting information, discussing and planning, providing and evaluating, and integrating into policy [104].

However, similarities can be found when comparing competencies in providing nursing care. Distinct characteristics are based on two main features: the ethical nature of patient need and resources present to meet the need [28]. Not as often, provision of spiritual care can face certain ethical challenges [66]. Foremost, spiritual care involves issues concerning the patient and a therapeutic relationship based on an ethical and human dimensions [28].

8.3.4 Nursing Care Within the Healthcare Multidisciplinary Team

Integration of spirituality in healthcare has been proven to have a positive impact not only on the patient but also on the multidisciplinary team and on the organizational culture [105]. Hence, the responsibility of providing spiritual care belongs to the entire multidisciplinary team [55], and therefore professionals, including nurses, chaplains or religious leaders, physicians, psychologists and social workers, among others, are not individually accountable for ensuring the quality of a spiritual and holistic care, but have a shared responsibility. It is profoundly important that all members within the healthcare team understand and be aware of each one's own limitations and boundaries, and that they realize that chaplains and spiritual leaders are recognized spiritual experts [106] to whom nurses should refer according to the patient's needs [55, 107]. A daily presence in a patient's life and involvement in the

Table 8.2 Spiritual nursing diagnoses in accordance with current nursing classifications

Nursing classifications	Diagnosis
NANDA—International (NANDA-I)—Taxonomy II http://www.nanda.org	**Domain 6: Self-perception** • *Class 1. Self-concept* – Readiness for enhanced hope (00185) – Hopelessness (00124) – Risk for compromised human dignity (00174) – Disturbed personal identity (00121) – Risk for disturbed personal identity (00225) – Readiness for enhanced self-concept (00167)
NANDA—International (NANDA-I)—Taxonomy II http://www.nanda.org	**Domain 9: Coping/stress tolerance** • *Class 2. Coping responses* – Ineffective activity planning (00199) – Risk for ineffective activity planning (00226) – Anxiety (00146) – Defensive coping (00071) – Ineffective coping (00069) – Readiness for enhanced coping (00158) – Ineffective community coping (00077) – Readiness for enhanced community coping (00076) – Compromised family coping (00074) – Disabled family coping (00073) – Readiness for enhanced family coping (00075) – Death anxiety (00147) – Ineffective denial (00072) – Fear (00148) – Grieving (00136) – Complicated grieving (00135) – Risk for complicated grieving (00172) – Impaired mood regulation (002419) – Readiness for enhanced power (00187) – Powerlessness (00125) – Risk for powerlessness (00152) – Impaired resilience (00210) – Readiness for enhanced resilience (002129) – Risk for impaired resilience (00211) – Chronic sorrow (00137) – Stress overload (00177)
NANDA—International (NANDA-I)—Taxonomy II http://www.nanda.org	**Domain 10: Life principles** • *Class 2. Beliefs* – Readiness for enhanced spiritual Well-being (000689) • *Class 3. Value/belief/action congruence* – Readiness for enhanced decision-making (00184) – Decisional conflict (00083) – Impaired emancipated decision-making (00242) – Readiness for enhanced emancipated decision-making (00243) – Risk for impaired emancipated decision-making (00244) – Moral distress (00175) – Impaired religiosity (00169) – Readiness for enhanced religiosity (00171) – Risk for impaired religiosity (00170) – Spiritual distress (00066) – Risk for spiritual distress (00067)

Nursing classifications	Diagnosis
NANDA—International (NANDA-I)—Taxonomy II http://www.nanda.org	**Domain 12: Comfort** • *Class 1. Physical comfort* – Impaired comfort (00214) – Readiness for enhanced comfort (00183) – Nausea (00134) – Acute pain (00132) – Chronic pain (00133 – Labor pain (00256) – Chronic pain syndrome (00255) • *Class 2. Environmental comfort* – Impaired comfort (00214) – Readiness for enhanced comfort (00183) • *Class 3. Social comfort* – Impaired comfort (00214) – Readiness for enhanced comfort (00183) – Risk for loneliness (00054) – Social isolation (00053)
International classification of functioning, disability and health (ICF) http://www.who.int/classifications/icf/en/ Or https://www.rehadat-icf.de/en/aktivitaeten-partizipation/d9/d930/d9300/index.html	**Part 2: Activities and participation:** **d9 community, social and civic life** • *d930 religion and spirituality* – d9300 organized religion – d9300 organized religion – d9301 spirituality – d9308 religion and spirituality, other specified – d9309 religion and spirituality, unspecified
International classification of functioning, disability and health (ICF) http://www.who.int/classifications/icf/en/ Or https://www.rehadat-icf.de/en/aktivitaeten-partizipation/d9/d930/d9300/index.html	**Part 3: Environmental factors** **e1 products and technology** • **e145 products and technology for the practice of religion and spirituality** – e1450 general products and technology for the practice of religion or spirituality – e1451 assistive products and technology for the practice of religion or spirituality – e1458 products and technology for the practice of religion or spirituality, other specified – e1459 products and technology for the practice of religion or spirituality, unspecified
International classification for nursing practice (ICNP®) http://www.icn.ch/what-we-do/international-classification-for-nursing-practice-icnpr/	**Negative diagnosis**
International classification for nursing practice (ICNP®) http://www.icn.ch/what-we-do/international-classification-for-nursing-practice-icnpr/	*Conflicting Religious Belief (10021757)*

(continued)

Table 8.2 (continued)

Nursing classifications	Diagnosis
International classification for nursing practice (ICNP®) http://www.icn.ch/what-we-do/international-classification-for-nursing-practice-icnpr/	*Difficulty Coping (10001120)* • Denial (10000624) – Denial about illness severity (10043850) • Difficulty coping with pain (10040731) • Impaired acceptance of health status (10029480) • Impaired adaptation (10022027) • Impaired community coping (10034817) • Impaired family coping (10034789) • Conflicting spiritual belief (10022769)
International classification for nursing practice (ICNP®) http://www.icn.ch/what-we-do/international-classification-for-nursing-practice-icnpr/	*Discomfort (10023066)*
International classification for nursing practice (ICNP®) http://www.icn.ch/what-we-do/international-classification-for-nursing-practice-icnpr/	*Emotional Problem (10029839)* • Ambivalence (10047209) • Anger (10045578) • Anxiety (10000477) – Death anxiety (10041017) – Reduced anxiety (10027858) • Depressed mood (10022402) – Decreased depressed mood (10027901) – Depressed mood during Post partum period (10029771) • Despair (10047056) – Decreased despair (10047444) • Dysfunctional grief (10001183) – Anticipatory grief (10000726) • Fatigue (10000695) – Reduced fatigue (10029390) – Treatment exhaustion (10022833) • Fear (10000703) – Fear about abandonment (10037823) • Fear about being a burden to others (10041671) – Fear about contagion (10037921) – Fear about death (10037834) – Fear about medication side effects (10043222) – Reduced fear (10027889) • Helplessness (10039952) • Hopelessness (10000742) • Lack of pride (10025693) • Lack of trust (10025947) – Lack of Trust in Health Care Provider (10025952) • Negative Euphoria (10047400) • Powerlessness (10001578) – Decreased powerlessness (10027120) • Sadness (10040662) – Chronic sadness (10000551) – Reduced chronic sadness (10027862) • Shame (10046761) • Spiritual distress (10001652) – Decreased spiritual distress (10027149) • Suffering (10025588)

Nursing classifications	Diagnosis
International classification for nursing practice (ICNP®) http://www.icn.ch/what-we-do/international-classification-for-nursing-practice-icnpr/	*Impaired Spiritual Status (10023336)*
International classification for nursing practice (ICNP®) http://www.icn.ch/what-we-do/international-classification-for-nursing-practice-icnpr/	*Lack of Meaning (10023423)*
International classification for nursing practice (ICNP®) http://www.icn.ch/what-we-do/international-classification-for-nursing-practice-icnpr/	*Lack of Resilience (10050439)*
International classification for nursing practice (ICNP®) http://www.icn.ch/what-we-do/international-classification-for-nursing-practice-icnpr/	*Potential for Risk (10017252)* • Risk for difficulty with coping (1,003,723) – Risk for impaired family coping (10032364) • Risk for situational low self esteem (10015180) • Risk for social isolation (10047213) • Risk for spiritual distress (10015325)
International classification for nursing practice (ICNP®) http://www.icn.ch/what-we-do/international-classification-for-nursing-practice-icnpr/	*Social Isolation (10001647)* • Decreased social isolation (10050070)

International classification for nursing practice (ICNP®) http://www.icn.ch/what-we-do/international-classification-for-nursing-practice-icnpr/	*Stress Overload (10021742)*
	• Caregiver stress (10027773)
	  – Reduced caregiver stress (10027794)
	• Decreased stress (10027929)
	  – Reduced caregiver stress (10027794)
	• Parental stress (10,001,385

International classification for nursing practice (ICNP®) http://www.icn.ch/what-we-do/international-classification-for-nursing-practice-icnpr/	**Positive diagnostic**

International classification for nursing practice (ICNP®) http://www.icn.ch/what-we-do/international-classification-for-nursing-practice-icnpr/	*Effective Coping (10022378)*
	• Acceptance of health status (10023499)
	  – Coping with pain (10040749)
	  – Effective caregiver coping (10034838)
	  – Effective community coping (10034801)
	  – Effective family coping (10034770)
	  – No denial (10044260)

International classification for nursing practice (ICNP®) http://www.icn.ch/what-we-do/international-classification-for-nursing-practice-icnpr/	*Effective Environmental Safety (10030233)*

(continued)

Table 8.2 (continued)

International classification for nursing practice (ICNP®) http://www.icn.ch/what-we-do/international-classification-for-nursing-practice-icnpr/	*Effective Family Process (10025232)* • Effective family coping (10034770) • Family grief (10038482)
International classification for nursing practice (ICNP®) http://www.icn.ch/what-we-do/international-classification-for-nursing-practice-icnpr/	*Effective Social Support (10045794)* • Effective spiritual status (10028529)
International classification for nursing practice (ICNP®) http://www.icn.ch/what-we-do/international-classification-for-nursing-practice-icnpr/	**Hope (10025780)**

International classification for nursing practice (ICNP®) http://www.icn.ch/what-we-do/international-classification-for-nursing-practice-icnpr/	*Positive Psychological Status (10038430)*
	• Anger control (10045699)
	• Good mood (10050015)
	  – Mood equilibrium (10035792)
	• Knowledge of psychosocial response to procedure (10033766)
	• Readiness for effective coping (10001469)
	  – Readiness for effective community coping (10001453)
	• Readiness for effective decision making (10025278)

International classification for nursing practice (ICNP®) http://www.icn.ch/what-we-do/international-classification-for-nursing-practice-icnpr/	*Positive Self Image (10027108)* • Positive body image (10028564) • 262 positive personal identity (10025664) • 263 positive self esteem (10025751)
International classification for nursing practice (ICNP®) http://www.icn.ch/what-we-do/international-classification-for-nursing-practice-icnpr/	*Readiness for Effective Spiritual Status (10033824)* • Resilient (10050441)

routines of care allow nurses an easier and closer access to patient needs. Compared to other professionals, nurses hold a privileged position for assessing spiritual distress [108].

Next, an example of a case study about spiritual distress is provided using NANDA-I. Further analysis allowed an insight to be presented on the role played by the healthcare team in an idealized multidisciplinary perspective and approach.

Case Study

S.J.H., a 55-year-old married woman, mother of three, Catholic, diagnosed with stage III right breast cancer, underwent radical mastectomy, currently undergoing the second cycle of chemotherapy, as an hospital inpatient.

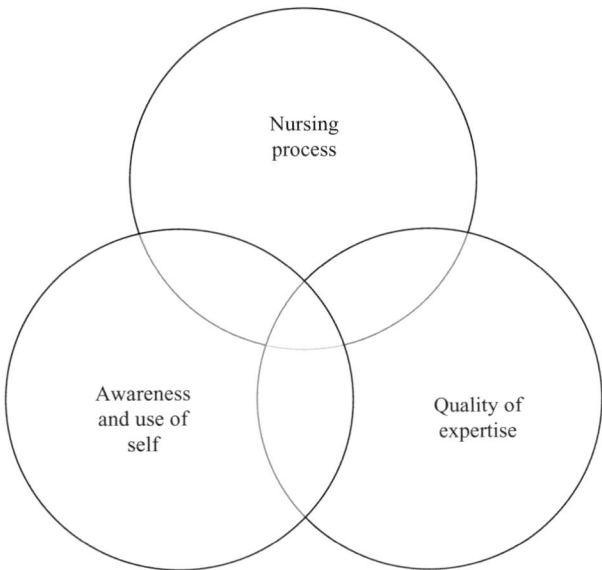

Fig. 8.1 Nurses competencies in three domains for providing spiritual care adaptation of van Leeuwen and Cusveller [104]

During hospitalization, patient has verbalized that she is Catholic but abandoned religious activities, referring that she lost faith in God and feels abandoned by "Him." Additionally, often describes fear of dying. Furthermore, refuses visits from her children, family and friends. The patient remarks she feels a lot of pain and the side effects of chemotherapy are difficult to handle (fatigue, nausea and vomiting) and added she is in a great suffering, is hopeless and lacks sense of meaning in life.

When analysing this clinical case, a multidisciplinary approach was required (Fig. 8.2), in which each element had a definite role within the limits of its competencies, aiming to provide patient-centered care in a holistic and individualized way.

Analysis and Synthesis of Case Study
- 55-year-oldold woman, married, three children, Catholic
- Pain
- Fear of dying
- Physical symptoms (fatigue, nausea and vomiting)
- Lack of meaning
- Suffering
- Hopeless
- Lost faith in god
- Refuses visits from her children, family and friends
- Abandoned religious activities

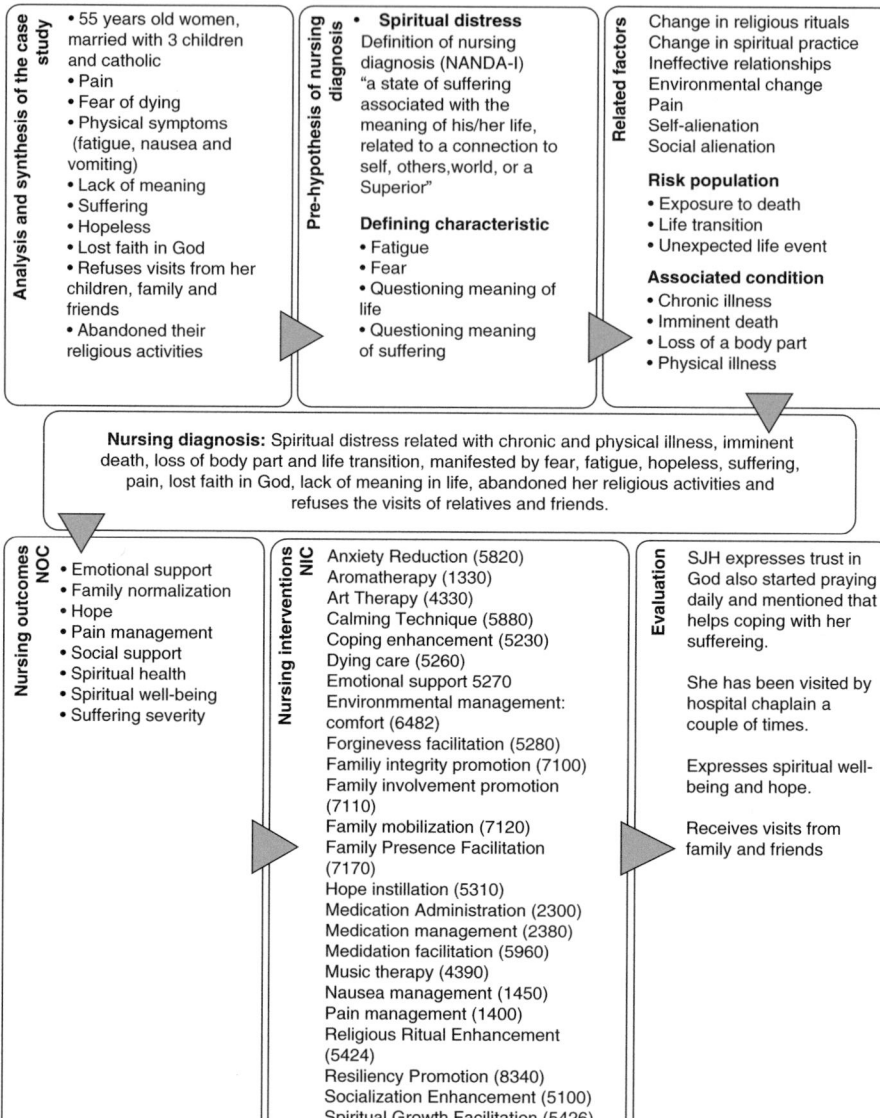

Fig. 8.2 Spiritual distress case study diagram, according to NANDA-I method in a multidisciplinary team approach

Pre-hypothesis of Nursing Diagnosis
- Spiritual distress

Definition of nursing diagnosis (NANDA-I): "A state of suffering associated with the meaning of his/her life, related to a connection to self, others, world, or a Superior" [2].

Spiritual Distress (00066) belongs to Domain 10 (Life principles) and Class 3 (Value/Belief/Action Congruence) (Approved 1978, revised 2002,2013,2017, level of evidence 2.1) [2].

Axis 1: diagnostic focus: spiritual distress.
Axis 2: subject of the diagnosis: individual.
Axis 3: judgment: risk.
Axis 4: location: non-applicable.
Axis 5: age: adult.
Axis 6: time: non-applicable.
Axis 7: status of the diagnosis: problem-focused.

Defining Characteristic
- Fatigue
- Fear
- Questioning meaning of life
- Questioning meaning of suffering

Related Factors
- Change in religious ritual
- Change in spiritual practice
- Ineffective relationships
- Environmental change
- Pain
- Self-alienation
- Social alienation

Risk Population
- Exposure to death
- Life transition
- Unexpected life event

Associated Condition
- Chronic illness
- Imminent death
- Loss of a body part
- Physical illness

Nursing Diagnosis
Spiritual distress related to chronic and physical illness, imminent death, loss of body part and life transition, manifested by fear, fatigue, hopeless, suffering, pain, lost faith in God, lack of meaning in life, abandoned her religious activities and refuses the visits of relatives and friends.

Nursing Outcomes (NOC)
- Emotional support
- Family normalization
- Hope
- Pain management
- Social support
- Spiritual health
- Spiritual well-being
- Suffering severity

Nursing Interventions (NIC)
- Anxiety reduction (5820)
- Aromatherapy (1330)
- Art therapy (4330)
- Calming technique (5880)
- Coping enhancement (5230)
- Dying care (5260)
- Emotional support 5270
- Environmental management: Comfort (6482)
- Forgiveness facilitation (5280)
- Family integrity promotion (7100)
- Family involvement promotion (7110)
- Family mobilization (7120)
- Family presence facilitation (7170)
- Hope instillation (5310)
- Medication administration (2300)
- Medication management (2380)
- Medication facilitation (5960)
- Music therapy (4390)
- Nausea management (1450)
- Pain management (1400)
- Religious ritual enhancement (5424)
- Resiliency promotion (8340)
- Socialization enhancement (5100)
- Spiritual growth facilitation (5426)
- Spiritual support (5420)

- Therapeutic touch 5465)
- Therapy group (5450)
- Touch (5460)
- Visitation facilitation (7560)

Role of other professionals of healthcare team in their approach to patient's spiritual distress:

The clinician assists in the symptomatic control of symptoms with therapeutic prescription in which the patient reports having pain and vomiting.

The psychologist contributes in helping the patient to preserve equilibrium and understanding of internal conflicts and reducing suffering.

The chaplain is the spiritual expert and can promote spiritual and religious assistance.

> **Nursing Diagnosis**
> Spiritual distress related with chronic and physical illness, imminent death, loss of body part and life transition, manifested by fear, fatigue, hopeless, suffering, pain, lost faith in God, lack of meaning in life, abandoned her religious activities and refuses the visits of relatives and friends.

8.4 Conclusion

To understand the origins of nursing one must go back in time to ancient civilizations, although it is argued that the essential elements that nursing provides were present at the beginning of humankind. Nevertheless, Florence Nightingale is considered the great promoter of modern nursing and responsible for a new professional era. From her time, great theoretical and scientific developments promoted the emergence of the fundamental paradigms that now ground the nursing discipline.

Nurses are a regular presence throughout the various stages of a patient's life transitions, regardless of conditions of health, cultural contexts or religiosity. Furthermore, nurse hold a privileged position within the multidisciplinary healthcare team since they are a *continuum* presence, by which they may facilitate the unique and deep nurse-patient connection. This relationship is essential for assessing an individual's needs and in providing a patient-centered, individualized care.

Spirituality is a dimension that contributes to the uniqueness of the individuals; it is a recognized therapeutic resource, associated with connection to others, possession of meaning in life and transcendence. Additionally, the patient uses the spiritual dimension to cope with illness and to overcome spiritual distress triggered by illness and other adverse events.

Delivery of spiritual care in nursing should be based on the nursing process. Moreover, nursing claims and embraces an ethical and human dimension, though serious gaps in nursing education and training compromises attention to spirituality.

The spiritual assessment is considered a fundamental step in the identification of patient spiritual distress. Several instruments are available to assist nurses in assessing the spiritual needs of patients. In addition, different nursing classifications allow accurate diagnoses and matching spiritual interventions in a truly holistic delivery of nursing care.

References

1. Henderson V. The concept of nursing. J Adv Nurs. 2006;53(1):21–31.
2. Herdman TH, Kamitsuru S. NANDA international nursing diagnoses: definitions and classification 2018–2020. Oxford: Wiley Blackwell; 2017.
3. McEvoy L, Duffy A. Holistic practice--a concept analysis. Nurse Educ Pract. 2008;8(6):412–9.
4. Papathanasiou I, Sklavou M, Kourkouta L. Holistic nursing care: theories and perspectives. Am J Nurs Sci. 2014;2(1):1.
5. Ramezani M, Ahmadi F, Mohammadi E, Kazemnejad A. Spiritual care in nursing: a concept analysis. Int Nurs Rev. 2014;61(2):211–9.
6. Drury C, Hunter J. The hole in holistic patient care. Open J Nurs. 2016;6:776–92.
7. Chirico F. Spiritual well-being in the 21st century: it's time yo review the current WHO's health definition? J Health Soc Sci. 2016;1(1):11–6.
8. Romeiro J, Caldeira S, Brady V, Hall J, Timmins F. The spiritual journey of infertile couples: discussing the opportunity for spiritual care. Religions. 2017;8(4):76.
9. Romeiro J, Caldeira S, Brady V, Timmins F, Hall J. Spiritual aspects of living with infertility: a synthesis of qualitative studies. J Clin Nurs. 2017;26:3917–35.
10. Crowther S, Hall J. Spirituality and childbirth: meaning and care at the start of life, vol. 204. New York: Routledge; 2017.
11. Monod S, Rochat E, Büla C, Spencer B. The spiritual needs model: spirituality assessment in the geriatric hospital setting. J Relig Spiritual Aging. 2010;22(4):271–82.
12. Caldeira S, Timmins F, de Carvalho EC, Vieira M. Nursing Diagnosis of "Spiritual Distress" in women with breast cancer: prevalence and major defining characteristics. Cancer Nurs. 2016;39(4):321–7.
13. Caldeira S, Timmins F, de Carvalho EC, Vieira M. Clinical validation of the nursing diagnosis spiritual distress in cancer patients undergoing chemotherapy. Int J Nurs Knowl. 2017;28(1):44–52.
14. Villagomeza LR. Spiritual distress in adult cancer patients: toward conceptual clarity. Holist Nurs Pract. 2005;19(6):285–94.
15. Carmody J, Reed G, Kristeller J, Merriam P. Mindfulness, spirituality, and health-related symptoms. J Psychosom Res. 2008;64(4):393–403.
16. Delgado C. A discussion of the concept of spirituality. Nurs Sci Q. 2005;18(2):157–62.
17. Caldeira S, Figueiredo AS, da Conceição AP, Ermel C, Mendes J, Chaves E, et al. Spirituality in the undergraduate curricula of nursing schools in Portugal and São Paulo-Brazil. Religions. 2016;7(134):1–9.
18. Attard J, Baldacchino DR, Camilleri L. Nurses' and midwives' acquisition of competency in spiritual care: a focus on education. Nurs Educ Today. 2014;34(12):1460–6.
19. Balboni MJ, Sullivan A, Enzinger AC, Epstein-Peterson ZD, Tseng YD, Mitchell C, et al. Nurse and physician barriers to spiritual care provision at the end of life. J Pain Symptom Manag. 2014;48(3):400–10.
20. Theofanidis D, Sapountzi-Krepia D. Nursing and caring: an historical overview from ancient Greek tradition to modern times. Int J Caring Sci. 2015;8(3):791–800.

21. Nursing definition [Internet]. Google. [cited 2018 Feb 21]. Available from: https://www.google.pt/search?dcr=0&ei=JT2KWt2iNYzrUuPxi_gJ&q=nursing+definition&oq=nursing+definition&gs_l=psy-ab.3..0j0i22i30k1l9.2935.5152.0.5831.11.5.0.6.6.0.138.654.0j5.5.0....0...1c.1.64.psy-ab..0.11.794...0i67k1.0.LrhGjOQ0zYg.
22. Infirm definition [Internet]. Google. [cited 2018 Feb 21]. Available from: https://www.google.pt/search?dcr=0&ei=LD2KWrjKM8HXU8qblfgI&q=infirm+definition&oq=infirm+definition&gs_l=psy-ab.3..0i7i30k1l10.51394.52240.0.52793.6.6.0.0.0.0.160.705.0j5.5.0....0...1c.1.64.psy-ab..2.4.581....0.5bY1wH4VoeI.
23. Nurse etymology [Internet]. Google. [cited 2018 Feb 21]. Available from: https://www.google.pt/search?dcr=0&ei=eT2KWs6vOsS0Ube7kvgJ&q=nurse+etymology&oq=nurse+etymologi&gs_l=psy-ab.3.0.0i19k1j0i13i5i30i19k1j0i8i13i30i19k1l2.11912.13848.0.15229.9.9.0.0.0.0.157.1287.0j9.9.0....0...1c.1.64.psy-ab..0.9.1276...0j0i22i30k1j0i22i10i30k1j0i22i30i19k1j0i22i10i30i19k1.0.uYunBoJ0x7U.
24. Johnson RW, Tilghman JS, Davis-Dick LR, Hamilton-Faison B. A historical overview of spirituality in nursing. ABNF J. 2006;17(2):60–2.
25. Nightingale F. Notes on nursing: what it is and what it is not. London: Harrison and Sons; 1860.
26. Kyle TV. The concept of caring: a review of the literature. J Adv Nurs. 1995;21(3):506–14.
27. George JB, Colaboradores. Teorias de Enfermagem. Os Fundamentos à Prática Profissional. 4th ed. Porto Alegre: Artmed Editora; 2000. 355 p.
28. Mesquita AC, Guilherme C, Caldeira S, Chaves E, de Carvalho EC. Espiritualidade e Sofrimento Espiritual como foco de atenção da Enfermagem. In: PRONANDA - Programa de Atualização em Diagnósticos de Enfermagem. 2nd ed. Porto Alegre: Artmed Panamericana Editors; 2014. p. 9–33.
29. Henderson V. The nature of nursing. Am J Nurs. 1964;64:62–8.
30. American Nurses Association. What is nursing? [Internet]. Maryland: American Nurses Association; 2018. [cited 2018 Feb 21]. Available from: http://www.nursingworld.org/EspeciallyForYou/What-is-Nursing.
31. International Council of Nurses. Definition of nursing [Internet]. Geneva: ICN; 2017. [cited 2018 Feb 21]. Available from: http://www.icn.ch/who-we-are/icn-definition-of-nursing/.
32. Royal College of Nursing. Defining nursing [Internet]. London: Royal College of Nursing; 2014. [cited 2018 Feb 2]. Available from: https://www.rcn.org.uk/professional-development/publications/pub-004768.
33. Shamian J. The role of nursing in health care. Rev Bras Enferm. 2014;67(6):867–8.
34. van Leeuwen R, Tiesinga LJ, Post D, Jochemsen H. Spiritual care: implications for nurses' professional responsibility. J Clin Nurs. 2006;15(7):875–84.
35. Frenk J, Chen L, Bhutta ZA, Cohen J, Crisp N, Evans T, et al. Health professionals for a new century: transforming education to strengthen health systems in an interdependent world. Lancet. 2010;376(9756):1923–58.
36. WHO. Framework for action on interprofessional education & collaborative practice. [Internet]. Geneva: WHO; 2010. [cited 2018 Feb 20]. 64 p. Available from: http://apps.who.int/iris/bitstream/10665/70185/1/WHO_HRH_HPN_10.3_eng.pdf?ua=1.
37. Yanez B, Edmondson D, Stanton AL, Park CL, Kwan L, Ganz PA, et al. Facets of spirituality as predictors of adjustment to cancer: relative contributions of having faith and finding meaning. J Consult Clin Psychol. 2009;77(4):730–41.
38. Lepherd L. Spirituality: everyone has it, but what is it? Int J Nurs Pract. 2015;21(5):566–74.
39. Martins AR, Pinto S, Caldeira S, Pimentel FL. Tradução e adaptação da spirituality and spiritual care rating scale em enfermeiros portugueses de cuidados paliativos. Rev Enferm Ref. 2015;serIV(4):89–97.
40. Barber C. Spirituality and religion: a brief definition. Br J Healthc Assist. 2012;6(8):378–81.
41. Catré MNC, Ferreira JA, Pessoa T, Catré A, Catré MC. Espiritualidade: Contributos para uma clarificação do conceito. Anál Psicol. 2016;34(1):31–46.
42. Mahlungulu SN, Uys LR. Spirituality in nursing: an analysis of the concept. Curationis. 2004;27(2):15–26.

43. Reinert KG, Koenig HG. Re-examining definitions of spirituality in nursing research. J Adv Nurs. 2013;69(12):2622–34.
44. McBrien B. A concept analysis of spirituality. Br J Nurs. 2006;15(1):42–5.
45. Sessanna L, Finnell D, Jezewski MA. Spirituality in nursing and health-related literature: a concept analysis. J Holist Nurs. 2007;25(4):252–62. discussion 263-264.
46. Jaberi A, Momennasab M, Yektatalab S, Ebadi A, Cheraghi MA. Spiritual health: a concept analysis. J Relig Health. 2017. https://doi.org/10.1007/s10943-017-0379-z.
47. Tanyi RA. Towards clarification of the meaning of spirituality. J Adv Nurs. 2002;39(5):500–9.
48. Vachon M, Fillion L, Achille M. A conceptual analysis of spirituality at the end of life. J Palliat Med. 2009;12(1):53–9.
49. Weathers E, McCarthy G, Coffey A. Concept analysis of spirituality: an evolutionary approach. Nurs Forum. 2016;51(2):79–96.
50. Nascimento LC, Santos T de FM, de Oliveira FCS, Pan R, Flória-Santos M, Rocha SMM. Espiritualidade e religiosidade na perspectiva de enfermeiros. Texto Contexto Enferm. 2013;22(1):52–60.
51. Balboni T, Balboni M, Paulk ME, Phelps A, Wright A, Peteet J, et al. Support of cancer patients' spiritual needs and associations with medical care costs at the end of life. Cancer. 2011;117(23):5383–91.
52. Natschke M. Holistic nurses know. Beginnings. 2017;37(3):5–22.
53. Hines ME. Turning words into action: advancing the role of advanced holistic nurses. J Holist Nurs. 2017;35(4):316–7.
54. Nursing RCo. Spirituality in nursing care: a pocket guide. London: Royal College of Nursing; 2011.
55. Timmins F, Caldeira S. Assessing the spiritual needs of patients. Nurs Stand. 2017;31(29):47–53.
56. Lutz K, Rowniak SR, Sandhu P. A contemporary paradigm: integrating spirituality in advance care planning. J Relig Health. 2017;57(2):662–71.
57. Rothman J. Spirituality: what we can teach and how we can teach it. J Relig Spiritual Soc Work. 2009;28(1/2):161.
58. Nurses ICo. Code of ethics for nurses. Geneva: ICN; 2012. p. 12.
59. McSherry W, Jamieson S. An online survey of nurses' perceptions of spirituality and spiritual care. J Clin Nurs. 2011;20(11–12):1757–67.
60. Deal B. A pilot study of nurses' experience of giving spiritual care. Qual Rep. 2010;15(4):852–63.
61. Cone PH, Giske T. Nurses' comfort level with spiritual assessment: a study among nurses working in diverse healthcare settings. J Clin Nurs. 2017;26(19–20):3125–36.
62. Ramezani M, Ahmadi F, Mohammadi E, Kazemnejad A. Catalysts to spiritual care delivery: a content analysis. Iran Red Crescent Med J [Internet]. 2016;18(3):e22420. [cited 2018 Mar 3] Available from: https://www.ncbi.nlm.nih.gov/pmc/articles/PMC4884212/
63. Caldeira S, Timmins F. Editorial: time as presence and opportunity: the key to spiritual care in contemporary nursing practice. J Clin Nurs. 2015;24:2355–6.
64. de Carvalho EC, Oliveira-Kumakura ARS, Morais SCRV. Clinical reasoning in nursing: teaching strategies and assessment tools. Rev Bras Enferm. 2017;70(3):662–8.
65. Koharchik L, Caputi L, Robb M, Culleiton AL. Fostering clinical reasoning in nursing students. Am J Nurs. 2015;115(1):58–61.
66. Caldeira S, Timmins F. Implementing spiritual care interventions. Nurs Stand. 2017;31(34):54–60.
67. Alfaro-LeFevre R. Nursing process and clinical reasoning. Nurs Educ Perspect. 2012;33(1):7.
68. Pesut B, Fowler M, Reimer-Kirkham S, Taylor EJ, Sawatzky R. Particularizing spirituality in points of tension: enriching the discourse. Nurs Inq. 2009;16(4):337–46.
69. Puchalski CM. Formal and informal spiritual assessment. Asian Pac J Cancer Prev. 2010;11(Suppl 1):51–7.
70. Balboni TA, Paulk ME, Balboni MJ, Phelps AC, Loggers ET, Wright AA, et al. Provision of spiritual care to patients with advanced cancer: associations with medical care and quality of life near death. J Clin Oncol. 2010;28(3):445–52.

71. Skalla KA, Ferrell B. Challenges in assessing spiritual distress in survivors of cancer. Clin J Oncol Nurs. 2015;19(1):99–104.
72. de Jager Meezenbroek E, Garssen B, van den Berg M, van Dierendonck D, Visser A, Schaufeli WB. Measuring spirituality as a universal human experience: a review of spirituality questionnaires. J Relig Health. 2012;51(2):336–54.
73. Hill PC, Hood RW. Measures of religiosity. Birmingham: Religious Education Press; 1999. p. 531.
74. MacDonald DA, Friedman HL, Kuentzel JG. A survey of measures of spiritual and transpersonal constructs: part one—research update. J Transpers Psychol. 1999;31(2):137–54.
75. MacDonald DA, Friedman HL, Kuentzel JG. A survey of measures of spiritual and transpersonal constructs: part two—additional instruments. J Transpers Psychol. 1999;31(2):155–77.
76. Shorkey C, Uebel M, Windsor LC. Measuring dimensions of spirituality in chemical dependence treatment and recovery: research and practice. Int J Ment Health Addict. 2008;6(3):286–305.
77. King JE, Crowther MR. The measurement of religiosity and spirituality: examples and issues from psychology. J Organ Chang Manag. 2004;17(1):83–101.
78. Howden JW. Development and psychometric characteristics of the spirituality assessment scale. Denton: Texas Woman's University; 1992. 310 p.
79. Kobylarz FA, Heath JM, Like RC. The ETHNIC(S) mnemonic: a clinical tool for ethnogeriatric education. J Am Geriatr Soc. 2002;50(9):1582–9.
80. McSherry W, Draper P, Kendrick D. The construct validity of a rating scale designed to assess spirituality and spiritual care. Int J Nurs Stud. 2002;39(7):723–34.
81. Delaney C. The spirituality scale: development and psychometric testing of a holistic instrument to assess the human spiritual dimension. J Holist Nurs. 2005;23(2):145–67. discussion 168-171.
82. Fisher J. Development and application of a spiritual well-being questionnaire called SHALOM. Religions. 2010;1(1):105–21.
83. Beck AT, Weissman A, Lester D, Trexler L. The measurement of pessimism: the hopelessness scale. J Consult Clin Psychol. 1974;42(6):861–5.
84. Maugans TA. The SPIRITual history. Arch Fam Med. 1996;5(1):11–6.
85. Mayers AM, Khoo S-T, Svartberg M. The existential loneliness questionnaire: background, development, and preliminary findings. J Clin Psychol. 2002;58(9):1183–93.
86. Steger MF, Frazier P, Oishi S, Kaler M. The meaning in life questionnaire: assessing the presence of and search for meaning in life. J Couns Psychol. 2006;53(1):80–93.
87. Ku Y-L, Kuo S-M, Yao C-Y. Establishing the validity of a spiritual distress scale for cancer patients hospitalized in southern Taiwan. Int J Palliat Nurs. 2010;16(3):134–8.
88. Hale-Smith A, Park CL, Edmondson D. Measuring beliefs about suffering: development of the views of suffering scale. Psychol Assess. 2012;24(4):855–66.
89. Hungelmann J, Kenkel-Rossi E, Klassen L, Stollenwerk R. Focus on spiritual well-being: harmonious interconnectedness of mind-body-spirit--use of the JAREL spiritual well-being scale. Geriatr Nurs. 1996;17(6):262–6.
90. Ellison CW. Spiritual well-being: conceptualization and measurement. J Psychol Theol. 1983;11:330–40.
91. Puchalski C, Romer AL. Taking a spiritual history allows clinicians to understand patients more fully. J Palliat Med. 2000;3(1):129–37.
92. Anandarajah G, Hight E. Spirituality and medical practice: using the HOPE questions as a practical tool for spiritual assessment. Am Fam Physician. 2001;63(1):81–9.
93. Peterman AH, Fitchett G, Brady MJ, Hernandez L, Cella D. Measuring spiritual well-being in people with cancer: the functional assessment of chronic illness therapy--spiritual well-being scale (FACIT-Sp). Ann Behav Med. 2002;24(1):49–58.
94. Gomez R, Fisher JW. Domains of spiritual well-being and development and validation of the spiritual well-being questionnaire. Personal Individ Differ. 2003;35:1975–91.
95. WHOQOL SRPB Group. A cross-cultural study of spirituality, religion, and personal beliefs as components of quality of life. Soc Sci Med. 2006;62(6):1486–97.

96. Pargament KI, Koenig HG, Perez LM. The many methods of religious coping: development and initial validation of the RCOPE. J Clin Psychol. 2000;56(4):519–43.
97. Baldacchino DR, Buhagiar A. Psychometric evaluation of the spiritual coping strategies scale in English, Maltese, back-translation and bilingual versions. J Adv Nurs. 2003;42(6):558–70.
98. Ai AL, Tice TN, Peterson C, Huang B. Prayers, spiritual support, and positive attitudes in coping with the September 11 national crisis. J Pers. 2005;73(3):763–91.
99. Büssing A, Matthiessen PF, Ostermann T. Engagement of patients in religious and spiritual practices: confirmatory results with the SpREUK-P 1.1 questionnaire as a tool of quality of life research. Health Qual Life Outcomes. 2005;3:53.
100. Nelson-Becker H. Development of a spiritual support scale for use with older adults. J Hum Behav Soc Environ. 2005;11(3–4):195–212.
101. Newlin K, Knafl K, Melkus GD. African-American spirituality: a concept analysis. ANS Adv Nurs Sci. 2002;25(2):57–70.
102. Mesquita AC, Caldeira S, Chaves E, de Carvalho EC. An analytical overview of spirituality in NANDA-I taxonomies. Int J Nurs Knowl. 2017;**29**(3):200–5.
103. Müller-Staub M, Lavin MA, Needham I, van Achterberg T. Meeting the criteria of a nursing diagnosis classification: evaluation of ICNP, ICF, NANDA and ZEFP. Int J Nurs Stud. 2007;44(5):702–13.
104. van Leeuwen R, Cusveller B. Nursing competencies for spiritual care. J Adv Nurs. 2004;48(3):234–46.
105. Brémault-Phillips S, Olson J, Brett-MacLean P, Oneschuk D, Sinclair S, Magnus R, et al. Integrating spirituality as a key component of patient care. Religions. 2015;6(2):476–98.
106. Puchalski CM. The role of spirituality in health care. Proc (Bayl Univ Med Cent). 2001;14(4):352–7.
107. Timmins F, Caldeira S. Understanding spirituality and spiritual care in nursing. Nurs Stand. 2017;31(22):50–7.
108. Fournier AL. Creating a sacred space in the intensive care unit at the end of life. Dimens Crit Care Nurs. 2017;36(2):110–5.

Loss and Grief in People with Intellectual Disability

Joy Powell

Abstract

This chapter on loss and grief in people with intellectual disability begins with the premise that loss and grief are normal integral aspects of life for all people and that people with intellectual disability do not differ from the general population in this. It is written from the perspective of a chaplain supporting people with intellectual disability through their grief journey. It acknowledges that grief is a normal part of life; it is not an event something to "get over" but rather a process that involves time, presence and deep listening skills, on the part of the chaplain or anyone who is supporting a person on the grief journey. What follows are some approaches to spiritual care provision among people with ID who are grieving. There are some examples from practice where people shared their stories with me; all names have been changed to protect identities.

Abbreviations

ID   Intellectual disability
NAHC   National Association of Healthcare Chaplains

9.1 Introduction

This chapter on loss and grief in people with intellectual disability (ID) begins with the premise that loss and grief are normal and integral aspects of life for all people and that people who are differently abled, that is, who have an ID, do not differ from the general

J. Powell (✉)
Saint John of God Hospitaller Ministries, Dublin, Ireland
e-mail: joy.powell@sjog.ie

population in this. Grieving is a process not an event, it is not something to "get *over*" but rather a process or journey which needs work and attention, and for people with an ID, because they may be lacking in the resilience of people more abled, they may need support during the process of the grief journey. I feel blessed to be supported in my work as a chaplain by being part of a multidisciplinary team of social care workers, nurses, doctors, psychologists, psychiatrist, speech and language and physiotherapists, occupational therapists, etc., all of who may make referrals to the Chaplaincy Department when a loss is imminent or when a death occurs. I am also supported in my work by a team of chaplains working across ID and mental health services. I am also supported in my work by the National Association of Healthcare Chaplains (NAHC), the Dublin Roman Catholic Hospital Chaplains and the Support Network of Catholic Health Care Chaplains.

What follows are some approaches to spiritual care provision among adults with ID who are grieving, who may live in supported residential settings or at home with family and who may also attend a day service or who work among the general population.

If we consider support for people who are grieving, in terms of a pyramid of supports, there are three levels with level 1 being information and support, level 2 extra support and level 3 professional therapy.

Chaplains in the intellectual disability sector offer support at levels one and two on this pyramid. In my professional capacity referrals for service users who are grieving can come from the person themselves, their family members, frontline staff or any of the above-listed disciplines.

It is often at the first level of information and support that we identify the role spirituality might take in building resilience needed to cope when grieving. The extra support often includes spiritual care.

For all of us it is natural to accumulate many losses over a lifetime.

"A lifetime is an accumulation of losses; these may play upon each other as triggers or may ignite what otherwise might be considered an inappropriate or excessive grief response. In addition, losses are often ignored or not validated, and unresolved losses are often found to be at the root of later mental health problems. Any given loss is set in a context of a lifetime and cannot be seen as an isolated event" ([1], p. VI). In the foreword of Caroline Lloyd's book *Grief Demystified*, Dr. Jennifer Dayes, a counselling psychologist, says that:

> we struggle to talk about death... and that society is hugely influenced by the idea that grief comes in stages, each identifiable, each to be worked through, yet this is not what [*she*] observed in her research or practice. The grief she saw in her therapy room did not come in such neat packages. No persons difficulties come as a single entity. They are situated in a web of past and current experiences and difficulties, a strand of which, sometimes overlooked is grief ([2], p. 11).

In the past many people with ID were not involved in the funeral or other rituals when a loved one died; this was I believe an attempt by families and organisations to protect the vulnerable person from the death of the significant person in their life. Therefore the loss of the loved one was never validated for them; sometimes it could be a long time before anyone informed them the person was dead. Breaking bad news is we now know a delicate task and involves professional skill. People with ID are not stupid; they pick up on the absence of a loved one over time and may be frustrated in their inability to communicate what is happening to them as they miss the absent person. We now know that it is the strength of the attachment to the person who has died which determines the level of grief, and to help alleviate the stress and anxiety associated with the loss, there is a need to normalise and validate the experience of that loss.

Thankfully this is changing, and more and more as chaplains working in ID services, we find ourselves supporting people, by breaking bad news in a compassionate and caring way and advocating for the person with ID to attend at the funeral or cremation. We offer ongoing support to the person and their family during these difficult transitions. Conversations now take place where we talk of the best way to break the bad news; it is never a question of not informing the person, but rather the decision to inform is based on the person' s right to know what has happened to their loved one. Generally wherever possible, chaplains are present when bad news is broken.

Over the past 12 years, I have worked as a healthcare chaplain with responsibility for the spiritual care of adults and children across the spectrum of intellectual disability, from profound, moderate to mild disability. I also support staff and families who are supporting people with ID.

Part of the role of being a healthcare chaplain with responsibility for people with ID is to accompany them in their search for meaning; many of the people I have supported through different categories of loss are influenced by their spiritual beliefs and practices. Their spirituality and spiritual activity help to give meaning to their lives. Spirituality pops up even in secular education programmes around grief, for example, in Seasons for Growth. It is quite common for a person experiencing the loss of a loved one to ask to see me and to invite me to say a prayer with them, light a candle or have a mass said (or even accompany them to mass or church or the funeral of a loved one or friend) for their loved one and speak about their loved one as being in heaven and free from suffering. I am often asked to accompany someone to the grave in the year after a loss as a process in helping the person let go and move on with their life.

Part of my role in supporting people with ID during the grieving process involves validating the loss by empathetic listening and supporting them to connect with whatever spiritual activity gives meaning to their life as Humphrey and Zimpfer suggest: "It is often observed that the spiritual realm is the only emotional anchor left for survival. Belief in an after life can provide a reason, for going on and hope for a reunion with a loved one" ([1], p. 13).

There are many theories and models about grief, loss and change; my experience in working with people with ID is to focus myself on the task model provided by William Worden. The reason Worden's model is my focus is because it is the one that the Seasons for Growth bereavement education programme is based on. (The Seasons for Growth programme is the one we use in the ID services.) I must reiterate though that while this is a theory with tasks and stages, I remind the reader that it is not linier. If we set the tasks or stages as benchmarks, we have already failed to accompany the grieving person; doing this may result in a person thinking they are not grieving properly or "getting over", "moving through" or "moving on from grief" fast enough and can in itself result in more stress and anxiety. I stress that it is not easy to be a grief worker especially in a society which is not one which normalises or even talks about grief and the behaviours associated with grieving. And in my work there is the added difficulty of intellectual disability to attend to.

William Worden (1991) building on the work of John Bowlby (*Attachment and Loss*) suggested not a new theory, but his intention was to provide some practical application of established theories to help people during counselling.

William Worden's four tasks for the grieving person are as follows (Worden 2001):

1. Accept the reality of the loss.
2. Work through the pain of grief.
3. Adjust to the environment in which the person is no longer present.
4. Emotionally letting go and reinvesting in life, p. 7.

By validating and acknowledging the reality of the change and loss, the person can begin to accept the reality of the loss. By learning about people's reactions to change and loss and each one's experience of these, as I listen to their story of loss, they are enabled to work through the pain of grief. We hope this will enable the person grieving to heal in body, mind and spirit as grief has emotional, cognitive, spiritual, physical and behavioural manifestations that can and often do overwhelm and debilitate the grieving person. I mention Worden's task because it is the theory behind the very practical education programme Seasons for Growth which is the one I have used in my practice for many years.

In my professional experience, healthcare chaplains working with people with ID often help people build resilience by developing skills to assist with processing their grief. It is empowering for the person to know that there are actions they can take and decisions they can make when they are grieving. It gives a sense of being in control (grief knocks us off-guard and makes us feel out of control/helpless) of how they act out of a feeling in a positive way. What we are trying to accomplish here is to enable the person adjust to the environment in which the person who died is no longer present. But it is also important for the person with ID to know who will be part of their circle of support as they grieve. The Seasons for Growth programme can assist people with ID in building resilience, and it very least provides peer support so the person knows they are not alone in their grief.

Chaplains explore with the person ways of dealing with their emotions by first being able to name them, linking thoughts and feelings and behaviour (emotional self-regulation), helping them to manage anxiety and stress and looking at what to do about their thoughts and what to do about their feelings. It is part of my experience that for many of the people I worked with, it can be that during these times the questions around spirituality and spiritual activity come up. Being part of a worshipping faith community offers some solace to many who find mass or Sunday worship the public place where neighbours and friends, family and staff can offer sympathy and validate their loss. When people with ID engage in the Seasons for

Growth education programmes (designed for young people who are grieving) which is not in itself a spiritual programme, it allows for the reflective space where people's spiritual needs emerge. They will speak of how prayer, visiting church buildings and religious objects give comfort and help with anxiety and stress; for some it is the walk in the park or by the sea; being in a natural setting which evokes a spiritual response can also bring calm. Equally for others it can be a visit to their church, lighting a candle, saying a prayer or attending a service which helps validate their loss and give comfort.

Over my years as a chaplain, I have learned that in order to be effective in this work, I need to care deeply about supporting adults with ID to understand and manage issues of change and loss. By developing empathetic listening skills, "seeking to understand before being understood", and hearing with the heart as well as the head, this skill/technique helps me connect emotionally as well as cognitively and spiritually with the person I am supporting.

I have learned the value of listening deeply, and it is hoped effectively, with both head and heart to the stories of each person. Respect for the uniqueness of each person's life story is paramount; I have learned to identify people's strengths in order to affirm them, reminding them that they are not alone and that grief is a normal part of life. I believe we are more resilient than we know, but grief and loss and the major changes they bring affect us like a tsunami wave that knocks us off course and most of us will need some support and time to process this in order to identify what gets us through.

To be effective in this work, I need to be able to ask questions sensitively and respect both silence and little idiosyncrasies and even what might be considered odd behaviours. Psychologist says that all behaviour is a way of communicating and if a person struggles cognitively or has difficulty expressing feelings with words, behaviour may be a coping mechanism; finding ways around challenging that behaviour into some creative way of expressing a feeling is a skill set in itself that the chaplain needs to develop within his- or herself. There is also a role for creative rituals here.

1. An example from practice:

One person I supported explained to me that 1 day shortly after the death of her father, she was in her kitchen drying dishes; for no apparent reason, she smashed a plate on the floor. She did not understand why she had done this; it was out of character for her. Over the course of many conversations, she could identify that she was thinking of her father when it happened. She identified feeling sad, angry and frustrated that he was gone. She said she missed him and that it felt good to smash the plate. It was a release. She also said that smashing the plate had upset some of the women she shares her home with; one was even frightened by her behaviour. She didn't feel good about that. My task was to listen non-judgementally and reflect on what the person was saying to me, responding not reacting.

Having discussed that feelings were neither good nor bad, they just are, they are normal and everybody has them, and it is ok/normal to feel sad, angry and frustrated that her dad was dead. We explored the fact feelings come and go and they change all the time, but we need to express them positively. We then explored what positive actions she could take to help when next time she feels sad, angry and frustrated about the loss of her dad before she acts out. I suggested that sometimes it helps to talk about it with another person you trust. I asked her to think about and name someone she would trust who would listen next time she was feeling like this and before she acts (smash the plate). She named her house staff and also a staff in her day service and her sister. We also explored some actions she could take on her own, by way of giving her some control over her actions.

As someone who liked to listen to music, she could go to her room and listen to her music or watch a favourite TV programme. She also agreed that she would like to make a memory box over time; she would put photos of family celebrations with her dad, a gardening magazine he used to read as he was a keen gardener, his glasses, his rosary beads and a cross. Going into the garden and being quiet and thinking about him made her feel better. Going to the church where they had worshipped together made her feel better. Going for a walk in the park was also a comfort. Sometimes when she engaged in the positive activities like walking in the park, sitting in the garden, going to church, or exploring her memory box, she found she would cry. Tears are also a normal response to grief like a river finds its end in the sea; tears are a gift that brings healing. Sometimes we all need to hear that it is ok to cry. Later she invited me to facilitate a short reflection/prayer service for her and her friends in her house as a way of validating before her friends how angry and sad she was at the loss of her father. Her friends were very sympathetic, and they spoke at length about the incident with the broken plate but also shared and prayed about some of their own losses.

Many people who I have supported over the years value the opportunity of making a memory box during the early stages of mourning; it provides them with a way of remembering an important person in their life who has died. Many of the memory boxes I have seen involve religious items like rosary beads, prayer books, crosses and holy pictures and medals. The box provides a way to explore memories which enable them to feel close and connected to the person who died. Some people like to show their memory box to people, e.g. staff or friends, who did not know their loved one; it works by way of giving the person an opportunity to be in charge of when and where they share their story of loss. To show their memory box to a trusted staff or volunteer is often an indication that they need to take time with someone to chat about what has happened, all part of the letting go process and giving opportunity to grieve. When people see the religious objects, they usually say things like "I will keep you in my prayers" or "can we say a prayer together" for the deceased and for the person grieving.

During the first 2 years of the mourning process, there is a delicate balance between the mutually conflicting demands of holding on to and letting go of the person who has died. However in order to move on and reinvest in life, there is a need to firstly have the loss validated which includes part of the past which has to be let go of eventually and the present which involves ongoing chances to grieve.

Other ways that people with ID deal with their losses are by telling their story of loss; this can be very empowering, helping to validate the loss by way of listening as they explore what happened when a significant person in their life has died.

I have learned never to take for granted the role of ritual in validating loss and helping people move through and make meaning.

2. Example from practice:

Mike (not his real name) is one of our older gentlemen who came from a large family many of who live abroad. Throughout his life they came to visit, or indeed he visited, often travelling abroad with them. As his siblings got older and died, the opportunity for family contact waned, and he grew a little melancholy. When the last of his sisters died abroad, the distance and logistics were unable to be overcome to enable him to attend her funeral. He asked to see me, and we agreed that he would like to have a prayer service in his local parish where he helped out as a volunteer. He wanted his friends and his staff to attend. He gave me a picture of his sister which we arranged in a sacred space with some flowers. We began by welcoming his friends and staff and acknowledging his sister's passing and how he needed to ritualise it in a way that would give meaning. It was a simple prayer service with music and Scripture readings and reflection on their life and the fun they shared growing up together. We had tea and coffee in the parish centre afterwards, and he met many parishioners who he was able to tell his story of loss to. People offering their condolences really moved him. Had we not done this simple ritual, no one would have known of his loss, and there would be no acknowledgement of his grief. I have a lovely thank you card from him for facilitating this ritual; my part however small meant something bigger for him. My learning is to never underestimate how a small act can help give meaning to a person grieving.

Those of us who have been privileged to spend time in the company of people with an intellectual disability have learned that the most important and often most challenging thing is to listen. When we listen to a personal story of loss, we acknowledge and validate not merely their experience but also their humanity. This type of encounter is both passionate and sublime. It is indeed a spiritual experience and a privilege to encounter. It is also egalitarian in that it is the gift of presence or being present for each other which touches the souls of both the listener and the one who shares their story.

Professor John McEvoy PhD who researches and lectures extensively on grief and loss in people with intellectual disability informs us of the need for person-centred planning and suggests ways of developing a support plan for persons with an ID and how to assess adaptation to loss.

He suggests there are five factors which contribute to the mourning process.

1. The physical and emotion and cognitive makeup of the person experiencing the loss. Can they recognise and express emotions? Do they understand the concept of death?

2. The specific nature of the lost relationship. What significance does the loss have on the person's family/social network?
3. The circumstances of the loss. Was it sudden or expected? Was the person involved in the funeral rites?
4. The frequency of other losses. Has the person experienced death and loss before? Do they understand the permanence of the situation?
5. The social environment, such as attitudes to expressions of grief. What levels of support are available?
    (course handbook: *Supporting people with ID through Bereavement and Loss* prof. John McEvoy PhD. Irish Hospice Foundation)

9.2 Conclusion

All of the above has informed my practice in supporting people with ID through the grieving process. With regard to the spiritual perspective if it is to provide hope and a reason to go on for many people, I have observed that spirituality though deeply personal has for many people an added community dimension is integrated within the web of relationships and the quality of those relationships to offer support to the person who is mourning. There are hints overtly and covertly of spiritual beliefs and the tenets of organised religion intertwined in the web of relationships. Spirituality can as Humphrey and Zimpfer suggest: "Make us aware of a dimension of our being that is not merely biological mechanical, or chemical, but by its very nature has about it already the element that transcends mortality by being in tune with the infinite and eternal…. It can expand our perspective so that while we are in this life we see beyond it" ([1], pp. 13–14).

My experience of working with people with ID for 12 years and supporting them through many of their losses and bereavement seems to concur with Humphrey and Zimpfer that "the spiritual realm can be a positive and emotional anchor for a person who is grieving" and that with the right kind of supports, a person with ID can manage emotions and feelings and behaviours during the grieving process.

I have learned the value of knowing how important it is that people know who to turn to for comfort, who will listen empathetically, and the value of rituals including funeral rituals in supporting people with intellectual disability.

Acknowledgement To Prof. John McEvoy PHD; Irish Hospice Foundation Dublin; Seasons for Growth, Margaret MacKillop Foundation, Sydney, Australia; Geraldine M. Humphrey and David G. Zimpfer; Caroline Lloyd; and the men and women whose stories are informed in this work, thank you.

References

1. Humphrey GM, Zimpfer DG. Counselling for grief and bereavement. London: Sage Publications; 2002.
2. Lloyd C. Grief demystified an introduction. London: Jessica Kingsley Publications; 2018. p. 11.

The Role of the Healthcare Chaplain: A Summary of the Contribution of Healthcare Chaplains to Modern Healthcare Practice

10

Chris Swift

Abstract

Spiritual care has become a more complex subject in the arena of health care. This chapter reviews the development of chaplaincy practice and its evolution in the context of social change. Key elements of the chaplain's work are identified, both for individual care and collective occasions. The distinction between the role of all health professions in spiritual care, and the specific function of the chaplain, is discussed.

10.1 Introduction

The Nursing and Midwifery Council (NMC) Code lays emphasis on the need to 'prioritize people' [1]. This includes the requirement to treat people as individuals and the need to listen to their concerns. The Code therefore recognizes that not all people are the same and consequently their preferences during care will vary and should never be standardized or assumed. There is ample evidence that for many people in healthcare, spiritual, pastoral and religious needs are significant [2]. The relative priority of this significance can fluctuate and change during an episode of care. While the need for spiritual care may be the thing furthest from someone's thoughts while things progress well, complications and a risk to life may draw issues of spirituality to the foreground. This can be seen in the context of pregnancy [3]. It should also be noted that the demographic of health service users is atypical of the general population in that people are both older and in need of healthcare. It is known from census returns that older people are more likely to identify with a form of religious belief. The provision of a professional chaplaincy service is one

C. Swift (✉)
MHA, Epworth House, Derby, UK
e-mail: Chris.Swift@mha.org.uk

© Springer Nature Switzerland AG 2019
F. Timmins, S. Caldeira (eds.), *Spirituality in Healthcare: Perspectives for Innovative Practice*, https://doi.org/10.1007/978-3-030-04420-6_10

way in which organizations prioritize people and ensure that dignity for a wide diversity of individuals is enhanced.

This chapter explores the way chaplains work in healthcare. Chaplains have been around a long-time in hospitals and other places of care, evolving their practice in response to a host of social and clinical changes [4]. Understandably people often have their own image of a chaplain and the way a chaplain works. It's important to test out whether these assumptions are correct or if they tell only part of the story. Before going on, it will be helpful for you to think about your own ideas concerning chaplains and see how this relates to the chapter as it unfolds.

 Before reading on, what do you think chaplains do today? Quickly put together a list of 4 or 5 things that you think chaplains do and leave this to one side until the end of the chapter.

> Before reading on, what do you think chaplains do today? Quickly put together a list of four or five things that you think chaplains do, and leave this to one side until the end of the chapter.

10.2 Background

In order to understand the modern concept of healthcare chaplaincy, it is necessary to explore how the profession has developed. Many of the stereotypes of hospital chaplains lie in the past, and it is important to recognize this legacy to appreciate its transformation. The role of the chaplain is as old as hospitals, and chaplains were the first group of professionally educated staff to work in Western healthcare institutions. While they were subject to change, along with the hospitals they served, little altered in the essential nature of their role. Chaplains were agents of the principal religion recognized in the locality, promoting the values of that religion and meeting the needs of patients within that framework of belief. Alongside the chaplain, these early places of care usually had a central chapel, for which the chaplain was responsible, where services would be led not only for patients but also for resident staff such as nurses. Until the middle of the twentieth century, the chaplain was understood to be an individual minister of religion working under the authority of, and was accountable to, a church. Often the chaplain's superior, such as a bishop, would be involved in the overall governance of the hospital alongside other dignitaries.

This situation meant that chaplains did not develop networks of professional association until modern times. The work of a chaplain was seen as neither clinical nor distinct from the activity of a church. Consequently, chaplains had a weak sense of professional identity or collective purpose. It was only as the twentieth-century developed that chaplains across the Western world began to examine their role and started to create a coherent community of practice. This emerging identity is what we call 'chaplaincy': a shared understanding of practice, theory and formation. This change has not yet evolved fully, and it is accurate to say that chaplaincy as it stands is a mixture of older and newer models. The extremities of these might be characterized on the one hand as 'religion serving the religious' and on the other as 'spirituality serving the community' [5].

Both the newer and older concepts of chaplaincy have grown to articulate their theory and practice to a wider audience. From the 1930s onwards, publications by chaplains emerged about the work of chaplaincy, and the rate of publication has increased in recent years. Alongside this, independent scholars have shown an interest in chaplaincy, and the role of the chaplain has been addressed in growing detail by policymakers [6] and health service administrations [7]. Some of the impetus for this has arisen in response to the politicized nature of state funded chaplaincy provision in the West.

It is important to note that one country in particular advanced the professional nature of chaplaincy by absorbing and adapting insights from the world of psychology. In the USA, and subsequently across many other countries, a system of education for chaplains was developed and utilized. 'Clinical Pastoral Education' (CPE) was a movement to strengthen the pastoral capabilities of chaplains through an approach of action-reflection. This typically involved the use of 'verbatim' (detailed narratives garnered from pastoral contacts) as a basis for individual and group reflection. As CPE is not explicitly aligned to a particular religion or culture, it has enjoyed considerable success in a landscape of widening religious diversity. It has effectively created a secular standard for chaplaincy which is not reliant on a single religious authority. Given the emphasis on the analysis of cases, it has also played a part in the growing publication of pastoral encounters in which chaplains are involved. CPE is now embedded as a standard for chaplaincy training in over a dozen countries.

10.3 Social Change and Chaplaincy

As the twentieth century progressed, Western societies began to change. In the last century, populations diversified, and the range of religions and spiritual beliefs in populations has broadened. While the pace of this has varied across the West, the underlying direction of travel has been the same. As the breadth of publicly articulated beliefs has grown the idea of a single dominant, spiritual tradition has waned. In turn this has challenged and changed the way chaplaincy is provided in healthcare settings. Matching the populations they serve, chaplaincy teams have diversified so that today it is possible to find a hospital served by Christian, Muslim, Sikh, Jewish, Hindu and Humanist chaplains.

At the same time as populations were changing, healthcare in the West was becoming more specialized. The range of treatments was expanding, and the number of people living into advanced older age has increased. As the population of those who do not identify with a single religious tradition has grown in the West, it has become more challenging to balance the specific needs of smaller communities alongside the needs of those unaligned to a single set of beliefs [8]. This has led to the emergence of humanist and/or non-religious chaplains who share the same, or similar, beliefs to a growing number of service users in healthcare [9].

In order to prioritise people we need to respect their needs. Think about how you would meet the needs of patients where some have specific religious requirements while others have less defined spiritual needs.

> In order to prioritize people, we need to respect their needs. Think about how you would meet the needs of patients where some have specific religious requirements while others have less defined spiritual needs.

As we consider the role of the chaplain, it is worth spending a moment reflecting on the challenges other staff can face in addressing questions of spirituality and belief.

10.4 "More Difficult to Ask About than Sex"

Religion and spirituality vary considerably in the level of significance people attach to them. For some people having a living relationship with God matters more than anything else. For others, religious and spiritual beliefs are seen to be irrelevant and do not feature explicitly in daily life. Given this gulf in the value placed on spirituality, not all healthcare staff feel comfortable in asking about a person's beliefs or spiritual practices. Furthermore, when spiritual beliefs are central to someone's life, they may regard this as precious and deeply intimate. Again, this can raise anxiety in staff when the option to record someone's beliefs is very limited and may come down to nothing more than ticking a box on an admission form. Healthcare staff do not want to disrespect the sincerity and importance beliefs can play in someone's life.

In order to support colleagues in working with issues of spirituality and religion, many chaplains are involved in training. This can be done in a variety of situations from bespoke sessions on a ward to a regular slot on corporate induction. Either way it's important that colleagues working in healthcare know that they can draw on the chaplain's support to improve the quality and accuracy of recording information about someone's spirituality. This is not only important for the individual but can also be significant for the organization when questions of equality arise. You cannot prove that care is provided equally for all religious and spiritual groups unless demographic data about beliefs is maintained. Nor can issues of inequality for a particular community be addressed unless there is data to identify and investigate any aspect of discrimination. When healthcare providers devise training about religion and belief, it can be helpful to draw together both chaplains and human resources staff to ensure the importance of this work is understood.

Part of the challenge in identifying spiritual needs lies not only in the potentially intimate nature of the topic but also in the labels attached to different elements of chaplaincy care. It will therefore be helpful to spend a moment looking at the three main categories of care used within chaplaincy. These are the terms: religious, spiritual and pastoral care. As these terms are sometimes used interchangeably, or, at the very least, seen to overlap, the following definitions may be helpful.

1. Pastoral Support/Care
   Pastoral care is used in many different contexts, including educational setting where it can refer to a 'pastoral tutor' as distinct from an 'academic tutor'. It implies supportive care which takes in the whole of the life of the individual, including issues which may seem outside of the immediate context but nevertheless impact on someone's well-being. It is generally viewed as less technically defined than psychological or counselling interventions and may be an accompaniment across an academic year or the entire time someone is with the institution. In a hospital, a member of staff (chaplain or not) may be said to have a pastoral care relationship if they have come to know the person receiving care and have a regard to their network of friends and family as well as other impactful issues pertinent to the individual. So, for example, knowing how a patient has previously felt about a medical procedure and recognizing (by sensitive conversation) that history when the procedure is repeated could be described as 'being pastoral'.

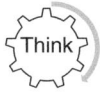 Can you think of an example of *pastoral* care you have seen or done? List a few ways you would describe why you see this as pastoral care.

> Can you think of an example of *pastoral* care you have seen or done? List a few ways you would describe why you see this as pastoral care.

2. Spiritual Support/Care
   This is often defined with reference to the concept of 'meaning' and meaning-making. It refers to care which recognizes or enables the particular convictions

of the person receiving care. For example, that nature connects us to a broader experience of creation and its importance; that participation in music has personal resonance and significance (a particular form of music or song); or that religious practices, texts or music provide spiritual support for the person. Within academic debate, this can generate some tension between a more cognitive 'meaning' focus and an understanding which links spirituality to ideas of the sacred. The latter can include the 'secular sacred' as defined by Gordon Lynch [10]. Some of those who identify as having spiritual needs will believe in a supreme power or authority, e.g. a God.

Can you think of an example of *spiritual* care you have seen or done? List a few ways you would describe why you see this as pastoral care.

Can you think of an example of *spiritual* care you have seen or done? List a few ways you would describe why you see this as pastoral care.

3. Religious Support/Care
   Religious care concerns the support of people who hold a shared attachment to a set of beliefs and practices which have significant common features and concern the transcendent (i.e. what is perceived to be beyond the material world). The root of the word religion means 'to bind', and this sharing of key doctrines and customs gives sufficient cohesion to a group to identify it as a religion. Beliefs often include reference to God and are likely to share an agreed narrative about the purpose of life and its conclusion. Religions will usually have a spirituality of their own which is recognized as the practice of a faith, e.g. Christian spirituality.

Can you think of an example of *religious* care you have seen or done? List a few ways you would describe why you see this as pastoral care.

Can you think of an example of *religious* care you have seen or done? List a few ways you would describe why you see this as pastoral care.

10.5 Identifying Spiritual Needs and Making Referrals

In recent years, many studies have identified the value spiritual beliefs can make to overall well-being. In particular, a coherent spirituality can provide considerable support when life-changing events are unfolding. Living with our finite physical nature is frequently a feature of religion and spirituality, and this has weight within the context of healthcare where even routine procedures can remind us of our mortality. Identifying the support someone may need to cope with a difficult diagnosis is highly relevant to their well-being. It follows that gaining some idea of a person's spiritual resources and needs may have a bearing on their overall health. However, as we have noted above, this is not always comfortable for staff, and it can be a considerable help to have tools which assist the discussion of spirituality. Equally, where staff feel competent to explore the issues, less formal approaches may help put a patient at ease during the discussion [11].

The first step in exploring someone's spiritual needs requires a screening tool. This helps staff identify whether the person has active spiritual beliefs and if these require support. There are a number of such tools available, including ones designed for use by nurses [12].

> **Tip** The significance of religion and spirituality may vary depending on context. It's a good idea when screening for spiritual needs to not only ask about a person's view at the time but also to ask 'has religion or spirituality *ever* been important for you?'. When someone enters a more reflective mode, they may recognize that spiritual care was significant at a previous point of crisis in their life and this may help them access the right support now.

Once spiritual need is identified, it is important to know how to respond. In order to offer effective support, staff also need to know the chaplaincy team and what it can offer. Usually chaplains are happy to visit a referred patient and spend time listening to the patient's story. This will lead the chaplain to work with the patient to see how beliefs or practices might be helpful as they cope with a current episode of poor health. The content of the conversation may touch on key relationships, personal beliefs and feelings about the future. Hopes and fears are likely to be discussed, and by the end of the encounter, the chaplain may have signposted other help, offered to see the patient again or provided all the necessary care in the session. Unlike disciplines such as psychology, the care provided by the chaplain is less regulated and defined. There is usually no set amount of time a chaplain will spend with a patient or a recognized series of contacts which would constitute a treatment or therapy. A central feature of chaplaincy is that the purpose of the episode of spiritual care tends to take shape during the encounter. On arriving at a bedside, the chaplain may have very limited information about the reason a referral was made. A skilled chaplain will discern during the conversation what kind of care might be offered and be most likely to succeed. This discernment will build on the issues identified from the screening tool by building up a more comprehensive spiritual history for the patient. Just as with screening tools, there are a range of templates for the taking of such a spiritual history.

Chaplains operate under the same expectations of safeguarding that apply to

How many places can you think of which might be described as having spiritual significance for someone? If you have chance visit a chapel in a hospital or other setting and see if there is a place for people to write a prayer or reflection. What kinds of things are mentioned?

> How many places can you think of which might be described as having spiritual significance for someone? If you have a chance, visit a chapel in a hospital or other setting, and see if there is a place for people to write a prayer or reflection. What kinds of things are mentioned?

other staff in healthcare. This means that they are bound to raise any concerns about a person's safety in the same way as any other member of staff. Furthermore, as part of the care team, they will want to work with healthcare colleagues to ensure the best care for the patient. In many instances, including end-of-life care, chaplains will attend meetings of the multidisciplinary team. This ensures that other staff are aware of what the chaplain can offer and also enables the chaplain to have a fuller picture of the challenges facing the patient.

10.6 The Contribution of the Chaplain

During a chaplain's pastoral work with a patient, the nature of the role can be witnessed and valued. It is not always easy to capture this fully in a statistical or data-based account of the chaplain's work. Most of the research about the way chaplains work lies in qualitative publications and case studies [13]. However, it may be helpful to examine the contribution of the chaplain through two modes of working: the individual and the collective.

10.7 Individual

Much of the time, chaplains are engaged in the support of individuals. This may take the form of one-to-one care, usually through conversation and listening. The role of the chaplain is to take a wide view of the person, and the way they are living with the reality of poor health. However, it is unusual for chaplains to work with people in complete isolation. Often chaplains will be liaising with healthcare staff about the patient's care as well as supporting members of a family. The implications of illness typically involve other people, and an effective chaplain will be mindful of this and seek to build appropriate relationships with those connected to the patient. For this reason, chaplains will sometimes be requested to participate in, or conduct, the funeral of someone for whom they have cared.

When a chaplain is engaged in one-to-one care, the following features of the encounter may be noted:

1. The chaplain is the guest of the patient. Permission must be sought for the contact to commence and continue, where the chaplain sits or stands in relation to the person and whether the encounter should (or can) take place in a confidential space.
2. The initial episode of care involves bridge-building with the patient. The chaplain will seek to establish trust and an awareness of the patient's spiritual history and present concerns.
3. Typically, the chaplain will use active listening and key questions to establish the needs of the person.
4. While the encounter may start in very general terms, the chaplain will be working to elicit the needs of the patient and decide what kind of response may help address those needs.
5. If the chaplain feels that further work with the patient may be helpful, permission and agreement will be requested from the patient for the timing and content of future contact.
6. In some cases, the patient might be leaving for another setting very soon. In such cases, the chaplain may see if the patient would like further support and ask for permission to make a referral to another chaplain.
7. Some record of the care given should be documented. Increasingly, this is done electronically, but in all events, a link to the patient's record should be made so that any multidisciplinary colleague can see that the chaplain is involved.

Some chaplains have a significant role in providing care to a number of people at once. This might take the form of an organization-wide occasion, such as a Christmas service or the memorial for a serving member of staff (Fig. 10.1). Many hospitals hold annual services of remembrance for people who have experienced the death of a baby. More often a chaplain may be involved in leading the funeral for a service user such as a patient or nursing home resident. When a chaplain is engaged in caring for a group of people, the following features may be noted:

1. The chaplain spends time speaking with those who have requested the event about their hopes, needs and expectations for the content and style of the occasion.
2. An effective chaplain will be alert to potential contradictions in the expectations of those likely to attend. For example, not all those who come to a funeral share the same view of the person being remembered.

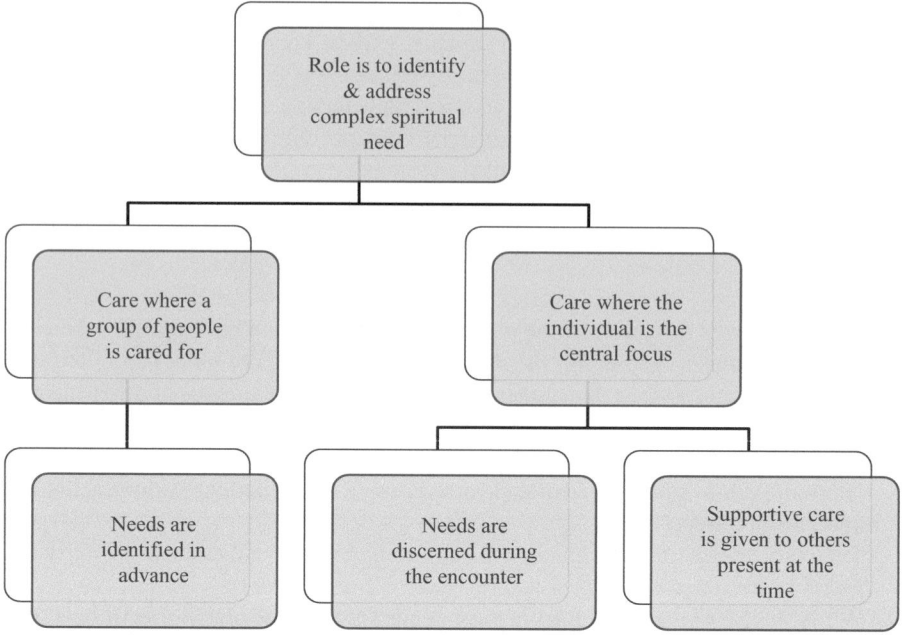

Fig. 10.1 The contribution of the chaplain is to both individuals and groups

3. Care is taken to test out the development of the event as preparations progress. The chaplain may offer support about content when people struggle to articulate what kind of occasion they wish it to be.
4. Appropriate materials are developed, such as an 'order of service'. The needs of those attending are anticipated and met. For example, are large print copies required or does the service need to be signed?
5. It is generally felt that opportunities for people to participate during the event are helpful. This can include the lighting of candles, the reading of names or another activity.

Feedback from service users and relatives can be invaluable and help illustrate the contribution the chaplain makes in situations where there may appear to be few tangible outcomes. Given the wide-ranging nature of chaplaincy, often operating across the full range of clinical settings, some areas have been the focus for more sustained academic attention and study. So, for example, end-of-life care and palliative care are areas with a growing body of research and peer-reviewed publication, some of which focuses on outcomes [14]. In a similar way, the Lothian PROM [15] marks an attempt to gather evidence from patients about the difference chaplaincy engagement has produced. These studies are accompanied by the emergence of work to classify chaplaincy interventions and generate a menu of activities which are recognizable by the profession [16]. This is now being tested in a selection of contexts to evaluate the similarities and differences relating to language and culture. Given the close relationships of spiritual care, culture and language, it would be surprising if spirituality could be tabulated in the same way for every context. However, this initial work in the USA has stimulated debate and provides a first step on the road to identifying with greater clarity the ingredients of effective chaplaincy spiritual care. The concept mapping done by Massey et al. [16] identifies 'active listening' as both the most frequently cited and most important element of the chaplain's contact with patients or clients. This is followed closely by 'pastoral presence' and demonstrating 'caring and concern'. Arguably all three elements are closely associated and might arise as descriptions of the same episode of spiritual care. With greater insight and a common language, the way has been opened for chaplains to develop care pathways, become more intentional in the way care is given and enable shared reflection based on a recognized vocabulary. However, there is still a long way to go before this can be realized as an international standard across cultures for the purposes of practice and research.

> **A Case Study**
> A 24-years-old male suffered a life-threatening head injury in a road traffic accident. He is in intensive care, and it has been determined that he will not recover and is expected to die when therapy is discontinued. Staff have spoken with his wife and other members of the family and mentioned the possibility of organ donation.
>
> While his wife is agreeable to this, his mother appears anxious and uncertain. In discussion with a nurse, it becomes clear that issues of religious belief are involved. The nurse asks if it would be helpful to speak with a chaplain. This is agreed.
>
> The chaplain visits the ward and is shown to a relatives' room where the patient's mother is sitting. After introductions, the chaplain listens to the concerns of the mother. These have arisen from conversations with the family of another patient on the ward, in a similar situation. Members of this family mentioned to the mother that they had also been asked about organ donation but, from their understanding of the Muslim faith, they did not feel able to agree to this. This led the mother to wonder, as a Christian, what the Christian faith had to say about organ donation.
>
> The chaplain explores the mother's feelings about this, and they share in a discussion about the life and teaching of Jesus and how that might be relevant to this situation. At the same time, the chaplain is mindful of the pastoral issues being faced by the mother not only with her son but also with her daughter-in-law who is next of kin.

10.8 Key Elements

Chaplaincy is practiced in a variety of ways. At times, specific assistance is required for someone, such as support with their religious faith or providing rituals at life events, such as bereavement. It is recognized that providing people with this support strengthens their sense of coherence and has positive impact in various ways, including mental health and psychological well-being. Both religion and spirituality can be linked to a person's sense of place in the world—a recognition of where things are heading and what life is for. When negative events occur, this can lead someone to question their beliefs, and a chaplain is trained to be an effective and impartial 'conversation partner' as people struggle to integrate events into their personal narrative. Using skills such as active listening, the chaplain enables a person to feel fully heard: to know that their dilemmas are recognized and respected. Sometimes chaplains will speak about this as a 'witnessing of suffering'. When people feel isolated and removed from their local community, the presence of the chaplain carries significance as a representative of a wider group, such as the people gathered round a particular mosque or synagogue. While this close community association can be valuable, it also places on chaplains a significant obligation for maintaining confidentiality. Sometimes chaplains will have a role both in a local health provider and a local church. It is vitally important that those in such dual roles have clear boundaries and maintain constant vigilance that confidentialities are not breached.

Chaplains also play a part in supporting staff. In the acute setting, they are usually a resource available to assist rapidly in urgent situations, including major incidents. At such times, chaplains work alongside other staff and participate in debriefing meetings at a later date. Some chaplaincies offer surgeries to staff who wish to come and speak with a chaplain. While typically employed in the organization, chaplains are nevertheless viewed as somewhat impartial. Conversations with chaplains will not normally be part of any record kept about the member of staff. For this reason, staff sometimes feel the chaplain is a more appropriate figure to speak with than more formal avenues of support. Chaplains need to ensure that those they speak with are made aware that chaplains are bound to report serious matters in the same way as anyone else but beyond this they can be a useful ear for those wishing to discuss a concern without it going any further.

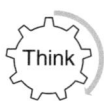

At the start of this chapter it was suggested you jot down your existing ideas about the work and impact of a chaplain working in healthcare. Has this chapter added anything to that understanding: if so, what? Might it change the way you interact with a chaplain in the future?

At the start of this chapter, it was suggested you jot down your existing ideas about the work and impact of a chaplain working in healthcare. Has this chapter added anything to that understanding: if so, what? Might it change the way you interact with a chaplain in the future?

10.9 Conclusion

Over the past 100 years, the story of spirituality in healthcare has featured two characteristics: firstly, that in the West religious practice has both diversified and, in its traditional forms, declined and, secondly, that in healthcare there has been a marked shift away from the institutional provision of religious care to the more individually determined application of spiritual support. In turn this has led to a widening of the range of practitioners involved in the explicit delivery of spiritual care. No longer does a single church dominate chaplaincy, but instead chaplains come from an ever-growing diversity of faiths and, most recently, those who have convictions and ethical beliefs unconnected to religious faith. This is especially true where chaplains are employed directly by the State or the health provider. Where chaplains are either volunteers or subcontracted from the church, etc., it is likely they will work with a particular focus on their own constituency. In such situations, unless care is taken to make other provision, those who do not identify with a particular faith will be those whose spiritual needs go unaddressed.

The current situation poses a dilemma for chaplaincy. On the one hand, the profession has been strengthened by an ever-widening group of practitioners. On the other hand, the common qualifications and training of chaplains have become more contested. Secularists object to a religious bar to the profession (i.e. that someone must be religious to become a chaplain), which still applies in many countries. The international movement of CPE offers a model of common qualification, but even here there are questions about research and academic rigor which are only now being addressed. Nor is CPE certification a universally required award for chaplaincy work.

Healthcare staff should expect chaplains to offer highly professional spiritual, pastoral and religious support to those in a clinical setting. Effective spiritual care involves everyone working in healthcare, but it is recognized that some staff and service users have complex spiritual needs which require a skilled professional to assist them. As societies in the West have diversified, people do not always present with the apparent clarity of belief and belonging which was once the case. People may be more eclectic in their beliefs, holding together convictions which would once have been seen to be at odds. As we saw in the case study, even where a faith is held, it may be influenced by different beliefs and practices. Chaplains have the knowledge and professional skill to enter such situations and work towards a meaningful outcome. In conjunction with other healthcare staff, especially nurses and midwives, the delivery of spiritual care described above ensures that people are recognized in all their diversity and that their dignity is honoured and supported.

References

1. Nursing and Midwifery Council (NMC). The code: professional standards of practice and behaviour for nurses and midwives. London: NMC; 2015.

2. Puchalski CM, Blatt B, Kogan M, Butler A. Spirituality and health: the development of a field. Acad Med. 2014;89(1):10–6.
3. Nuzum D, Meaney S, O'Donoghue K. The spiritual and theological challenges of stillbirth for bereaved parents. J Relig Health. 2017;56(3):1081–95.
4. Swift C. Hospital chaplaincy in the twenty-first century: the crisis of spiritual care on the NHS. London: Routledge; 2016.
5. Swift C. Does chaplaincy for all amount to chaplaincy for none? Pluralism and particularity in spiritual care. Normal Autton Lecture. https://www.researchgate.net/publication/268210577_Does_chaplaincy_for_all_amount_to_chaplaincy_for_none_Pluralism_and_particularity_in_spiritual_care. Accessed 05 Nov 2017.
6. Timmins F, Caldeira S, Murphy M, Pujol N, Sheaf G, Weathers E, Whelan J, Flanagan B. An Exploration of current approaches to and facilities for spiritual care provision in the Republic of Ireland. J Pastoral Care Counsel. 2017;71(2):122–31.
7. Swift C. NHS Chaplaincy guidelines 2015: promoting excellence in pastoral, spiritual and religious care. London: NHS England; 2015.
8. Woodhead L. The rise of "no religion": towards an explanation. Sociol Relig. 2017;78(3):247–62.
9. Swift C, Handzo G, Cohen J. Health care chaplaincy. A handbook of chaplaincy studies: understanding spiritual care in public places. London: Ashgate Publishing; 2016. p. 163.
10. Lynch G. On the sacred. London: Routledge; 2014.
11. Timmins F, Caldeira S. Assessing the spiritual needs of patients. Nurs Stand. 2017;31(29):47–53.
12. Vlasblom JP, Van Der Steen JT, Walton MN, Jochemsen H. Effects of nurses' screening of spiritual needs of hospitalized patients on consultation and perceived nurses' support and patients' spiritual well-being. Holist Nurs Pract. 2015;29(6):346–56.
13. Fitchett G, Nolan S. Spiritual care in practice. London: Jessica Kingsley Publishers; 2015.
14. Kestenbaum A, Shields M, James J, Hocker W, Morgan S, Karve S, Rabow MW, Dunn LB. What impact do chaplains have? A pilot study of spiritual aim for advanced cancer patients in Woodhead L. The rise of "no religion": towards an explanation. Sociol Relig. 2017;78(3):247–62.
15. Snowden A, Telfer I. Patient reported outcome measure of spiritual care as delivered by chaplains. J Health Care Chaplain. 2017;23(4):131–55.
16. Massey K, Barnes MJ, Villines D, Goldstein JD, Pierson ALH, Scherer C, Vander Laan B, Summerfelt WT. What do I do? Developing a taxonomy of chaplaincy activities and interventions for spiritual care in intensive care unit palliative care. BMC Palliat Care. 2015;14(1):10.

Teaching and Learning About Spirituality in Healthcare Practice Settings

Jacqueline Whelan

Abstract

This chapter considers the importance of contemporary teaching and learning approaches to spirituality within healthcare practice drawing on international evidence. The chapter integrates recent systematic literature challenges and issues that relate to its integration. Spirituality is recognised as a standard for good practice; attention is drawn to research that outlines guidance arising from international standards, guidelines, professional codes of practice and competency frameworks and key competency skills across healthcare. A consensus definition of spirituality is offered to understand spirituality within healthcare practice. Spiritual awareness, meaning making and respecting patient's worldviews are recognised as core spiritual care competencies. Spiritual care needs, undertaking a spiritual history, formal and informal spiritual assessment methods, spiritual distress and timely referral are established as core spiritual care competencies. It is acknowledged that humanistic compassionate person-centred approaches grounded in connection are warranted to transform the educational process for the patient, student and practitioner experiences in healthcare.

Abbreviations

ACP - ASIM	American College of Physicians and American Society of Internal Medicine
CSI Memo Spiritual History	**C**omfort **S**tress **I**nfluence **M**em (Member) **O**ther spiritual needs
ETHNICS	**E**xplanation **T**reatment **H**ealers **N**egotiate **I**ntervention **C**ollaborate **S**pirituality

J. Whelan (✉)
School of Nursing and Midwifery, Trinity College, Dublin, Ireland
e-mail: whelanj1@tcd.ie

© Springer Nature Switzerland AG 2019
F. Timmins, S. Caldeira (eds.), *Spirituality in Healthcare: Perspectives for Innovative Practice*, https://doi.org/10.1007/978-3-030-04420-6_11

FICA Spiritual History	**F**aith, **I**mportance and Influence, **C**ommunity and **A**ddress
FAITH	**F** Faith **A** Application **I** Influence/importance **T** Talk/terminal events planning **H** Help
HCN	Healthcare Chaplaincy Network
HOPE	**H** Sources of Hope, meaning comfort, strength, peace love and connection **O** Organised religion **P** Personal Spirituality and Practices **E** Effects on medical care and end of life issues
NANDA	**N**orth **A**merican **N**ursing **D**iagnostic **A**ssociation
SHALOM	Spiritual Health and Life - Orientation Measure
SPIRITual History	**S**piritual Belief System **P**ersonal Spirituality **I**ntegration with a spiritual community **I**ntegration with a spiritual community **R**itualised Practice's and Restrictions **I**mplications for Medical Care **T**erminal Event Planning
RCN	**R**oyal **C**ollege of **N**ursing
2Q-SAM	**2T**wo **Q**question **S**piritual **A**ssessment **M**odel

11.1 Introduction

Consider the following:

> Why is spirituality currently trending in contemporary healthcare practice?

Spirituality is a distinct science within the professional landscape of healthcare today [1–3]. Contemporary evidence views spirituality as an innate genuine aspect of who we are, an important integral aspect of holistic person-centred care that values authenticity, dignity, respect and compassion [4–9]. Political, legislative, professional and societal changes have generated an increased focus on spirituality within healthcare from national, European and global perspectives to ensure that patients cannot be discriminated against on the premise of beliefs and religion [10].

The teaching and learning of spirituality and spiritual care provision concern all healthcare educators, students, practitioners and multidisciplinary team members, as people receiving healthcare have a right to spiritual care and wish to have spiritual and/or religious needs addressed [11–16]. Evidence clearly demonstrates positive linkages between spirituality and physical health, contributing to patient's needs, well-being, response, improved outcomes, increased coping, mental health, recovery time and quality of life [17–21]. Evidence also highlights the value of spiritual care to patients [22–25]. However, healthcare practitioners lack essential values, knowledge, skills, competence and understanding of patients' religious foundations to support patients' spiritual needs, due to poor spirituality education in healthcare programmes, thus minimising patient distress and experience of spiritual care with increasing health-related costs [13, 26–28].

The importance of spirituality related to healthcare and well-being is acknowledged as a distinct professional practice concern which has been subject to revolutionary debate that questions the inclusion and validity of spirituality in healthcare curricula [29–33]. Spirituality contextualises a patient's view of their life world amongst many existential challenges that life brings [34]. Disparate worldviews exist that hold spiritual and scientific realms to be incompatible with one another; however the healthcare practice environment is precisely where both realms meet, thus requiring educators to reconcile the value of spirituality as a protective health factor in patient care [35, 36]. Given the commodification of healthcare driven by outcomes and decreasing resources, recent reports have challenged the crisis in compassion that exists in healthcare [12, 37, 38] as 'neglect of spirituality and a conflicted spirit can obstruct good practice and result in poor quality health care' ([39], p. 14).

Historically the subject has been avoided which minimises the opportunity for students and practitioners to examine the spiritual domain aligned to the patient experience [40]. The concepts of spirituality and spiritual care lacks clarity, consensus, standardisation, bias and are inconsistently applied which questions educators' capacity to professionalise spiritual care by developing students' capacity to care holistically [41–44]. Additional challenges exist for educators in both university and practice settings that are influenced by positivist reductionist approaches which fragment rather than prepare students to deal with a patient's spiritual, religious and diverse faith needs, existential crises and distress [45–49]. Educators are faced with significant challenges in teaching and learning of spirituality that mitigate teaching the subject; lack of time to advance student skill sets; availability of appropriate mentoring for students; and workloads and management issues aligned to limited resources which have still to be reconciled [50–53].

Given that the primary aim of spiritual care education is 'to broaden the scope of professional responsibility', this chapter is concerned with effective modes of preparation in teaching and learning about spirituality in healthcare in order to provide practical help to students and practitioners to advance knowledge, skills, attitudes, values, competence and spiritual literacy and to prepare and sensitise students and nurses to all personal and professional interdisciplinary aspects that ultimately benefit the care that patients receive [54].

11.2 Standards, Professional Codes and Guidelines

Professional practice demands that spiritual care be regarded as a standard for 'good healthcare practice' (p. 110) [55–60]. Internationally, spirituality and spiritual care provision has been highlighted as a standard, endorsed by key academics and multiple professional bodies such as the Royal College of Nursing (UK) [61, 62] and Healthcare Chaplaincy Network (USA) across healthcare that include nursing, medicine, chaplaincy, social work, occupational therapy, psychology and other allied health practitioners [63–67].

Fundamentally all professional standards acknowledge the significance of spiritual care as a constituent of whole person-centred care approaches, respecting patient's individual worldviews and experience of spirituality, stressing the need for inclusive multifaith cultural competent standards that relate to spiritual provision which we need to pay attention to [55, 57–59, 66, 68–74]. Professional standards *view assessment of a patient's spiritual, religious and well-being as distinct quality care elements across contexts and healthcare practitioners* [75, 76] and demand that *spiritual assessment* be undertaken as a standard patient care practice [77–79] as such requirements are only partially maintained through chaplaincy provision [80]. Standards draw attentions to the practitioners' role in respect of assessment whilst equally demanding that ethical approaches be adopted that reconcile both patients and multidisciplinary perspectives. The North American Nursing Diagnosis Association (NANDA) for Nanda International, Inc. has recognised the *importance of acknowledging patient's spiritual needs* by establishing specific nursing diagnoses as standards, 'spiritual distress' [70] amongst others. Despite the availability of such standards, codes and guidelines, research findings demonstrate a distinct lack of educational preparation and spiritual integration as a standard in healthcare curricula [8, 47, 61, 81].

11.3 Contemporary Issues in Teaching and Learning Spirituality in Healthcare

Evidence suggests that a positive relationship exists between spiritual care education, student- and staff-related attitudes, delivery and outcomes [82–84]. However the process of embedding spirituality and spiritual care into practice to manage the patient care experience is complex due to its 'Trojan Horse' base and the demands of multiple ways of knowing [85–88]. Attempts to define and determine the what, when, structure, timing, form, content, standards, competencies and outcomes; how it should be taught, assessed and applied and by whom; and what approaches genuinely work to impart care of a person's spirit in practice are broad and lack consensus in the literature [71]. There is a dearth of healthcare texts that seek to address spiritual awareness thus hampering educational efforts further [89, 90]. Healthcare educators need to coherently develop holistic person-centred curricula (knowledge, skills, attitudes, values and ways of being) to prepare students and practitioners to safely enter the emotional landscape of meeting both patient and student spiritual needs in practice. This is essential in order to align healthcare students and practitioners to their professional roles, responsibilities in addressing patient's illness, existential concerns and suffering with a view to developing fully competent practitioners and shaping the kind of practitioner they need to be to serve the diverse needs of society at large [48, 91–93].

Snowden and Ali [88] argue that traditional principles of teaching and learning within the university sector are predominantly teacher-led grounded in passive 'hierarchical dyadic' approaches to education that favour the educator as expert and minimise the student's involvement and ability to learn. For authentic education to occur, new expanded integrated spiritual models and curricular paths are warranted shaped by dynamic creative and innovative approaches to foster the application of holistic person-centred advances that are student-led, directed towards new thinking to facilitate active student engagement and create essential space to design learning that fits the changing world of healthcare [94]. Dall'Alba and Barnett [95, 96] suggest that there is a need to orientate healthcare programmes 'towards an ontological turn' and to philosophically 'reconfigure professional education as a process of becoming' (p. 649). What this means in real terms is that educators need to move beyond theorising and conceptualising spirituality to creating ontological 'being' spaces for students to learn who they are by taking account of their internal being. This can be achieved through expanding and examining epistemological knowing (multiple worldviews and the self), ontological knowing (assumptions, values, attitudes, being and behaviours) and how students interact (through practical knowing, skill and experience). Such ways of knowing help students to think about patients humanity, with a view to developing effective resources that relates to a patients narrative and health situation [88, 97, 98]. This ontological wave is aligned to the theory of heutagogy underpinned by solution, peer and mentor learning approaches which provide a creative holistic option for positioning students at the centre of the learning process, for students to determine what they want to learn, to foster their capabilities in practice and institute change by 'taking effective action, explaining what they are about, work effectively with others, continue to learn from their experiences… in real time' (p. 438) [88, 99].

A mixed methods explorative study on healthcare teaching staff's perspectives of spirituality reinforces this practical knowing dimension with findings advocating where teaching and learning need to be strengthened through self-awareness, reflection, empathy and compassion and teacher role modelling [47]. These being approaches give fundamental direction in handling the complexity of spirituality within curricula and practice to defining the concept, knowing and meeting the needs of society and institution/s whilst developing new learning spaces that assimilate growth and transformation of the student and the healthcare practitioner through self-determination.

11.4 Professional Spiritual Competency Development in Healthcare Practice

The need to develop holistic spiritual care competences in healthcare education and practice is mandated for and required by professional bodies from theoretical and clinical perspectives to effectively prepare students and practitioners to undertake comprehensive assessment of patient's spiritual and cultural needs and to implement spiritual care provision to recognise patient's spiritual issues as integral aspects of person-centred care [8, 56, 58, 59, 100, 101]. A recent definition of spiritual competent practice in healthcare clarifies exactly what spiritually competent practice encompasses and means:

> involves compassionate engagement with the whole person as a
> > unique human being, in ways which will provide them with a sense of meaning and purpose, where
> > > appropriate connecting or reconnecting with a community where they experience a sense of wellbeing,
> > > > addressing suffering and developing coping strategies to improve their quality of life. This
> > > > > includes the practitioner accepting a person's beliefs and values, whether they are religious in foundation
> > > > > > or not, and practising with cultural competency. ([102], p. 3)

Internationally spiritual competency frameworks facilitate the development of competences within healthcare professions and from interdisciplinary perspectives to permit practitioners to acknowledge spirituality, meaning, appropriate interventions and capacity required for spiritual care delivery [60, 66, 100, 103–111]. Such frameworks share core understandings of knowledge, skills and attitudes, aligned to professional spiritual care that helps educators to establish a grounding to navigate the field of teaching spiritual care. Three core competency perspectives are evident across all frameworks linked to the student or practitioner discerning their individual worldview and beliefs of spirituality, the need to *accommodate patient's diverse worldviews and experience* and to enable *relevant actions* that *fit with patient's frames of reference and needs* ([66], p. 38).

Competent spiritual practice implies that students need to be helped through enhancing personal resources with increased self-awareness and reflection, developing therapeutic collaborative communication skills, practicing from an ethical base and understanding the professional chaplaincy role, combined with providing supportive healthcare systems and quality standards [112–115]. Key competency skills prioritised in research literature to date include students and practitioners undertaking a spiritual history, knowledge of spiritual assessment process, ability to undertake a spiritual assessment, the capacity to ascertain patient's spiritual and religious needs and therapeutic presencing care and the capacity to know when to make effective referrals to chaplains and other specialists [13, 116, 117]. In spite of recent developments in establishing standards, guidelines and competency frameworks, the problem of adopting a consistent gold standard approach to practice remains.

11.5 Towards a Definition and Understanding of Spirituality in Healthcare

Reflective Think Point

> How would you describe your understandings of spirituality?

How spirituality is defined within healthcare, and how it is understood makes it simpler for students and practitioners to clarify its central importance for inclusive healthcare practice [118]. Swinton [119] illuminates the benefits and constraints of examining spirituality and its associated meanings through generic, biological and religion approaches (p. 17–35). Studies have attempted to broadly debate, define and describe the abstractness and nature of spirituality from multiple perspectives, philosophical, existential, humanistic, religious, relational, transcendent and meaning perspectives that can be difficult for practitioners and students to navigate [120–126].

Spirituality is a human phenomenon that is essential to our lives, which is shaped by our individual worldviews [91]. It is a need that is felt of being valued with unique subjective interpretations that are subject to change related to a person's individual life experience of ill health, suffering or death [91]. McSherry [127], p. 34 developed a taxonomy that classifies the diverse nature of spirituality using eight descriptions: 'theistic, religious, language, cultural political and ideologies, phenomenological, existential, quality of life, mystical.' This is a good starting point for giving literacy to the varied nature of the subject in accordance with a person's worldviews, thus making it more tangible.

Activity—Pick two papers of your choice from the above-listed authors, and compare and contrast differences in descriptions of spirituality from your own understandings of spirituality.

When teaching about spirituality, there is a definitive need to differentiate spirituality separately from religion as they are often misconstrued as being synonymous with one another in order to ascertain patient needs [117, 128]. Religion is community focused and restricted to organised religion that focus on a God aligned to a particular system of belief, whereas spirituality is individually orientated towards understanding broader personal and transcendent aspects of existence as an existential search for 'meaning, purpose and fulfilment' [129] coupled with central matters of 'hope, connectedness and values' shaped through our relationships with others ([39], p. 2–63).

One way of understanding spirituality is through examining a consensus approach provided such an approach exists. Puchalski et al. [130] offer an expert international consensus approach in defining spirituality as 'the dynamic dimension of human life that relates to the way persons (individual and community) experience, express and/or seek meaning, purpose and transcendence, and the way they connect to the moment, to self, to others, to nature, to the significant, and/or the sacred' (p. 887). More recently, Weathers et al. [131] undertook a detailed empirical and concept analysis of spirituality utilising 47 studies from interdisciplinary health literature (nursing, social work, psychology, theology and other health-related fields) between 2002 and 2013. This comprehensive analysis concluded by offering another definition of spirituality 'as a way of being in the world in which a person feels a sense of connectedness to self, others, and/or higher power or nature; a sense of meaning in life; and transcendence beyond self, everyday living and suffering'.

Both contemporary definitions are particularly useful as they consider the multidimensional nature of spirituality and acknowledge core secular challenges and values in addition to religious foundations underpinning the spiritual dimensions in healthcare. These definitions stress the importance of understanding of the self, personhood and meaning whilst recognising that an experiential element of how spirituality is understood is required ([47], p. 4). As such, this provides an initial common ground for the development of teaching and learning content in healthcare education. However, it cannot be assumed that such thematic elements represent the patient's subjective perspective entirely [132], which demands the adoption of a humanities-based approach to education that values knowing the person and understanding unique diverse perspectives of a patient's spirituality [133]. Additional spiritual concepts allied to the teaching and learning of spirituality have also been identified in the literature that need to be explored to understand the patient experience, religion, belief, needs, distress culture, care and caring, coping, hope and suffering as these aspects have the potential to impact on patients' physical and mental health which is beyond the scope of this chapter [117, 134]. A priority identified in the systematic literature is concerned with expanding sensitivities in advancing personal spiritual awareness in students and practitioner in order to understand the everyday reality of patient experience in practice.

11.6 Towards an Understanding of Spiritual Awareness in Healthcare

Self-Reflective Exercise Consider the following questions:

> Reflect on your spiritual beliefs, values, wants and needs…what is significant to you?
> How do your beliefs and values impact on your attitude and/or behaviours towards others?
> What has influenced and challenged your development of beliefs most?

Evidence has clearly demonstrated that the single most significant determinant of spiritual care and its provision in practice relates to how students and practitioners views and personal experience of spirituality can be raised [71, 135]. How practitioners think about spirituality in practice determines how they will sense and develop self-awareness, behave, feel, act, respond and relate to patients' and families' expressions of spirituality [136]. Spiritual awareness is essential to developing safe empathetic compassionate practice, to comprehend safe professional and patient ethical boundaries, understanding the need for consent, when referral is necessary, and to discriminate issues to uphold rather than conflate patient's spiritual needs. Clarity is required regarding what healthcare worker's beliefs, value sets, biases they hold, strengths and limitations and how these may be borne out through behaviours and decisions in practice [115, 137, 138]. This challenges educators to include spiritual awareness in the teaching and learning of spirituality as a precursor to 'develop sensitivity' through experiential learning [54] in practitioners in order to ascertain and understand patient's spiritual needs in the context of spiritual care provision [139]. Once student's personal values, beliefs, feelings, assumption and prejudices have been clarified and differentiated out from patients' needs, students will be better positioned to have the capacity to promote, integrate and support spiritual patient care as aspects of growth [93, 140, 141].

Taylor's seminal workbook 'What do I Say' [142] proposes a model framework and acts as an evidence-based resource for all healthcare educators and practitioners (which requires ten hours of work) for supporting a practitioners and patient's spiritual well-being and healing through increasing *three dimensions of spiritual awareness: cognitive, emotional and bodily aspects.* Cognitive awareness is recognised through the development of a number of micro skills, for example, by developing rapport with patients, utilising restatements, asking patient's questions openly, use of self-disclosure and listening and reflecting on patient's narratives ([143], p. 8). Emotional awareness is manifest through consideration of patient needs and feelings, understanding empathy, using effective open responses and instituting religious ethical rituals to promote spiritual healing. Spiritual bodily awareness is concerned with the macro skill of reflecting and listening to the body's signals and responses for the patient to focus with a view to developing resilient resources ([144], p. 91). Taylor further proposes a series of six exercises that healthcare professionals can undertake, one of which includes 'practicing soul enquiry'([144], p. 11). Based on the work of Stairs [145], this practice necessitates consideration of nine separate expressions with a view to opening the practitioner's heart up to increased spiritual awareness, for example, 'What is dying in me is...', 'This death is an intrusion in my life because', 'What I want to scream about is', 'My faith is challenged because', 'I weep for', 'What I need to be unbound from is', 'What paralyses me, makes me indecisive is', 'What embitters me is' and 'What I fear losing control of most is' ([144], p. 11). Taylor uses the metaphor of the 'wounded healer' and argues that health practitioners need to be sensitised to their own personal hurt in order to be open to and respond to patients' needs and to reconcile patients healing.

Time Out Activity: Reflect on any past and current hurts in your life, and consider their impact on practice....how you can best support and take care of your spiritual self?

Kearney and Weininger [146], argue the importance and relevance of 'understanding the dynamics of the frightened ego' to minimise practitioners from engaging in distancing behaviours and to gain ego control to allow the development of empathetic meaningful caring relationships with patients. The significance of harvesting a soul care programme of education is further suggested to help practitioners to become more consciously aware and to introspect using four therapeutic aspects: 'self-knowledge, self-empathy, mindful awareness and contemplative awareness' ([146], p. 276–277). Mindfulness practice is an awareness intervention by drawing attention to the breadth, which generates space for students and practitioners 'being' to come alive in the present, with a view to developing intrapersonal and interpersonal connections ([146], p. 276). The work of Thich Nhat Hanh is crucial in increasing spiritual sensitivity which few practitioners and educators are qualified in [147]. Implicit in increasing spiritual awareness is the need for students and practitioners to develop compassionate multicultural care, awareness and appropriate cultural literacy and to understand how culture impacts on people's values, needs and behaviours [148].

Activity: Observe Cultural Awareness for Healthcare Professionals (English version) video.

http://www.youtube.com/watch?v=Gxp_7aRA_tQ

A number of models are available for the purposes of developing culturally compassionate competent professionals and becoming a skilled intercultural communicator [149, 150]. Studies support the use of strategies such as case studies, reflection, reflective journaling, reflective exercises to progress personal development aspects and critical reflection with a view to increasing spiritual awareness in the clinical environment [151–153]. These approaches challenge us to develop new ways of seeing and being as a means of developing spiritual awareness in healthcare.

11.7 Towards an Understanding of Meaning Making in Healthcare

Reflection Points

> How do you wish to live your life?
> How do you make sense of things that occur in your life?
> Is your life and work meaningful and fulfilling to you?
> What is the significance of your life map to date?
> What does spirituality mean to you and what does it represent for you?

Acute, chronic and terminal illnesses threaten a patient's lifespan and challenge patients to question their sense of well-being, life experience, identity, purpose and meaning in life which raise existential issues relating to the existential domain in healthcare practice [154]. When confronted with adverse pain, illness, suffering, loss, grief or death, a patients security is threatened, which may result in anxiety, distress, meaninglessness and hopelessness or conflict which culminates in expressions of existential concerns and needs [155]. For La Cour and Hvidt, existential concerns are ordinarily related to 'meaning, the value of life, personal values, freedom, responsibility, loneliness' [156]. There is a definitive need for healthcare practitioners to address such matters without being fearful as they correlate with quality of life. However, significant knowledge deficits exist regarding patients existential needs, well-being and understanding these broad concepts, what characterises an existential issue and how best to address patients concerns that arise from existential questions such as 'Why me?' [157, 158].

Meaning making is significant in healthcare as it provides understandings of how patients' lives, suffering and existential pain are experienced, expressed and valued subjectively through religious or nonreligious dimensions [159]. From a teaching perspective, La Cour and Hvidt [156] propose a framework for meaning making in the context of existence, illness and secularisation that is beneficial to educators in addressing secular, spiritual and religious realms aligned to cognitive, psychomotor and affective domains in healthcare with examples of questions to ascertaining practitioners attitudes.

Frankl's [160] in man's search for meaning and theory of logotherapy and existential analysis offers another possible framework for practitioners to contextualise meaning in existence as it represents healing through meaning. Frankl's theory is comprised of three central tenets: that we are primarily free to exercise and choose our attitude, that we are free to choose how we respond to life and that the spiritual dimension (represented by freedom and responsibility) wills and motivates us to learn and understand our purpose in life without condition.

> A man who becomes conscious of the responsibility he bears towards a human being will never be able to throw his life away. He knows the why for his existence and will be able to bear almost any how. ([161], p. 3)

Educators have a responsibility to prepare, sensitise and support practitioners to assess, understand, engage and respond positively to patient's perceptions and existential needs through eliciting meanings of the patient experience in a caring dignified manner in order to meet patients' needs and to decrease emotional labour and burden on staff [134, 162]. The importance of recognising and discerning patients emotions created through loss of meaning, suffering and the grieving process is essential without making reactive attempts to hasten the process with quick fixes [163]. Seven universal emotions have been identified to be present amidst cultures: anger, fear, sadness, disgust, surprise, contempt and happiness [164].

Activity
Download http://atlasofemotions.org/.
Work through the interactive tool that addresses all seven emotions.
Observe video developing global compassion.
Watch https://www.paulekman.com/resources/micro-expressions/.
What have you learned?

Burkhart and Schmidt [165] stress the need for student and practitioner learning concerning how to engage meaningful in spiritual conversations. Taylors [166] work offers such an approach and (citing the work of Clinebell [167]) articulates the need to actively listen for spiritual themes and to 'make sense of what you hear' (p. 45) within patient conversations and to consider how patients feel using seven indicators: *feeling words; emotion in the voice; emotion expressed in face or body; protesting too much; self-contraindications which indicate inner conflict; discussion of parental or other crucial need-satisfying relationship; and recognising negative feelings* ([168], p. 29–30). The concept of presence needs to be taught and understood to underpin all these activities which require the healthcare practitioner to be open, adaptable, flexible and committed to intentionally developing and supporting a therapeutic relationship built on empathy, congruence and unconditional positive regard in order to preserve an individual's holistic well-being when existential vacuum arises [169]. Moreover, an increased awareness and knowledge of existential concerns through religious, nonreligious, communicative and reflective education is warranted especially towards practitioners who have difficulty engaging meaningfully in order to serve diverse needs of all patients [155, 163].

Ultimately the key to providing spiritual care is to understand what spirituality means to the person you are caring for [170].

11.8 Towards an Understanding of Spiritual Care and Spiritual Care Provision in Healthcare

> How have you experienced spirituality in the workplace?
> How do you support patient's spirituality in practice?

Education in spiritual care provision for practice is concerned with 'the application of person centred approaches' [39, 171] underpinned by interpersonal knowing based on Rogers 'core principles of empathy, unconditional positive regard and congruence' ([39], p. 15) for students to support patients' health needs during illness. Modelling and clarification of spirituality by educators is warranted, for students to integrate spiritual care in practice to supporting patient's spiritual resources [47, 172]. This raises the question as to how spiritual care is defined. According to NHS for Scotland, spiritual care is defined as ([173], p. 6):

> That care which recognises and responds to the needs of the human
> Spirit when faced with trauma, ill health or sadness and can include the
> needs for meaning, for self-worth, to express oneself, for faith support,
> perhaps for rites or prayer or sacrament, or simply a sensitive listener.
> Spiritual care begins with encouraging human contact in compassionate
> Relationship, and moves in whatever direction need requires.

From this definition, it can be seen that the aim of spiritual care practice is 'uniquely different' ([13], p. 74) from normal physical care provision. Spiritual care provision is in essence concerned with 'meeting people at the point of deepest need' ([174], p. 213), establishment of trust, presence, facilitation of a supportive environment and 'being with' the patient in order to connect and respond to patients fears, pain and spiritual needs that stem from the transcendent [13, 175]. Sharp and Nash [176] suggest that spiritual care teaching can only start by helping students to see the 'person-centred image of the human being' (p. 149) that is grounded in the teachings of personhood before facilitating the 'being' aspects of practice [70, 71]. Recent calls have been made for the incorporation of being, concept of presence and the principles of *availability, vulnerability, hospitality* and *narrative therapy skills* [177], p. 52 to be integrated into spiritually competent practice in healthcare.

Qualitative findings from a number of research studies reveal spiritual care aspects, determining and respecting patients' and families' dignity and spiritual needs, adopting a compassionate approach to care, addressing a patient's suffering, communicating by making time, listening to patients and networking with family contacts, being present with patients, providing appropriate interventions, knowing when to intervene and referral to support resources and promoting hope, with the aim of assisting patients to locate inner resources of strength with practitioner support [141, 178, 179].

The task of education therefore is to clarify the distinct role of spirituality within healthcare and to develop students' and practitioners' cues and to be spiritually competent when encountering patients with specific skill sets using a person-centred care approach, ability to undertake a spiritual history, development of spiritual assessment skills, identification and assessment of spiritual needs, self-knowledge when addressing spiritual needs, appropriate times and methods of making referrals to pastoral care or clients' ministers and knowing when to include religious practices or prayer [8, 101, 135, 165, 180–182]. Caring and active listening skills have been identified as a crucial skills for spiritual care whilst using the integrative bio-psycho-socio-spiritual integrative model during patients' management [183]. Overall these studies highlighted that the health sciences students could be assisted to enhance their knowledge on how to plan, execute, guard and evaluate the spiritual care of the patient in association with other disciplines. Ultimately the key to providing spiritual care is to understand what spirituality means to the person you are caring for [184, 185].

11.9 Towards an Understanding of Patients Spiritual Needs and Distress

> How would you describe patients spirituality needs in your area of practice?
> How do patients' needs differ from carers and or family needs?

Patients have expectations to have their spiritual needs met. Studies report that patient needs are not addressed sufficiently and continue to be largely unmet [186–191]. Identifying patients' spiritual care needs, resources and distress is recognised as a significant core aspect of compassionate person-centred healthcare internationally in order to support and care for patients' well-being, effect better patient care quality outcomes, minimise distress and help patients cope [131, 135, 186, 187, 192–196].

Spiritual care needs are culturally diverse and differ across the lifespan pending a patient's health illness continuum. Descriptive and classification approaches to understanding spiritual needs are suggested [197–199], p. 39 which are also useful in framing the topic: theistic, religious, existential, psychological, social, relational, mystical, normative, comparative, felt and expressed need dimensions. Qualitative differences exist regarding how US and UK spiritual needs are interpreted and referred to, for example, in the USA patient views are more aligned to religious aspects, whilst in the UK needs are understood broadly from a human perspective [200]. The manner in which patients perceive and interpret illness is subject to change over time and impinges on how spiritual care needs are actually expressed and requires a differential approach [193, 201]. A recent systematic report cites that the (UK) Standards for Hospice and Palliative Care Chaplaincy offers a possible way forward in eliciting patients spiritual needs by suggesting it involves:

exploring attitudes, beliefs, ideas, values and concerns around life and death issues; affirming life and worth by encouraging reminiscence about the past; exploring the individual's
hopes and fears regarding the present and future for themselves and their families/carers; exploring
the why questions in relation to life death and suffering. ([200], p. 23)

This understanding unpacks aspects of patients' spiritual care needs for practitioners to participate in decision-making processes in practice. The work of Seager et al. [36] highlights the need to understand five universally accepted needs that relate to every one of us whether a giver or indeed a recipient of care, being loved, being heard, belonging, making a difference and having meaning and purpose, which position us to understand the extent and reality of needs. Multiple studies outline that patient needs are specific and contextually bound to palliative care, chronic illness and elderly patients' cross-cultural dimensions [13, 194, 202, 203], differentiating patient spiritual needs from carers needs. Puchalski et al. [204] propose an interdisciplinary model that allows collaborative effort of multidisciplinary team members to work together to maximise patient and family care.

A chaplaincy survey in England and Wales [205] examined hospice services in addition to hospitals and found that patients are preoccupied with adversity related to suffering coupled with familial concerns as distinct from transcendent concerns. Paradoxically, patients' needs within hospitals are centred on religious concerns as distinct from hospices. More recently Selman et al. [191] utilised an international sample of 74 patients and 71 carers across 9 countries to ascertain spiritual care needs taking account of the patient experience and expressed preferences. Five themes emerged which highlighted a significant number of concerns across existential, psychological, religious and social realms, culminating in insufficient care.

The need to identify, know and understand spiritual distress and patient signals are stressed as a means of providing compassionate person-centred care. Spiritual distress is defined as:

A state of suffering related to impaired ability to experience meaning in life through connectedness with self, others, world or superior being. [70]

Whilst this definition broadly articulates the characteristics of spiritual distress, specific patient concerns or behaviours are not apparent. Puchalski citing the work of Liebert ([206], p. 202) provides a complex list of spiritual concerns that requires chaplaincy intervention and referral when ordinary interventions do not work: 'existential concerns, abandonment by God (lack of love, loneliness) and others, anger at God and others, concerns about relationship with deity, conflicted or challenged belief systems, despair/hopelessness, grief/loss, guilt/shame, reconciliation, isolation, religious/spiritual struggle'. It is incumbent upon the healthcare practitioner to develop communication skills, to listen for themes within stated concerns and to dialogue with the patient in order to manage and support where feasible [206].

Fundamentally all patient needs are concerned with manifesting a need for human connection, for community, a need to maintain an identity, need to being acknowledged and valued, meaning, purpose, hope, having the ability to face death, engaging in rituals religious practices and professional staff interactions in order to address patients and family concerns. The subtleties involved are wholly dependent upon how sensitised the practitioner and student are, coupled with awareness, picking up cues, maturity and the ability to discern [207] to accompany the patient on their life journey.

11.10 Towards an Understanding of Spiritual Assessment, Interventions and Barriers

Spiritual assessment is a measure of the difference between the patients' experience and their expectancies which demands a compassionate qualitative approach by practitioners and students alike [208, 209]. There are noted ambiguities and inconsistencies relating to expectations and engagement of nursing professionals with assessment processes due to differing professional mandates [196]. However a generic agreement exists which identifies spiritual assessment as an integral aspect of person-centred care, thus rendering the process as everybody's business 'spiritual care generalists' (nurses, doctors, social workers, physiotherapists, etc.) and not just the sole domain of role of chaplaincy 'spiritual care specialist' and pastoral care services [63, 200]. Practitioners need to appreciate that spiritual assessment involves every multidisciplinary team member taking responsibility for attending to the spiritual dimension of patients care (within proficiency levels and limitations of competence) and necessitates understanding individual roles of team members and the exact nature of the assessment process. Spiritual assessment demands a coordinated effort and evidenced-based approach centred around three distinct levels of enquiry to promote an integrative approach to care, spiritual care screening, spiritual history taking followed by a detailed spiritual assessment [210].

There is a need for practitioners to understand the rationale, principles, purposes, aims and the how of undertaking initial spiritual screening, to ensure 'safe, inclusive and nonintrusive' assessment approaches, to determine whether patient or familial distress is present through asking open-ended questions and whether a more detailed assessment or referral is warranted [70, 211, 212]. The primary aims of screening are twofold, to establish whether a chaplain is required for emergency purposes and to ascertain patients who require a comprehensive chaplaincy assessment [213]. Students and practitioners need to be aware of both narrative and quantitative questioning protocols, the need to explain why such tools are being used and the need to seek consent and to document care [13, 196]. Puchalski [213] draws on Fitchetts' work to give examples of spiritual screening questions that include one and/or two-item questions, for example, (1) 'Are there any spiritual beliefs that you want to have discussed in your care with us here?

Similarly, there is a need for practitioners to understand the rationale, principles, purpose, goals and frequency and when to undertake a spiritual history, the role of patient's beliefs in illness and impact of beliefs on decisions required for care and to determine level of patient supports required [13]. Recommendations for advancing history taking include the use of validated instrument assessment tools, to monitor for spiritual distress and to understand the chaplain's role [214] in formalised spiritual assessments, rationale for referral and designated timeline regarding point of referral [213]. A significant range of tools are available for the purposes of undertaking a formal assessment; however practitioners and students need to know how to conduct these assessments. Three brief spiritual tools are utilised in medicine; CSI Memo Spiritual History by JAMA, ACP Spiritual History developed by consensus by the American College of Physicians and American Society of Internal Medicine and pneumonic FICA Spiritual History are outlined by Koenig [13] all posing four questions based on evidence. For example,

1. Faith—What is your faith tradition?
2. Importance—How important is your faith to you?
3. Church—What is your church community of faith?
4. Address—How might we address your spiritual needs?

Other assessment tools such as HOPE, ETHNIC(S) and SHALOM and their use are highlighted [196]. Luchetti et al. [215] undertook a systematic analysis of 25 spiritual history tools and concluded that FICA Spiritual History, FAITH, HOPE and Royal College of Psychiatrists scored more significantly over other tools analysed. The RUSH protocol is utilised widely in the USA by asking a series of three questions [216], whereas three narrative aspects predominate in the UK [78, 217, 218]. Specific resources are available through the National Center for Cultural Competence in Georgetown University, Washington, at https://nccc.georgetown.edu/index.php.

Responding to the praxis needs of clinical environments, Ross and McSherry [219] have recently developed an innovative pragmatic two-question model (2Q-SAM) with a person-centred focus that is easy to understand, encouraging patients to reveal their identity, desires and stresses without being subjected to a broad range of questions that they may find taxing.

> What's most important to you now?
> How can we help?

There is a need for healthcare professionals to know and understand spiritual assessment methods which demands an individualised person-centred approach that is practical, in keeping with time available, patient friendly and aligned to context to respect the patients' belief system and to negotiate relational caring with patients as a means of advancing spiritual care interventions [220, 221]. Spiritual care interventions are concerned with the being and doing aspects of person-centred care [222]. Puchalski [213] cites the work of Liebert who categorises three spiritual health interventions such as therapeutic communication techniques, therapy and self-care which stress the importance of negotiating commitment and involvement in the practitioner-patient relationship underpinned by reflective practice [223].

Practitioners who personally engage in interventions may be positioned to progress compassionate care practices further [224].

Multiple barriers have been identified in the literature which mitigate against the inclusion of spirituality in curricula [222]. Koenig ([13], p. 23) suggests specific barrier aspects that need to be taught and understood using both lecture and discursive techniques to advance practitioner thinking and to minimise practitioner-patient problems from occurring; what stops healthcare workers from engaging in spiritual history taking, communication difficulties relating to spirituality in patient-practitioner encounters, examine matters concerning patient choice, isolation from religious support and to concentrate on secular objectives, boundary recognition, handling challenging situations.

11.11 Conclusion

Healthcare provisions are mandated to move beyond spirituality that is merely 'caught' rather than 'taught' [225] formalising contemporary teaching approaches with a view to supporting student's awareness and being with essential knowledge, skills, attitudes and competence required for the actual reality of spiritual care provision in undergraduate education programmes and for newly qualified staff. Given that the primary aim of spiritual care education is 'to broaden the scope of professional responsibility', we need to open ourselves to humanities in addition to evidence-based practice to guide future relational development of educators, practitioners and students alike. In so doing we will attempt to connect and communicate meaningfully with our patients; hold the sacred space for the mystery of life of another in our hands that cannot be abandoned, isolated or alienated; and orientate ourselves towards compassionate care, spiritual care competencies and responsibilities, to promote patient well-being, to alleviate patient suffering and to help patients cope [221, 226].

Resources

Health Care Chaplaincy White Papers
Spiritual Care: What It Means, Why It Matters in Health Care https://spiritualcare-association.org/docs/resources/spirituality.pdf
Spiritual Care and Nursing: A Nurse's Contribution and Practice https://spiritual-careassociation.org/docs/resources/nurses_spiritual_care_white_paper_3_22_2017.pdf
Spiritual Care and Physicians: Understanding Spirituality in Medical Practice https://spiritualcareassociation.org/docs/resources/hccn_whitepaper_spirituality_and_physicians.pdf
Spiritual Care and Social Work https://www.healthcarechaplaincy.org/docs/about/spiritual_care_and_social_work.pdf

Handbook Patients Spiritual and Cultural Values for Health Care Professionals https://www.healthcarechaplaincy.org/docs/publications/landing_page/cultural_ sensitivity_handbook_from_healthcare_chaplaincy_network_11_11_2015.pdf

Cultural and Spiritual Sensitivity; A Learning Module for Healthcare Professionals https://www.healthcarechaplaincy.org/docs/publications/landing_page/cultural_ spiritual_sensitivity_learning_Module_7_10_09.pdf

Spiritual Care Resources for Health Care Professionals

Chaplains https://spiritualcareassociation.org/docs/spiritual_care_resources/chaplains_flyer_5_1_18.pdf

Nurses https://spiritualcareassociation.org/docs/spiritual_care_resources/nursing_flyer_4_15_18.pdf

Social Workers https://www.healthcarechaplaincy.org/docs/spiritual_care_resources/social_workers_flyer_5_1_18.pdf

https://www.theberylinstitute.org/news/264925/The-Critical-Role-of-Spirituality-in-Patient-Experience-Explored-by-The-Beryl-Institute-.htm

Associations, Centres, Foundations, Institutes, Organisations, Research Groups and Centres of Excellence

British Association for the Study of Spirituality: www.basspirituality.org.uk

The Association for Children's Spirituality: www.childrenspirituality.org

Centre for Cultural Competence https://nccc.georgetown.edu/index.php http://spiritualcareassociation.org/resources.html

Centre for Spirituality, Health & Disability: www.abdn.ac.uk/cshad

Foundation for Workplace Spirituality: www.workplacespirituality.org.uk/

John Templeton Foundation https://www.templeton.org/

Fetzer Institute http://fetzer.org/

George Washington Institute for Spirituality and Health https://smhs.gwu.edu/gwish/

Research Institute for Spirituality and Health: www.rish.ch

spIRE Spirituality Institute for Research and Education and http://spiritualityinstitute.ie/

Viktor Frankl Institute Ireland https://viktorfranklireland.com/

World Health Organisation: www.who.int

Spirituality and Research Innovation Group (SRIG) Trinity College Dublin http://nursing-midwifery.tcd.ie/SRIG/

The Royal College of Psychiatrists Spirituality and Psychiatry Special Interest Group https://www.rcpsych.ac.uk/members/specialinterestgroups/spirituality.aspx

Dr. Daniel Goleman – Expert in Emotional Intelligence http://www.danielgoleman.info/

Dr. Kristin Neff – Expert in Self Compassion Website www. http://www.self-compassion.org/

Test how self compassionate you are http://www.self-compassion.org/test-your-self-compassion-level.html Self Compassion Exercises http://www.self-compas-

sion.org/self_compassion_exercise.pdf Watch TED video The Space Between Self-Esteem and Self Compassion accessible on website.
Royal College of Nursing (UK) Online Resource 2011 https://www.rcn.org.uk/professional-development/publications/pub-003887
Dr. Jean Watson Expert in Caring Science Website https://www.watsoncaringscience.org/
The Centre for Compassion and Altruism and Education Research http://ccare.stanford.edu/
Greater Good Science Centre at Berkeley https://greatergood.berkeley.edu/

References

1. Steinhauser K, Balboni T. State of the science of spirituality and palliative care research: research landscape and future directions. J Pain Symptom Manage. 2017;54:426–7.
2. Steinhauser KE, Fitchett G, Handzo GF, Johnson KS, Koenig HG, Pargament KI, Puchalski C, Sinclair S, Taylor EJ, Balboni TA. State of the science of spirituality and palliative care research. Part 1: definitions, measurement and outcomes. J Pain Symptom Manage. 2017;54:428–40.
3. Balboni TA, Fitchett G, Handzo GF, Johnson KS, Koenig HG, Pargament KI, Puchalski CM, Sinclair S, Taylor EJ, Steinhauser KE. State of the science of spirituality and palliative care research part I: definitions, measurement, and outcomes. J Pain Symptom Manage. 2017;54:441–53.
4. Pesut B, Taylor EJ, Reimer Kirkham S, Sawatzky R. Conceptualising spirituality and religion for healthcare. J Clin Nurs. 2007;17:2803–10.
5. Timmins F, Egan R, Flanagan B, Muldowney Y, OBoyle C, Brady V, Whelan J, Neenan K, McSherry W. Special issue "international conference of spirituality in healthcare. Nurturing the spirit"—Trinity College Dublin 2016. Religions. 2017;8:204. https://doi.org/10.3390/rel8100204.
6. Attard J, Baldacchino DR, Camilleri L. Nurses' and midwives' acquisition of competency in spiritual care: a focus on education. Nurse Educ Today. 2014;34:1460–6.
7. Ross L, Van Leeuwen R, Baldacchino D, Giske T, McSherry W, Narayanasamy A, Downes C, Jarvis P, Schep-Akkerman A. Student nurses perceptions of spirituality and competence in delivering spiritual care: a European pilot study. Nurse Educ Today. 2014;34:697–702.
8. Lucchetti G, Lamas A, Lucchetti G, Puchalski CM. Spirituality in medical education: global reality? J Relig Health. 2012;51:3–19.
9. Puchalski CM, Ferrell B, Virani R, Otis-Green S, Baird P, Bull J, Chochinov H, Handzo G, Nelson-Becker H, Prince-Paul M, Pugliese K, Sulmasy D. Improving the quality of spiritual care as a dimension of palliative care: the report of the Consensus Conference. J Palliat Med. 2009;12:885–904.
10. Ross L. Why the increasing interest in spirituality within healthcare? In: McSherry W, Ross L, editors. Spiritual assessment in healthcare practice. Cumbria: M & K Publishing; 2014. reprint pp. 5–17.
11. World Health Organisation. The world health report 1998 - life in the 21st century: a vision for all. Geneva: WHO; 1998.
12. Health Information and Quality Authority (HIQA). Standards for safer better healthcare in the Irish healthcare system. Dublin: Health Information and Quality Authority; 2012.
13. Koenig HG. Spirituality in patient care why, how, when, and what. 3rd ed. West Conshohocken: Templeton Press; 2013.
14. Ellis MR, Campbell JD. Patients' views about discussing spiritual issues with primary care physicians. South Med J. 2004;97:1158–64.

15. Burkhardt L, Hogan W. Measuring effectiveness of spiritual care pedagogy in nursing education. J Prof Nurs. 2012;28:315–21.
16. D'Souza R. The importance of spirituality in medicine and its application to clinical practice. Med J Aust. 2007;186(Suppl 10):57–9.
17. Cohen AB, Koening HG. Religion, religiosity and spirituality in the biopsychosocial model of health and ageing. Ageing Int. 2003;28:215–41.
18. Koenig HG, Larson DB, Larson SS. Religion and coping with serious illness. Ann Pharmacother. 2001;35:352–9.
19. Fitchett G, Murphy PE, Kim J, Gibbons JL, Cameron JR, Davis JA. Religious struggle: prevalence, correlates and mental health risks in diabetic, congestive heart failure, and oncology patients. Int J Psychiatry Med. 2004;4:179–96.
20. Balboni TAL, Vanderwerker LC, Block SD, Paulik ME, Lathan CS, Peteet JR, Prigerson HG. Religiousness and spiritual support among advanced cancer patients and associations with end-of-life treatment preferences and quality of life. J Clini Oncol. 2007;25: 555–60.
21. Balboni TA, Nilsson M, Macjejewski PK, Phelps AC, Schrag D, Trice E, Paul E, Wright AA, Prigerson HG, Block SD, Peteet JR. Religious coping and use of intensive life prolonging care near death in patients with advanced cancer. JAMA. 2009;341:1147–0.
22. Murray SA, Kendall M, Boyd K, Worth A, Benton TF. Exploring the spiritual needs of people dying of lung cancer or heart failure: a prospective qualitative interview study of patients and their carers. Palliat Med. 2004;18(1):39–45.
23. Ross L. Spiritual care in nursing: an overview of the research to date. J Clin Nurs. 2006;157:852–62.
24. Cockell N, McSherry W. Spiritual care in nursing: an overview of published international research. J Nurs Manag. 2012;20:958–69.
25. Ross L, Austin J. Spiritual needs and spiritual support preferences of people with end stage heart failure and their carers: implications for nurse managers. J Nurs Manag. 2013;23:87–95.
26. Astrow AB, Wexler A, Texeira K, He MK, Sulmasy DP. Is failure to meet spiritual needs associated with cancer patients perceptions of quality of care and their satisfaction 2007. J Clin Oncol. 2007;25:5753–7.
27. Puchalski CM, et al. Improving the spiritual dimension of whole person care: reaching national and international consensus. J Palliat Med. 2014;17:642–56.
28. Paal P, Helo Y, Frick E. Spiritual care training provided to healthcare professionals: a systematic review. J Pastoral Care Counsel. 2015;20:1757–67.
29. Stranahan S. Spiritual perception, attitudes about spiritual care, and spiritual care practices among nurse practitioners. West J Nurs Res. 2001;23(1):90–104.
30. McSherry W. The principles components model: a model for advancing spirituality and spiritual care within nursing and health practice. J Clin Nurs. 2006;15:905–17.
31. Ross L. Why the increasing interest in spirituality within healthcare? In: Mcsherry W, Ross L, editors. Spiritual assessment in healthcare practice. Cumbria: M & K Publishing; 2013.
32. McSherry W, Jamieson S. An online survey of nurse's perceptions of spirituality and spiritual care. J Clin Nurs. 2011;20:1757–67.
33. Paley J. Spirituality and secularization: nursing and the sociology of religion. J Clin Nurs. 2008;17:175–86.
34. Carroll B. A phenomenological enquiry of the nature of spirituality and spiritual care. Mortality. 2001;6:81–98.
35. Koenig HG. Religion, spirituality and health: the research and clinical implications. ISRN Psychiatry. 2012;2012:278730. https://doi.org/10.5402/2012/278730.
36. Seager M, Bush M. Supporting the practitioner. In: Wattis J, Curran S, Rogers M, editors. Spiritually competent practice in health care. London: CRC Press; 2017. p. 99–114.
37. Willis P. Quality with compassion: the future of nursing education. Report of the Willis Commission on Nursing Education 2012. London: Royal College of Nursing; 2012.
38. Francis R. Report on the Mid Staffordshire NHS Foundation Trust public inquiry. London: The Stationary Office; 2013.

39. Wattis J, Curran S, Rogers M. What does spirituality mean for patients, practitioners and health care organisations. In: Wattis J, Curran S, Rogers M, editors. Spiritually competent practice in health care. New York: CRC Press; 2017. p. 99-1141-7.
40. Narayansamy A. Learning spiritual dimensions of care from a historical perspective. Nurs Educ Today. 1999;19:386–95.
41. Cooper K, Chang E, Sheehan A, Johnson A. The impact of spiritual education upon preparing undergraduate nursing learners to provide spiritual care. Nurs Educ Today. 2013;33:1057–61.
42. Mthembu TG, et al. Teaching spirituality and spiritual care in health sciences education: a systematic review. Afr J Phys Act Health Sci. 2016;22:1036–57.
43. Best M, Butow P, Olver I. Do patients want doctors to talk about spirituality: a systematic review. Patient Educ Couns. 2015;98:1320–8.
44. Schonfeld T, Schmid K, Boucher-Payne D. Incorporating spirituality into health sciences education. J Relig Health. 2016;55:85–96.
45. Benner P, Sutphen M, Leonard V, Day L. Educating nurses: a call for radical transformation. Chichester: Jossey-Bass/Carnegie Foundation for the Advancement of Teaching; 2010.
46. Barss K. Building bridges an interpretive phenomenological analysis of nurse educators clinical experience of building the Trust model of inclusive spiritual care. Int J Nurs Educ Scholarsh. 2012;9:1–15.
47. Prentis S, Rogers M, Wattis J, Jones J, Stephenson J. Healthcare lecturers perceptions of spirituality in education. Nurs Stand. 2014;29:44–52.
48. Yilmaz M, Gurler H. The efficacy of integrating spirituality into undergraduate nursing curricula. Nurs Ethics. 2014;21:929–45.
49. Ali G, Wattis J, Snowden M. Why are spiritual aspects so hard to address in nursing education? A literature revie (1993-2015). Int J Multidiscip Comp Stud. 2015;2:7–31.
50. McSherry W, Draper P. The spiritual dimension why the absences within nursing curricula. Nurs Educ Today. 1997;17:413–7.
51. McSherry W. Making sense of spirituality in nursing and healthcare practice. 2nd ed. London: Jessica Kingsley; 2006.
52. Lucchetti G, Lucchetti AL, Puchalski CM. Spirituality in medical education: global reality? J Relig Health. 2012a;51(1):3–19.
53. Monareng LV. An exploration of how spiritual care is applied in nursing practice. Health SA Gesondheid. 2013;18:a635. https://doi.org/10.4102/hsag.v18i1.635.
54. Paal P, Helo Y, Frick E. Spiritual care training provided to healthcare professionals systematic review. J Pastoral Care Counsel. 2015;20:1757–67.
55. Nursing and Midwifery Council. NMC competence domain; 2009. tinyurl.com/px5luaj.
56. Nursing and Midwifery Council. NMC standards for preregistration nursing education. London: NMC; 2010.
57. Nursing and Midwifery Council. The code: professional standards of practice and behaviour for nurses and midwives; 2015. www.nmc.org.uk/standards/code.
58. International Council of Nurses. The ICN code of ethics for nurses. Geneva: ICN; 2012.
59. Nursing and Midwifery Board of Ireland. Code of professional conduct and ethics for nurses and midwives. Dublin: NMBI; 2014.
60. Jones J, Smith J, McSherry W. Spiritually competent practice in health care: what is it and what does it look like? In: Wattis J, Curran S, Rogers M, editors. Spiritually competent practice in health care. New York: CRC Press; 2017. p. p35–52.
61. The Royal College of Nursing (UK). RCN spiritual survey. London: RCN; 2011.
62. The Royal College of Nursing (UK). Spirituality in nursing care: a pocket guide. London: RCN; 2012.
63. Healthcare Chaplaincy Network. Spiritual care and nursing: a nurses's contribution and practice (White Paper); 2017.
64. Jones J, Topping A, Wattis J, Smith J. A concept analysis of spirituality in occupational therapy practice. J Study Spirituality. 2016;6:38–57.
65. Carey LB, Mathison BA. Spiritual care for allied health practice. London: Jessica Kingsley; 2018.

66. Hodge DR, Bushfield S. Developing spiritual competence in practice. J Ethn Cult Divers Soc Work. 2007;15:101–27.
67. Furman LD, Benson PW, Canda ER, Grimwood C. Comparative international analysis of religion and spirituality in social work: a survey of UK and US social workers. Soc Work Educ. 2005;8:101–24.
68. Hodge D. Spirituality and religion among the general public: implications for social work discourse. Social Work. 2015;60(3):219–27.
69. Timmins F, Neill F, Murphy MA, Begley T, Sheaf G. Spiritual care competence for contemporary nursing practice: a quantitative exploration of the guidance provided by fundamental nursing textbooks. Nurse Educ Pract. 2015;15:485–91.
70. Caldeira S, Carvalho E, Vieira M. Spiritual distress: proposing a new definition of defining characteristics. Int J Nurs Knowl. 2013;24:77–84.
71. Baldacchino D. Spiritual care education of health care professionals. Religions. 2015;6:594–613.
72. American Nurses Association. Code of ethics with interpretative statements. Silver Spring, MD: American Nurses Association; 2015. http://www.nursingworld.org/MainMenuCategories/EthicsStandards/CodeofEthicsforNurses/Code-of-Ethics-For-Nurses.html.
73. Nursing and Midwifery Council. NMC standards for preregistration nursing education. London: NMC; 2009.
74. Malta code of ethics for nurses and midwives. https://deputyprimeminister.gov.mt/en/phc/pdu/Documents/maltese_code_of_ethics_nurses.pdf.
75. The American Association of Medical Colleges (AAMC). Learning objectives for medical student education guidelines for medical schools: report 1 of the Medical School Objectives Project. Acad Med. 1999;74:13–8.
76. Institute of Medicine and Royal College of Psychiatrists Position Statement (PS03/2011).
77. Joint Commission on Accreditation of Health Care Organisations. Spiritual assessment standards CAHO; 2008. https://www.jointcommission.org/standards_information/jcfaq.aspx?ProgramId=0&ChapterId=0&IsFeatured=False&IsNew=False&Keyword=spiritual%20assessment&print=y
78. The Royal College of Nursing (UK). RCN spiritual survey; 2011. London: RCN.
79. The Royal College of Nursing (UK). Spirituality in nursing care: a pocket guide; 2012. London: RCN.
80. Hughes BP, et al. Spiritual care and nursing: a nurses contribution and practice. New York: Healthcare Chaplaincy Network; 2017.
81. Neely D, Minford EJ. Current status of teaching spirituality in UK medical schools. Med Educ. 2008;42(2):176–82.
82. Ross L. Spiritual care in nursing : an overview of the research to date. J Clin Nurs. 2006;15:852–62.
83. Lovanio K, Wallace M. Promoting spiritual knowledge and attitudes: a student nurse education project. Holist Nurs Pract. 2007;21:42–7.
84. Van Leeuwen R, Tiesinga LJ, Middel B, Post D, Jochensen H. The effectiveness of an educational programme for nursing students on developing competence in the provision of spiritual care. J Clin Nurs. 2008;17:2768–81.
85. Pulchaiski CM, Cobb M, Rumbold B. Curriculum development courses, and CPE. Part 1: curriculum development in spirituality and health in the health professions. In: Cobb M, Pulchaiski CM, Rumbold B, editors. Oxford textbook of spirituality in healthcare. New York: Oxford University Press; 2014. p. 417–27.
86. McSherry W. Making sense of spirituality in nursing practice : an interactive approach. London: Churchill Livingstone; 2000.
87. Monareng LV. An exploration of how spiritual care is applied in nursing practice. Health SA Gesondheid. 2013;18:1–11.
88. Snowden M, Ali G. How can spirituality be integrated into in undergraduate and post graduate education. In: Wattis J, Curran S, Rogers M, editors. Spiritually competent practice in health care. New York: CRC Press; 2017. p. 71–5.

89. Pesut B, Fowler M, Taylor EJ, Reimer-Kirkham S. Spirituality and spiritual care in nursing fundamentals textbooks. J Nurs Educ. 2008;47:167–73.
90. Timmins F, Murphy M, Neill F, Begley T, Sheaf G. An exploration of the extent of inclusion of spirituality and spiritual care concepts in core nursing textbooks. Nurs Educ Today. 2015;35:277–82.
91. Pesut B. Developing spirituality in the curriculum: worldviews, intrapersonal connectedness, interpersonal connectedness. Nurs Educ Perspect. 2003;6:290–4.
92. McSherry W. Making sense of spirituality in nursing and health care practice: an interactive approach. 2nd ed. London: Jessica Kingsley; 2006.
93. Ross L, van Leewen R, Baldacchion D, Giske T, McSherry W, Narayanasamy A, Downes C, Jarvis P, Schep-Akkermann A. Student nurses perceptions of spirituality and competence in delivering spiritual care. A European pilot study. Nurs Educ Today. 2014;34:697–702.
94. Dall'Alba G, Barnacle R. An ontological turn for higher education. Stud High Educ. 2007;32:679–91.
95. Dall'Alba G. Learning professional ways of being: ambiguities of becoming. Educ Philos Theory. 2009;41:34–45.
96. Barnett R, Coates K. Engaging the curriculum in higher education. Buckinghamshire: SRHE and Open University Press; 2005.
97. Lennon-Dearing RL, Florence JA, Halvorson H, Pollard JP. An interprofessional educational approach to teaching spiritual assessment journal of healthcare chaplaincy 2012. J Healthc Chaplain. 2012;18:121–32.
98. Swinton J. Spirituality in healthcare: just because it may be 'made up' does not mean that it is not real and does not matter (Keynote 5). J Study Spirituality. 2014;4:162–73.
99. Kelly E. Competences in spiritual care education and training. In: Cobb M, Pulchaiski CM, Rumbold B, editors. Oxford textbook of spirituality in healthcare. New York: Oxford University Press; 2014. p. 435–42.
100. Gordon T, Mitchell D. Competency model for the assessment and delivery of spiritual care. Palliat Med. 2004;18:646–51.
101. Neely D, Minford EJ. Current status of teaching on spirituality in UK medical schools. Med Educ. 2008;42:176–82.
102. Wattis J, Curran S, Rogers M. What does spirituality mean for patients, practitioners and health care organisations. In: Wattis J, Curran S, Rogers M, editors. Spiritually competent practice in health care. New York: CRC Press; 2017. p. 3.
103. The Marie Curie Cancer Care Framework. Spiritual and religious care competencies for specialist palliative care. London: Marie Curie Cancer Care; 2003.
104. McSherry W. The principle components model: a model for advancing spirituality and spiritual care within nursing and health care practice. J Clin Nursing. 2006;15(7):905–17.
105. Van Leeuwen R, Cusveller's B. Nursing competencies for spiritual care in undergraduate nursing programmes. J Adv Nurs. 2004;48:234–46.
106. Timmins F, Caldeira S, Murphy MA, Pujol N, Sheaf G, Weathers E, Whelan J, Healthcare Chaplaincy. An exploration of current in hospital spiritual care resources in the republic of Ireland and review of international chaplaincy standards (report). Trinity College Dublin, The University of Dublin.
107. NHS Education for Scotland. Standards for NHS Chaplaincy services. Edinburgh: NHS Education for Scotland; 2007.
108. NHS Education for Scotland. Spiritual and religious care capabilities and competencies for healthcare chaplains. Edinburgh: NHS Education for Scotland; 2008.
109. Standards of practice for chaplaincy in acute settings. 2011. http://www.professionalchaplains.org/files/professional_standards/standards_of_practice/standards_practice_professional_chaplains_acute_care.pdf.
110. Standards of practice for chaplaincy in long term care. http://www.professionalchaplains.org/files/professional_standards/standards_of_practice/sop_longtermcare.pdf.
111. Vieten C, et al. Spiritual and religious competencies for psychologists. Psychol Relig Spiritual. 2013;5:129–44.

112. Baldacchino D. Nursing competencies for spiritual care. J Adv Nurs. 2006;15:885–96.
113. Attard J, Baldacchino DR, Camilleri L. Nurses' and midwives' acquisition of competency in spiritual care: a focus on education. Nurs Educ Today. 2014;34:1460–6.
114. Van Leeuwen R, Cusveller V. Nursing competencies for spiritual care. J Adv Nurs. 2004;48:234–96.
115. Biro AL. Creating conditions for good nursing by attending to the spiritual. J Nurs Manag. 2012;20:47–53.
116. Rankin EA, DeLashmutt MB. Finding spirituality and nursing presence: the students challenge. J Holist Nurs. 2006;24:282–8.
117. Mthembu TG, Wegner L, Roman NV. Teaching spirituality and spiritual care in health sciences education: a systematic review. Afr J Phys Act Health Sci. 2016;22:1036–57.
118. Wattis J. What does spirituality mean for patients, practitioners and health care organisations. In: Wattis J, Curran S, Rogers M, editors. Spiritually competent practice in health care; 2017. p. 1–18.
119. Swinton J. The meanings of spirituality a multi – perspective approach to 'the spiritual'. In: McSherry W, Ross L, editors. Spiritual assessment in healthcare practice. Keswick: M&K Update; 2013. p. 17–36.
120. Narayanasamy A. Spiritual care: a practical guide for nurses and healthcare practitioners. London: Quay Books; 2001.
121. McSherry W, Cash K. The language of spirituality: an emerging taxonomy. Int J Nurs Stud. 2004;41:151–61.
122. Hill PC, Pargament K. Advances in the conceptualisation and measurement of religion: implications for physical and mental research. Psychol Relig Spiritual. 2008;S(1):3–17.
123. Baldacchino DR, Borg J, Muscat C. Psychology and theology meet: illness appraisal and spiritual coping. West J Nurs Res. 2012;34:818–47.
124. Swinton J, Pattison S. Moving beyond clarity: towards a thin, vague, and useful understanding of spirituality in nursing care. Nurs Philos. 2010;11:226–37.
125. Pike J. Spirituality in nursing: a systematic review of the literature from 2006-2010. Br J Nurs. 2011;20:743. https://doi.org/10.12968/bjon.2011.20.12.743.
126. Reinert K, Koenig H. Re-examining definitions of spirituality in nursing research. J Adv Nurs. 2013;69:2622–34.
127. McSherry W. What we know about spirituality. In: The meaning of spirituality and spiritual care within nursing and health care practice. London: Quay Books; 2013. p. 19–94.
128. Miller WR, Thoresen CE. Spirituality, religion, and health. An emerging research field. Am Psychol. 2003;58:24–35.
129. McSherry W, Smith J. Spiritual care. In: McSherry W, Mcsherry R, Watson R, editors. Care in nursing principles, values and skills. Oxford: Oxford University Press; 2012. p. 117–28.
130. Nolan S, Saltmarsh P, Leget C. Spiritual care in palliative care. Eur J Palliat Care. 2011;18:86–9.
131. Weathers E, McCarthy G, Coffey A. Concept analysis of spirituality: an evolutionary approach. Nurs Forum. 2015;51:79–96.
132. McSherry W, Cash W, Ross L. Meaning of spirituality: implications for nursing practice. J Clin Nurs. 2004;13:934–41.
133. Sharpiro J, Coulehan J, Wear D, Montello M. Medical humanities and their discontents: definitions, critiques and implications. Acad Med. 2009;84:192–8.
134. Ferrell B, Del Ferraro C. Suffering. In: Cobb M, Pulchaiski CM, Rumbold B, editors. Oxford textbook of spirituality in healthcare. New York: Oxford University Press; 2014. p. 158–68.
135. Vlasblom JP, van der Steen J, Jochamsen H. Effects of a spiritual care training for nurses. Nurse Educ Today. 2011;31(8):790–6.
136. Wagner AL, Seymour MA. A model of caring mentorship. J Nurses Prof Dev. 2007;23(5):201–11.
137. Baillie L, Black S. Professional values in nursing. New York: CRC Press; 2015.
138. Keith P, Rogers R. Spirituality in the primary care setting. In: Wattis J, Curran S, Rogers M, editors. Spiritually competent practice in health care; 2017. p. 129–44.

139. Mitchell DL, Bennett MJ, Manfrin-Ledet L. Spiritual development of nursing students: developing competence to provide spiritual care to patients at the end of life. J Nurs Educ. 2006;45:365–70.
140. Bennett V, Thompson ML. Teaching spirituality to student nurses. J Nurs Educ Pract. 2015;5. https://doi.org/10.5430/jnep.v5n2p26.
141. Jones J. Spirituality in acute health care settings. In: Wattis J, Curran S, Rogers M, editors. Spiritually competent practice in health care. London: CRC Press; 2017. p. 99–114.
142. Taylor EJ. Let's begin. In: What do I say? Talking with patients about spirituality. Philadelphia: Templeton Press; 2007. p. 1–8.
143. Taylor EJ. Verbal responses to spiritual pain. In: What do I say? Talking with patients about spirituality. Philadelphia, PA: Templeton Press; 2007. p. 53–100.
144. Taylor EJ. Preparing the healer. In: What do I say? Talking with patients about spirituality. Philadelphia, PA: Templeton Press; 2007. p. 9–24.
145. Stairs J. Listening for the soul pastoral care and spiritual direction. Minneapolis: Fortess; 2000.
146. Kearney M, Weininger R. Care of the soul. In: Cobb M, Pulchaiski CM, Rumbold B, editors. Oxford textbook of spirituality in healthcare. New York: Oxford University Press; 2014. p. 274–8.
147. Sitzman K, Watson J. Caring science, mindful practice implementing Watsons human caring theory. New York: Springer; 2016.
148. Bach S, Grant A. Communication and interpersonal skills in nursing. London: Sage; 2011.
149. Papadoupoulos I. The Papadoupoulos Tilki and Taylor model of developing cultural competence. In: Papadopoulos I, editor. Transcultural health and social care: development of culturally competent practitioners. London: Churchill Livingstone, Elsevier; 2006. p. 7–24.
150. Baughan J, Smith P. Compassion, caring and communication skills for nursing practice. 2nd ed. London: Routledge; 2011.
151. Giske T, Cone P. Opening up to learning spiritual care of patients: a grounded theory study of nursing students. J Clin Nurs. 2012;21:2006–15.
152. Cone T, Giske P. Teaching spiritual care – a grounded theory study among undergraduate nursing educators. J Clin Nurs. 2013;22:1951–60.
153. Baldacchino D. Teaching on spiritual care: the perceived impact on qualified nurses. Nurs Educ Pract. 2011;11:47–53.
154. Langle A. The search for meaning in life and the existential fundamental motivations. Int J Existent Psychol Psychother. 2007;1:1708–696.
155. Udo C. The concept and relevance of existential issues in nursing. Eur J Oncol Nurs. 2014;18:347–54.
156. La Cour P, Hvidt NG. Research on meaning-making and health in secular society: secular, spiritual and religious existential orientations. Soc Sci Med. 2010;71:1292–9.
157. Henoch I, Danielson E. Existential concerns among patient with cancer and interventions to meet them: an integrative review. Psycho-Oncology. 2008;18:225–36.
158. Browall M, Danielson E, Henoch I. Health care staff's opinions about existential issues among patients with cancer. Palliat Support Care. 2010;8:5968.
159. Sessana L, Finnell D, Jezewski MA. Spirituality in nursing and health related literature: a concept analysis. J Holist Nurs. 2007;25:252–62.
160. Frankl V. Psychotherapy and existentialism: selected papers on logotherapy. New York: Simon & Schuster; 1967. p. 3.
161. Frankl VE. Man's search for meaning an introduction to logotherapy. London: Hodder & Stoughton; 1987.
162. Strang S, Henoch I, Danieson E, Browall M, Melin-Johansson C. Communication about existential issues with patients close to death – nurses reflections on content, process and meaning. Psycho-Oncology. 2014;23(5):562–8.
163. Le May K, Wilson KG. Treatment of existential distress in life threatening illness: a review of interventions. Clin Psychol Rev. 2008;28:472–93.

164. Ekmann P. What scientists who study emotion agree about. Perspect Psychol Sci. 2016;11:31–4.
165. Burkhart L, Schmidt W. Measuring effectiveness of a spiritual care pedagogy in nursing education. J Prof Nurs. 2012;28:315–21.
166. Taylor EJ. Making sense of what you hear. In: What do I say? Talking with patients about spirituality. Philadelphia, PA: Templeton Press; 2007. p. 41–52.
167. Clinebell HJ. Basic types of pastoral counselling. Nashville: Abington; 1966.
168. Taylor EJ. Listening – beginning the healing response. In: What do I say? Talking with patients about spirituality. Philadelphia, PA: Templeton Press; 2007. p. 25–39.
169. Finfgeld-Connett D. Metasynthesis of presence in nursing. J Adv Nurs. 2006;55:708–14.
170. Gordon J, Watts C. Applying skills and knowledge: principle of nursing practice F. Nurs Stand. 2011;25:35–7.
171. Harbinson MT, Bell D. How should teaching on whole person medicine including spiritual issues be delivered in the undergraduate medical curriculum in the United Kingdom? BMC Med Educ. 2015;15:96.
172. McSherry W, Ross L. A spiritual shortfall? Nurs Stand. 2015;29:22.
173. NHS Scotland. Spiritual care matters: an introductory resource for all NHS Scotland Staff. Edinburgh: NHS Education for Scotland; 2009. p. 6.
174. McSherry W, Ross L. Nursing. In: Cobb M, Pulchaiski CM, Rumbold B, editors. Oxford textbook of spirituality in healthcare. New York: Oxford University Press; 2014. p. 213.
175. Puchalski CM, Romer AL. Taking a spiritual history allows clinicians to understand patients more fully. J Palliat Med. 2000;3:129–37.
176. Sharp J, Nash S. Spiritual teamwork within end of life care. In: Wattis J, Curran S, Rogers M, editors. Spiritually competent practice in health care. New York: CRC Press; 2017. p. 145–60.
177. Rogers M, Beres L. How two practitioners conceptualise spiritually competent practice. In: Wattis J, Curran S, Rogers M, editors. Spiritually competent practice in health care. New York: CRC Press; 2017. p. 52–69.
178. Sawatzky R, Pesut B. Attributes of spiritual care in nursing practice. J Holist Nurs. 2005;23:19–33.
179. McSherry W, Jamieson S. The qualitative findings from an online survey investigating nurses' perceptions of spirituality and spiritual. J Clin Nurs. 2013;22(21-22):3170–82.
180. Costello M, Atinaja-Faller J, Hedberg M. The use of simulation to instruct students on the provision of spiritual care: a pilot study. J Holist Nurs. 2012;30:277–81.
181. King DE, Crisp MD. Spirituality and health care education in family medicine residency programs. Fam Med. 2005;37:399–40.
182. Lemmer C. Reflections on teaching "spirituality in the healthcare environment". J Holist Nurs. 2010;28(2):145–9.
183. Watson J. Human caring science: a theory of nursing. 2nd ed. Sudbury: Jones & Bartlett Learning; 2012.
184. Ousager J, Johannessen H. Humanities in undergraduate education: a literature review. Acad Med. 2010;85:988–98.
185. Gordon JJ. Medical humanities: state of the art. Med Educ. 2008;43:333–7.
186. Balboni TAL, Vanderwerker LC, Block SD, Paulik ME, Lathan CS, Peteet JR, Prigerson HG. Religiousness and spiritual support among advanced cancer patients and associations with end-of-life treatment preferences and quality of life. J Clin Oncol. 2007;25:555–60.
187. Astrow AB, Wexler A, Texeira K, He MK, Sulmasy DP. Is failure to meet spiritual needs associated with cancer patients perceptions of quality of care and their satisfaction. J Clin Oncol. 2007;25:5753–7.
188. Ross L, Austin J. Spiritual needs and spiritual support preferences of people with end-stage heart failure and their carers: implications for nurse managers. J Nurs Manag. 2015;23:87–95.
189. Balboni MJ. The relationship between medicine, spirituality and religion: three models for integration. J Relig Health. 2014;53:1586–98.

190. Caldeira S, Timmins F. Time as presence and opportunity: the key to spiritual care in contemporary nursing practice. J Clin Nurs. 2015;24(17-18):2355.
191. Selman L, Brighton LJ, Sinclair S, et al. Patients' and caregivers needs, experiences, preferences and research priorities in spiritual care. A focus group study across nine countries. Palliat Med. 2018;32:216.
192. Lin HR, Bauer-Wu SM. Psycho-spiritual well-being in patients with advanced cancer: an integrative review of the literature. J Adv Nurs. 2003;44:69–80.
193. Bussing A, Koenig HG. Spiritual needs of patients with chronic diseases. Religions. 2010;1:18–27.
194. Hodge DR, Horvath VE. Spiritual needs in health care settings: a qualitative meta-synthesis of clients perspectives. Soc Work. 2011;56:4.
195. Ellman MS, Schulman-Green D, Blatt L, Asher S, Viveiros D, Clark J, Bia M. Using online learning and interactive stimulation to teach spiritual and cultural aspects of palliative care to interprofessional students. J Palliat Care. 2012;15:1240–7.
196. Timmins F, Caldeira S. Assessing the spiritual needs of patients. Nurs Stand. 2017;31:47–53.
197. Swinton J. Spirituality in mental health care: rediscovering the forgotten dimension. London: Jessica Kingsley; 2001.
198. McSherry W. What we know about spirituality. In: The meaning of spirituality and spiritual care within nursing and health care practice. London: Quay Books; 2007. p. 19–94.
199. Narayanansamy A. Recognising spiritual needs. In: McSherry W, Ross L, editors. Spiritual assessment in healthcare practice. Keswick: M&K Update; 2013. p. 57–78.
200. Holloway M, Adamson S, McSherry W, Swinton J. Spiritual care at the end of life: a systematic review of the literature. London: Department of Health; 2009.
201. Selman L, Young T. Research priorities in spiritual care: an international survey of palliative care researchers and clinicians. J Pain Symptom Manage. 2014;48:518–31.
202. Monod S, Rochat E, Bula C, Spencer B. The spiritual needs model: spirituality as assessment in the geriatric hospital setting. J Relig Spiritual Aging. 2010;22:271–82.
203. Selman L, Siegert R, Harding R, Gysels M, Speck P, Irene MA, Higginson J. A psychometric evaluation of measures of spirituality validated in culturally diverse palliative care populations. J Pain Symptom Manage. 2011;28:315–21.
204. Puchalski CM, Lunsford B, Harris M, Miller RT. Interdisciplinary spiritual care for seriously ill and dying patients palliative and supportive care: a collaborative model. Cancer J. 2006;12:398–416.
205. Kernohens WG, Waldron M, McAfee C, Cochrane B, Hasson F. An evidence base for a palliative care chaplaincy service in Northern Ireland. Palliat Med. 2007;21(6):510.
206. Puchalski CM, Lunsford B, Miller T. Interdisciplinary spiritual care for seriously ill and dying patients: a collaborative model. Cancer J. 2006;12:398–413.
207. Ross L. Spiritual aspects of nursing. J Adv Nurs. 1994;15:439–47.
208. Bonevski R, Sanson-Fisher A, Girgis L, Burton P, Cook A. Evaluation of an instrument to assess the needs of patients with cancer. Supportive Care Review Group. Cancer. 2000;88:217–25.
209. Draper P. An integrative review of spiritual assessment: implications for nursing management. J Nurs Manag. 2012;20:970–80.
210. Fitchett G, Risk JL. Screening for spiritual struggle. J Pastoral Care Counsel. 2009;63(1-2):1–12.
211. McSherry W. Spiritual assessment definition, categorisation and features. In: McSherry W, Ross L, editors. Spiritual assessment in healthcare practice. Keswick: M&K Update; 2013. p. 57–78.
212. Healthcare Chaplaincy Network. Spiritual care and nursing: a nurse's contribution and practice; 2017. https://spiritualcareassociation.org/docs/resources/nurses_spiritual_care_white_paper.
213. Puchalski CM. Restorative medicine. In: Cobb M, Puchalski CM, Rumbold B, editors. Oxford textbook of spirituality in healthcare. New York: Oxford University Press; 2014. p. 197–210.

214. Timmins F, Caldeira S, Pujol N, Weathers E, Whelan J, Flanagan B. The role of the healthcare chaplain. J Health Care Chaplain. 2018;24:87–106.
215. Luchetti G, et al. Taking a spiritual history in clinical practice: a systematic review of instruments. Explore. 2013;9:159–70.
216. Healthcare Chaplaincy Network. Spiritual care and nursing: a nurses's contribution and practice (White Paper); 2017. https://spiritualcareassociation.org/docs/resources/nurses_spiritual_care_white_paper.
217. Tanyi RA. Spirituality and family nursing assessment spiritual assessment and interventions for families. J Adv Nurs. 2006;53:287–94.
218. JCAHO. http://www.uphs.upenn.edu/pastoral/resed/jcahorefs.html.
219. Ross L, McSherry W. Two questions that ensure person centred spiritual care. Nursing Standard [Internet]. 2018. Available from: https://rcni.com/nursing-standard/features/two-questionsensure-person-centred-spiritual-care-137261.
220. Watson J. Nursing: the philosophy and science of caring. In: Smith MC, Turkel MC, Wolf ZR, editors. Caring in nursing classics: an essential resource. New York: Springer; 2013. p. 143–53.
221. Whelan J. The caring imperative: a hallmark in nursing education. In: Lee SM, Palmeiri PA, Watson J, editors. Global advances in human caring literacy. New York: Springer; Watson Science Caring Institute; 2017. p. 33–42.
222. Caldeira S, Timmins F. Implementing spiritual care interventions. Nurs Stand. 2017;31:54–60.
223. Morse J. Negotiating commitment and involvement in the nurse-patient relationship. J Adv Nurs. 1991;16:455–68.
224. Pulchaski CM, Lunsford B. The relationship of spirituality and compassion in health care (White Paper). Kalamazoo: Fetzer Institute; 2008.
225. Bradshaw A. Teaching spiritual care to nurses: an alternative approach. Int J Palliat Nurs. 1997;3:51–7.
226. Watson J. Caring science as sacred science. Philadelphia PA: F. A. Davis; 2005.

Working with Diversity: An Overview of Diversity in Contemporary Society and the Effect of This on Healthcare Situations

12

Gayatri Nambiar-Greenwood

Abstract

In this age of digital and social media, there is a need for a consideration of individual spiritual needs within the infinite forms of diversities found within any population in today's globalised world. Faced with the endless range of individualities, this chapter considers concepts, such as development of individual identities of culture, the dominant influences of cultural perception (such as media and politics) and the personal experience of intersectional processes in shaping personal needs, wants and notions of spirituality.

Abbreviations

BAME Black and Minority Ethnic Groups
UK   United Kingdom
UNHCR United Nations High Commission for Refugees
WHO   World Health Organization

12.1 Introduction

The fundamental ethos behind encompassing spirituality within holistic nursing and all forms of healthcare is its focus on individuality and what has been described as a unique 'inner, intangible dimension' ([1], p. 1140) in which a person finds personal meaning and self-purpose. There is concern, however, that patients being

G. Nambiar-Greenwood (✉)
Faculty of Health, Psychology and Social Care, Manchester Metropolitan University, Manchester, UK
e-mail: G.Nambiar-Greenwood@mmu.ac.uk

© Springer Nature Switzerland AG 2019
F. Timmins, S. Caldeira (eds.), *Spirituality in Healthcare: Perspectives for Innovative Practice*, https://doi.org/10.1007/978-3-030-04420-6_12

admitted to hospital are not having their spirituality or faith needs met and may be suffering personal consequences as a result. In an increasingly diverse and complex environment, healthcare staff may find themselves not prepared for the resourcefulness such a role requires of them.

The consideration of the spiritual needs for the varying forms of diversities found within any population in today's globalised world, however, requires a mind shift from limiting identifications and conversations regarding cultural care. In order to grapple with the infinite range of individualities, a number of concepts, such as personal identities of culture, the dominant influences of cultural perception and the personal experience of intersectional processes, need to be considered in order to show their inextricable link in shaping human behaviour and self-identity.

12.2 Personal Identities of Culture

In order to understand any patient, a fundamental place to begin the process needs to occur within the nurses, themselves. By understanding how each one of us is part of our diverse population and how our cultural individualities develop and co-exist, it provides a basis of a more open and less judgemental perspective to seeing how we perceive our patients and their diversities.

12.2.1 Defining One's Cultural Self

The ideas around culture, regardless of their various definitions and purposes, all have in common a number of shared characteristics that add to the inescapability and complexity of the concept for each one of us. Culture is expressed through multiple layers of complexity. This complexity is often variably addressed in terms of 'levels' in sociological and anthropological literature. One example of this is by the seminal writer on culture [2].

At one level, tertiary culture occurs when it is recognisable and evident as an observable appearance. Ideas such as a dress code, a regional dialect, fashionable trends in healthy food or the manner in which people address each other [3] would be considered tertiary culture.

At the secondary level, culture is demonstrated when values are expressed by individuals and in their rationalisations as to why they behave the way they do. The core reasons for a certain person's behaviour will be either unconscious or purposefully hidden; despite what they may express are the intentions or rationalisations for that behaviour or what they would preferably like those reasons to be [4]. At this secondary level, culture becomes less explicit but manifests as underlying rules, such as those of jargon or the colloquial way a common language is spoken. It tends to be known to members of a group but not shared with outsiders.

The final manifestation of culture, the primary level, can be associated to basic underlying assumptions [5]. Underlying assumptions are an unconscious revelation of culture, and it is that which actually determines how individuals or groups perceive, think and feel about themselves and 'Others'.[1] At this most implicit level, rules are embedded and taken for granted and, at times, even unexplainable by even that person or group. It is rarely spoken about, yet known to that entire group.

All the different levels of culture together influence an individual's behaviour and the interpretations of that same behaviour by 'Others'. Tsai [6] makes an important argument that although certain aspects of culture are overtly visible, their related meanings and reasoning remain invisible. Figure 12.1 illustrates the complexity of an individuals' culture by comparing it to an iceberg, in that what can be seen on the outside is restricted and does not reflect the values and personal historical influences that a person has experienced. This seminal idea of comparing a person's culture to an iceberg was originally utilised by Hall [2] but has incorporated some concepts around faith and spirituality for the purpose of this chapter.

So, a certain stance, behaviour or gesture in one society, which is deemed friendly, may be considered rude in another, as the underlying reason for the action is unknown to those who may find it offensive. In addition, Hofstede [7] also suggests that how we perceive ourselves, express and behave culturally is also influenced by the dimensions of individualism-collectivism within our own group. The idea of individualism-collectivism is the range of feelings, beliefs and behavioural intentions intrinsic within a group, related to the degree of independence or solidarity and expressed degrees of concern for others [8]. Therefore, some communities may see their individual role or place within the identity of a wider group, rather than as a singular experience.

However, ideas around personal or cultural self-identity are interchangeable either being an individual construct or a social construct. Cultural self-identity reveals itself as an interchangeable collective set of characteristics by which a person is recognisable or known [9]. These may be behavioural or a personal characteristic founded on the notion that it mimics someone else's characteristic.

Bringing the various 'levels' of culture together, in conversation, the individual cultural construct gives meaning to 'I' or 'me', while a more social identity supports that meaning and allows a person to speak of the 'we'. This supports the fact that an individual's cultural 'self-identity' is mainly unconscious and constructed by the context they find themselves in at that time. In other words, our behaviour and expressions of our cultural self are dependent on whom we are with, at that moment. It is sometimes overtly obvious but mainly subtle.

Our social identity also changes, modifies and adapts over time by being influenced at a personal level, genetically and socially [10], and externally, through history and politics and by the media [11]. The culture of an individual or group is never a static experience. Your understanding of the personal attributes you hold of yourself in society can be at times accepting or non-accepting of yourself and of 'Others' within your environment. The aspect of cultural self-identity that an individual chooses to identify their self with could be selected interchangeably, among others, from a social, psychological, ethnic, powerful or helpless persona or through

---

[1] 'Others' here represents anyone who we see differently from our group we are operating within at that moment. Thus, it could be personal, professional, ethnic, nationalistic, etc.

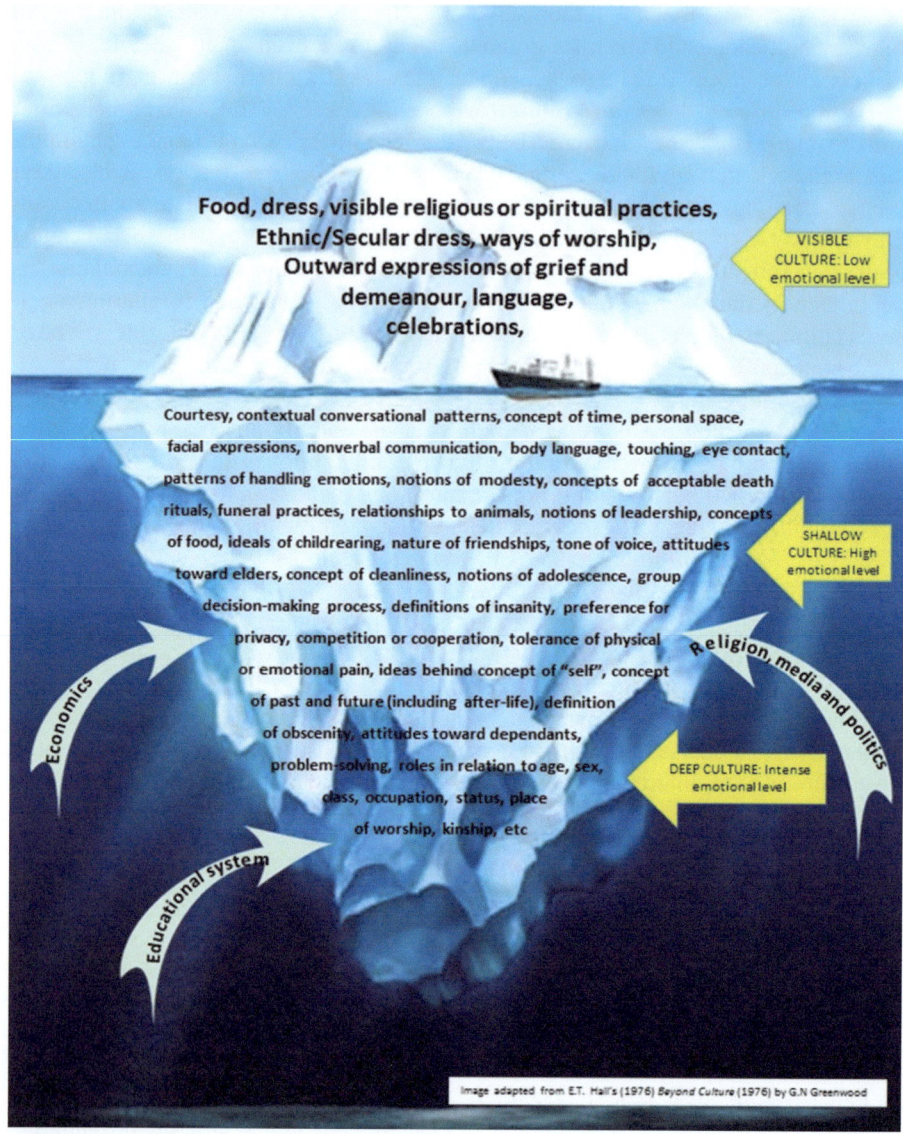

Fig. 12.1 Cultural Iceberg: visualisation of a person's visible and invincible culture

a gender or class label at the same time [12]. In addition, individuals and communities, due to the persistence of derogatory labels from external sources and stigma, can also, over time, internalise and adopt the negative self-identities assigned to them [13, 14]. An example of this can be seen in groupings such as 'gang culture'.

However, culture, in whatever form it takes or academic representation it originates from, is never an autonomous whole, uniquely distinctive or idiosyncratic.

Culture and cultural self-identity is porous. Factors such as the diffuse notions of identity [15]; the de-territorialised links between members of a group through resettlement [16]; and the varieties of rules, regulations and norms that guide verbal and non-verbal communication [17] together ensure its malleability to the individual person, at a point in time.

It is imperative to note that groups that appear overtly similar in terms of language and appearance cannot genuinely be considered monocultural because of the varying subtleties of the culture for each person. In any diverse and multicultural country, culture cannot only be a feature of Black, Asian and Minority Ethnic (BAME) groups [18] but the countless differences within the Majority population and groups beyond the limitations of race and ethnicity [19]. As early as 1958, Williams [20] was already expressing the intricacy of the nature of culture within all our everyday lives and stated that 'culture is ordinary': so ordinary that we do not see it until we are, one way or another, challenged by differences in what we expect and accept as the norm.

Another aspect that would cause the failure of addressing the spiritual needs of a diverse population is the lack of inclusion of the Majority population outside those who are considered to be diverse and at times, without cultural needs. It is too simplistic to look at changes in culture only from the perspective of changes to the BAME population, as people from all backgrounds adapt, change and evolve socially and culturally through time [21]. For example, since the 1950s, the Majority population in the United Kingdom (UK) has undergone a transformation in the way they see themselves culturally, among others, through a process of formalised legal changes in the country [22]. At that time, abortion and homosexuality became legal, capital punishment ended and measures were taken to improve the position of women and other minorities, economically, socially and politically. Regional cultures, habits and preferences, such as dialects, had previously been 'taught away' in schools [23] and rejected by the wider media. However, these idiosyncrasies have now developed into something to be proud of, reducing the perpetuation of the idea of cultural homogeneity or monoculturalism of the Majority population [24, 25]. Over a period of five decades, there has been a continued selection and adaptation of choices in customs or everyday practices such as food or festivals, between migrants and the Majority population, which has resulted in a form of 'hybridisation' of cultures [26].

12.2.2 Factors Influencing Culture

Generally, considerations around diversity and culture tend to be narrowed down to ethnicity, race, organised faith or religion and migrants [27]. This persisting narrative negatively affects discussions around diversity and on equality and fairness in healthcare.

The strongest influencers of culture are politics and history and are then perpetuated by the mass media [11]. Everyday political, mass media and historical conversations regarding culture tend to focus on BAME populations and their differences from a unknown collective of 'us', mainly relating such comparisons to the Majority population.

Having considered the concepts that influence the diffuse notions of cultural self-identity, this section will look at how this awareness then affects how we consciously and unconsciously perceive those outside our cultural location. Also, the notion of the cultural 'Other' is necessary within this chapter, as the perceptions around this concept affect the way individuals distinguish between different forms of cultural identities, needs and associated social activity. Within this, nurses and patients perceiving each other as the cultural 'Other' will impact the relationship they will have and the expectations and delivery of spiritual care.

Piller [28] states that the sense of belonging (or otherwise) to a community has an effect on the way individuals or groups 'culturally' behave, perceive and communicate with each other. This cultural behaviour is part of the Majority population's self-identities and not just BAME populations. They also expressed that the question of difference is emotive: it promotes ideas about 'them' and 'us'; a sense of belonging or otherwise; membership or ostracisation from groups; and how to define 'us' in relation to others or the 'Other'. From this, we get ideas about communities, sometimes-imagined communities and even ethno-national boundaries.

The notion of the cultural 'Other' comes from an imagined idea of difference, either superior or inferior, to the cultural self-identity or social identities that may represent the norm [29]. Discussion about this concept is normally found in literature regarding racism [30], gender perceptions [31] and observations regarding disability [32], to name a few. The idea of 'Otherness' is central to the analyses of how Majority and BAME identities are constructed [33].

In childhood, identifying with the cultural 'Other' is a natural process of choice, towards those familiar and those our families identify and feel safe with. As we grow, the process of constructing or perpetuating a cultural 'Other' is amplified by subjective feelings of insecurity, chaos and vulnerability. Cleveland et al. [34] state that as a rule, the negative subjective feelings that are caused by social, economic and political concerns regarding 'Others' coming into a familiar group always result in some form of tension. These unconscious biases result in the ensuing struggles acted out by these groups or in the mass media and by politicians, with arguments inevitably being reconstructed around differences in cultural identities. Not unique to any community, from this emerges ideas that are ethnocentric, which is the root of racism. Ethnocentrism is the belief that your cultural or ethnic group remains superior to all other cultural and ethnic groups. With ethnocentrism, the acceptance or perception of all 'Other' cultural practices is compared negatively to your own. These challenges and arguments that surround cultural self-identity will be then made meaningful by a dependence on religious or ideological values, beliefs, myths and narratives and become framed within a general moral gauge of 'good' or 'evil' [35].

Another form of ethnocentrism is for a group to distinguish themselves as 'cultureless', thus normal. The personal perception that culture is 'exotic' and seen only through the lens of festivals and different foods reduces the understanding of the intrinsic everyday feature of culture and diversity.

Although politically, in Western societies, the role of religion as a central certainty has been considered to have lost its cultural relevancy, it has, over the past few decades, become reimagined as a cultural symbol of identity, which further perpetuates the construction of 'self' and 'Others' [36].

With the massive acceleration of globalising trends in the past decade, including changes to economic interdependence and fears around mass migration, nations and national identities have been subject to considerable transformations that affect intercultural communications and behaviour [37]. Gallagher [38] feels that the construction of the cultural 'Other' had worsened in the past decade because of manipulation by politicians and a sensationalist media. Society, at large, looks for targets to vent their worsening frustrations on during times of economic stress. Studies as early as 2003, such as Miles and Brown [39], the UNHCR report [40] and, more recently, the UK 2014 National Social Attitude survey [41], had noted that it remains commonplace for politicians and the mass media to adopt a more nationalistic stance of intolerance, often to increase electoral popularity or to increase sales of publications through sensationalism.

Some examples of these have become apparent since the most recent European economic downturn of the past decade. It has become more familiar for politicians across the political spectrum and the media to make unguarded and unsubstantiated comments for their own gain [42, 43]. With this, the negative targeting of some British-born groups who share a variety of extrinsic traits with those undergoing this widely broadcasted negative scrutiny has been emerging, as they report experiences of a newer emerging discrimination previously not seen by them [44, 45]. Reese and Lewis [46] and Legault et al. [47] argued that this rhetoric becomes instrumental in our internalisation of what we see as the truth over a period of time and with it, our internalisation of what makes up the cultural identity of 'Others' and ourselves. McCroskey [48] referred to this as 'intercultural communication apprehension', where a fear or anxiety associated with either real or anticipated communication with people from different groups, especially cultural and/or ethnic groups' ([48], p. 148), becomes ingrained with a persistent rhetoric from politics and the media. In essence, people who have high levels of intercultural communication apprehension will innately have communication problems stemming from their fear or anxiety and limit communication with those who fit the idea of the 'Other'. The fears around intercultural communication, however, will be blamed upon society becoming more politically correct.

12.3 The Two-Way Process of Intercultural Communication

Theories of cultural care can often frame conversations with patients in an 'etic' way. An 'etic' slant to learning about diversity and culture utilises the worldview that would have originated from outside the culture being studied, looking inward towards the patient approach. Taking into account the discussion in the previous section regarding the perception of how we may see ourselves dependent on what 'Others' may think of us, with an etic approach to appreciating diversities, the nurse remains outside the experience of providing spiritual care from his or her perspective, not the patients'.

What is more effective would be for the nurse to be aware with the impact of authority and establishment of trust as being crucial to the ease at which the communication process takes place, in a more 'emic' approach. Central to an 'emic' approach to the communication process is the aptitude of the nurse to be reflective, culturally self-aware and have the ability to listen to the patient's narrative in a non-ethnocentric manner. The nurse also needs to consider the impact of social and organise structures in enabling or inhibiting communication, cultural practices and health lifestyles. As such, they consider the provision of effective spiritual care, with the nurse keeping in mind individual differences, as opposed to providing care regardless of individual differences and seeing the 'Other' only as a member of a bigger group. Cultural care theories such as Papadopoulos' [49] transcultural health and social care model and Ramsden's [50] model of cultural safety specifically developed these 'emic' ideas within their frameworks, ensuring the nurse understands his or her role in inhibiting or promoting effective cultural conversations.

In addition to those aspects discussed in the last section that provide the characteristics of individuals' culture, there are two significant intersubjective factors that influence how we behave and interact with others. At one level, the varying determinants of health have a role in deciding the choices we are able to make to live our life in a certain way. Interconnected to this are our intersectional experiences of the determinants, which together influence how our patients are choose to interact with us.

12.3.1 The Social Determinants of Our Health

WHO [51] describes the social determinants of health as the conditions in which people are born, grow up, live, work and age and the systems put in place by their country, in order to deal with health and illness. As shown by the arrows underneath the iceberg in Fig. 12.1 which are the wider influencing factors, these circumstances are in turn shaped by a wider set of forces: economics, social policies and the political ethos of a country at varying points.

The way society at international, national or local level organises its matters gives rise to systems of social position and hierarchy. Although not unique, populations generally tend to organise itself according to income, education, employment, gender and ethnicity, among others. Where people are in the social hierarchy, this can affect the conditions in which they then grow, learn, and live and also their understanding, susceptibility and the consequences of ill health. All of these influence how they live culturally, how they perceive themselves and how they are perceived by others.

12.3.2 Intersectionality/Intersectional Processes

Intersectionality refers to those coinciding or intersecting shared identities and the experience of interconnected structures of discrimination that all of us may experience. Together, this can cause multiple layers of exclusion and influences the culture an individual adopts or exists within [52]. During any interaction, the nurse and patients' social and professional positions (such as gender, ethnicity, immigration status, personal journey, political and professional beliefs, biases, to emotional responses to patients, among others) unconsciously influence the way a two-way conversation takes place. This moves ideas around learning or caring for people in a diverse community, from just asking questions about personal preferences to a more therapeutic person-centred interaction.

Scollon et al. [53] and McIntosh et al. [54] found that health professionals needed to be aware of these intersubjective issues when communicating with a patient of any culture. They expressed the need for the nurse to listen without making pre-judgements to them while being aware of issues around authority, hierarchy, status, and subordination and appreciating the symbolic and contextual impact of the conversation to the outcome of the meeting for it to be successful.

All communication encounters dynamically move between these areas in one conversation, as symbols and contexts of communication represent different things to those involved in the conversation [55]. However, considering all conversations involved more than one person, a nurse's exercise of authority, at times, could also work in the patients' favour where a conversation is stilted due to the participants' previous experiences. Reciprocal conversations, as Lindgren [56] stated, need to be productive and mutual, with the understanding that both sides bring their own histories with them.

12.4 Becoming Aware of Ethnocentricity and Intercultural Communication Apprehension

Developing cultural self-awareness is the foundation to reducing ethnocentricity and dealing with intercultural communication apprehension. A consideration of self-awareness 'crucially contributes towards one's understanding of the nature and construction of their cultural identity' ([49], p. 10). Engaging in a reflexive self-awareness, however, can be an uncomfortable exercise for anyone, as it requires people to be honest about previous errors, their ethnocentricities and personally held prejudices. Nurses with a lack of self-awareness about their own ethnocentric views or paternalistic attitudes can immediately stifle the communication process from being a mutually beneficial experience [57]. In addition, the belief that by just working in a multiethnic environment can develop the affective constructs such as cultural sensitivity, competence and desire could fail to manifest, if the management support for such an environment is absent [58].

The first thing to remember in this situation is that ethnocentricity and prejudice are universal behaviours: not unique to any community, country nor group of people. We are all innately prejudiced. However, the lack of awareness of our strongly held worldviews, as superior to others has the potential to do unspeakable emotional and psychological harm to our patients. There needs to be a clear and honest discussion around how our professional values are affected by our personal values. Professional values may be the guiding beliefs and principles that influence work behaviour; however, it is inevitable our personal values and those ideas we have grown up with influence the conversations we choose to have or ignore the patient by.

It is important to note the completion of statutory strategies regarding diversity and equality cannot be seen as solution enough for improving our understanding about diversity. For example, diversity and equality training that is now compulsory for all UK National Health Service staff consists of the utilisation of online courses that concentrate on the law around equality and diversity. However, these online exercises do not take into account that completing a tool about being fair to 'Others' could add to intercultural communication apprehension as those participating can feel they are being judged, instead of a more time-consuming safe space to deliberate the origins of all our learnt prejudices.

Despite the personal responsibility of reducing ethnocentricity and becoming aware of intercultural communication apprehension, there needs to be a supportive, strong, safe environment and leadership for it to be effective in terms of patient care [59]. Within this, there needs to be awareness that reflection as a process can result in a greater suppressed self-determined 'prejudice regulation' if it not facilitated or managed effectively and done just as a 'tick-box' activity [60]. It results in nurses providing socially desirable or politically correct responses so as not to appear biased or prejudiced without any real critical reflection [61, 62]. Duffy [63] and Jirwe et al. [64] have found that nurses, nurse educators and health and social care professionals often avoid any form of analyses that challenge the dominance of Western political and cultural systems. Encouraging a safe atmosphere to reflect on the origins of our prejudices, which are present in everyone's behaviour, provides a more neutral starting place for all nurses.

Research by Nambiar-Greenwood [65] found that for both the participants from her study (from both the Majority and BAME populations) voiced their concern over how nurses, in their previous experiences, had unconsciously stereotyped or assumed their needs (or lack of need) by outward appearances or regional accents. The patients from the Majority population were not asked if they had any specific needs and the BAME participants in particular expressed the homogenisation of their overall culture.

Another factor that the participants of this study felt would influence the success or failure of understanding diversity was related to sensitivities surrounding conversations around culture in Western societies. All the participants from the BAME groups expressed that nurses are needed to be less anxious and be interested in questioning aspects of their culture that may be deemed sensitive, as a way of improving their illness experience. For example, two South Asian, Muslim participants expressed that nurses had adopted an oversensitive politically correct stance, avoided questioning and made assumptions about their needs, which then made the provision of spiritual care for them ineffective.

This avoidance and anxiety of questioning is connected to the perpetuation of the mass media regarding BAME communities apparently becoming overly sensitive. This is where real or anticipated communication with people from different groups, especially cultural and/or ethnic groups, results in avoidance or stereotyping. These fears and anxieties could also be related either to personal fears of appearing offensive or discriminatory, perpetuated by the mass media [66], or to ethnocentricity [67].

According to Van Boven [68], the pressure to appear politically correct can have important consequences for the way people conduct intercultural communication. Despite private doubts, in order not to appear racist, sexist or culturally insensitive, a person (or community) could adopt a more defensive but socially acceptable reaction to what has come to be perceived as socially charged incidences. This pressure could lead to 'pluralistic ignorance': a situation in which a majority of group members may privately reject a norm, but incorrectly assume that most others accept it, and therefore go along with it [69]. The danger remains that this apprehension will reduce the ability of nurses to really listen or hear the patients' needs due to long-term held ethnocentricities and stereotyping prejudices.

Another issue with the ideas perpetuated around intercultural communication apprehension was that, as a reaction to not wanting to be perceived as racist or discriminatory, the nurse feels unable to challenge any behaviours of the service user, even if it is harmful to them [70] or unlawful [71]. Consequently, in some societies that have had more exposure to the notions of political correctness and the development of anti-discriminatory legislation, there is an experience of people feeling judged and fearful of being blamed for potentially sensitive subjects [72]. Individuals from both sides worry about how 'Others' view them as representatives of their social identity groups. They also feel inhibited and afraid to address even the most banal issues directly, such as questions about the correct pronunciation of the other person's name or culture. As a consequence, without really listening to service user's stories, private conclusions are drawn based on stereotypes, previous judgements and ideas perpetuated by the media, among others; then unconfirmed, these assumptions become immutable [73] and part of the information we use to care.

Central to challenging the insecurities surrounding the negative interpretation of political correctness or intercultural communication apprehension remains the art of effective questioning and listening. The assessment process at admission, despite having to pay attention to the immediate reasons for hospitalisation, needs to take into account their associated anxieties, their ideas of support and the factors beyond that illness that defined how they see themselves at that point.

Intercultural communication apprehension and ethnocentricity is, however, never a one-way process. Intercultural communication apprehension from the perspective of the service user also has an impact on the success of CAC being successful. Service users themselves, as unique individuals with unique horizons, bring with them their socialised or learnt apprehension to sharing their needs with the nurse. As Taylor et al. [74] stressed individuals from a more collectivist community, whatever their ethnicity may not be as willing to share their needs or problems with

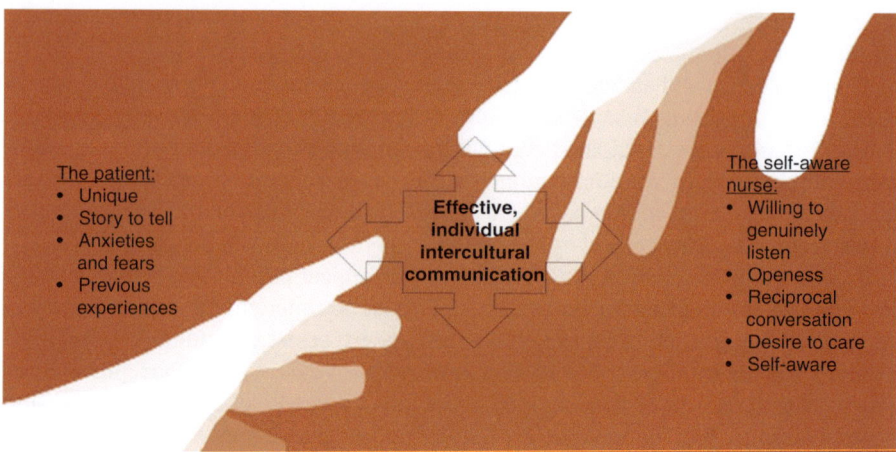

Fig. 12.2 A two-way reciprocal intercultural communication

the nurse. This may be because the person normally, within their community context, avoids bringing their personal problems to the attention of others or seeking support because of the perception that such an act can weaken the harmony of their bigger social group.

In dealing with our long-held ethnocentricities, and being aware of where our apprehensions in intercultural communication influence the way we communicate with a diverse society, it provides us with a more neutral foundation for effective intercultural communication. It allows us to hear our patients, with open mind to what they might have to say, need and want from spiritual care (Fig. 12.2).

12.5 Conclusion

Having an appreciation for diversity is not an experience or perspective that can be limited to extrinsic visible differences in individuals. The ability to provide effective spiritual care to a diverse community needs nurses and nurse educators to perceive it as a fundamental idea that has the ability to open up a holistic way of thinking about delivering individualistic care. The nurse needs to be able to see patterns of human behaviour beyond racial, ethnic, religious or social groupings. The nurse must be able to 'see' groupings culture in age, generation, disability, body image or varying types of mental illness. Within this, they also need to maintain flexibility by appreciating the construct of subcultures. Assessing diverse needs should not be extra or for 'special people'. It is not successful just by learning about 'Other' BAME groups' needs in terms of diet or prayer. This does not excuse the nurse from not learning about the differences and main tenets of the communities within which she or he works, but ultimately, the provision of spiritual care needs to be based on fairness and compassion for all patients, as we all have certain wants, needs and preferences during an illness experience.

Appendix: Scenarios

Travelling Family

Milly Smith is a 66-year-old woman who has just arrived in the A&E department with an exacerbation of her long-term chronic lung condition (chronic obstructive pulmonary disease), with a high temperature and dangerously low oxygen saturation levels (a pyrexia of 38.7 and saturated oxygen of 88%). She requires admission, for IV antibiotics and further care and investigations. Milly has been a heavy smoker (20–30 cigarettes a day) since the age of 10. She was diagnosed with this terminal condition approximately 10 years ago, and it has been recommended by a number of previous consultants that she access end-of-live palliative care services. Due to the transient nature of their lives, Milly has been unable to do so.

A devout Catholic, Milly was born into a travelling community and has moved around the United Kingdom and Western Europe throughout her lifetime. She and her family are currently based on an illegal campsite in the North West of England, and the local council is trying to evict the community from here in the next few days. She has 15 supportive adult children, between the ages of 24 and 51, the first child being born when Edna was 16. A widow of 4 years, Milly is very much a matriarch within her family and local community. She is accompanied in A&E by five adult daughters who are very concerned about their mum but express concern about her being admitted as it is likely that they will be moved on by the council in the next day or two. She is also distressed as they worship together on Sundays, in a shared communal way. The eldest daughter explains that her father died in hospital and the family experienced negative and racist treatment from the hospital staff.

1. What are the main issues that individuals and families who choose not to have a permanent address face in accessing healthcare? What can be done to facilitate her spiritual needs in this instance that makes her feel valued?
2. What are the differences between Gypsies, Roma, Travellers and New Age Travellers?
3. What issues may inhibit or limit how freely Milly and her family communicate with you?
4. How do programmes like 'My Big Fat American Gypsy Weddings' or other programmes that denigrate gypsy and traveller families influence our unconscious bias regarding Milly and her family?

Jewish Community

Joel Abrahams is a 48-year-old Orthodox Jewish man who has been admitted to a local psychiatric inpatient service due to an exacerbation of his enduring episodes of clinical depression. The nurses are reporting him not to be cooperative with any organised group work as he does show any interest in taking part in the activities provided by the unit, such as watching movies, playing pool or the weekly exercise group. He is also particularly uncomfortable in taking part in any mixed gender group activity.

Joel has, during one of his previous admissions, mistakenly been diagnosed as having obsessive-compulsive disorder due to the psychiatrist not appreciating his religious practice of the concept of 'scrupulosity' and his desire for repetitive prayer throughout the day, accompanied by chanting and swaying. He also only dresses in the traditional religious manner of his community.

1. What are the factors that may reduce Joel's ability to communicate freely and effectively with health and social care staff?
2. What actions can be taken in relation to balancing Joel's religious or spiritual needs and the needs for the service for him to engage in activities that are alien to him and his daily life, his privacy and his dignity?
3. How does knowing about Joel's previous diagnosis of obsessive-compulsive disorder influence our unconscious behaviour/bias towards him?
4. What are the intersectional factors from Joel's perspective that influence his health?

References

1. Narayanasamy A. The puzzle of spirituality for nursing: a guide to practical assessment. Br J Nurs. 2004;13(19):1140–4.
2. Hall ET. Beyond culture. New York: Anchor Book; 1976.
3. Nakai M. Social differentiation of cultural taste and practice in contemporary Japan: nonhierarchical asymmetric cluster analysis. In: Data science. Cham: Springer; 2017. p. 149–59.
4. Spencer-Oatey H. Culturally speaking: culture, communication and politeness theory. London: Bloomsbury Publishing; 2008.
5. Applebaum RP, Carr D, Duneir M, Giddens A. Conformity, deviance, and crime. In: Introduction to sociology. New York: W. W. Norton & Company, Inc; 2009.
6. Tsai JL. Ideal affect: cultural causes and behavioral consequences. Perspect Psychol Sci. 2007;2(3):242–59.
7. Hofstede G. Culture's consequences: comparing values, behaviors, institutions, and organizations across nations. 2nd ed. Thousand Oaks: Sage; 2001.
8. Brewer MB, Chen YR. Where (who) are collectives in collectivism? Toward conceptual clarification of individualism and collectivism. Psychol Rev. 2007;114(1):133.
9. Hodos T. Local and global perspectives in the study of social and cultural identities. In: Hales S, Hodos T, editors. Material culture and social identities in the Ancient World. Cambridge: Cambridge University Press; 2010.
10. Clarke S. Culture and identity: the Sage handbook of cultural analysis. London: Sage; 2008.
11. Triandis HC, Trafimow D. Culture and its implications for intergroup behaviour. In: Brown SL, editor. Blackwell handbook of social psychology: Intergroup processes, vol. 3; 2001. p. 367–85.
12. Fiske ST, Taylor SE. Social cognition: from brains to culture. London: Sage; 2013.
13. Rew L, Arheart KL, Johnson K, Spoden M. Changes in ethnic identity and competence in middle adolescents. J Transcult Nurs. 2015;26(3):227–33.
14. Yap SCY, Anusic I, Donnellan MB, Lucas RE. Evidence of self-informant agreement in ethnic identity. Soc Psychol Personal Sci. 2014;5(8):865–72.

15. Berry JW. Acculturation: living successfully in two cultures. Int J Intercult Relat. 2005;29(6):697–712.
16. Papastergiadis N. The turbulence of migration: globalization, deterritorialization and hybridity. 2nd ed. Cambridge: Polity Press; 2013.
17. Carbaugh D. Cultural communication and intercultural contact. East Sussex: Routledge; 2013.
18. Cortis JD. Culture, values and racism: application to nursing. Int Nurs Rev. 2003;50:55–64.
19. Hunt LM. Beyond cultural competence: applying humility to cultural settings. Park Ridge Cent Bull. 2001;24:3–4.
20. William R. Culture is ordinary. In: Szeman I, Kaposy T, editors. Cultural theory: an anthology. West Sussex: Wiley-Blackwell; 1958. p. 92–100.
21. Ghosh B. Cultural changes in the era of globalisation. J Dev Soc. 2011;27(2):173–5.
22. Black. Britain since the seventies. Edinburgh: Reaktion Books; 2004.
23. Trudghill P. Social differentiation in Norwich. Cambridge: Cambridge University Press; 1974.
24. Bassi C. Multiculturalism, racism and class. Workers Libery Online; 2007.
25. Gunew S. Haunted nations: The colonial dimensions of multiculturalism. London: Routledge; 2004.
26. Nedeerveen-Pieterse J. Oriental globalisation: past and present. In: Delanty G, editor. Europe and Asia beyond east and west: towards a new cosmopolitanism. London: Routledge; 2006.
27. Horsti K, Titley G, Hulten G. National conversations: public service media and cultural diversity in Europe. Bristol: Intellect Books; 2014.
28. Piller I. Intercultural communication: a critical introduction. Edinburgh: Edinburgh University Press Ltd; 2011.
29. Miller J. Otherness. In: The SAGE Encyclopaedia of qualitative research methods. London: Sage; 2008.
30. Pon G. Cultural competency as new racism: an ontology of forgetting. J Progress Hum Serv. 2009;20(1):59–71.
31. Ghosh SR. The woman's body as cultural other: an Indian perspective. [Online]. n.d. www.brunel.ac.uk/Sumana-R.-Ghosh-The-Womans-Body-as-Cultural-Other.pdf. Accessed 10 Jan 2015.
32. O'Hara J. Learning disabilities and ethnicity: achieving cultural competence. Adv Psychiatr Treat. 2003;9(3):166–74.
33. Zevallos Z. What is otherness? [Online]. 2011. http://othersociologist.com. Accessed 6 June 2015.
34. Cleveland M, Laroche M, Pons F, Kastoun R. Acculturation and consumption: textures of cultural adaptation. Int J Intercult Relat. 2009;33(3):196–212.
35. Chen YW. Public engagement exercises with racial and cultural "others": some thoughts, questions, and considerations. J Publ Deliberation. 2014;10(1):14.
36. Goodwin M. UKIP shares more with the far right than it admits. The Guardian [Online]. 2012. https://www.theguardian.com/commentisfree/2012/mar/12/ukip-far-right-bnp. Accessed 13 Mar 2012.
37. Young M, Zuelow E, Sturm A. Nationalism in a global era: The persistence of nations. Abingdon: Routledge; 2007.
38. Gallagher CA. Blacks, Jews, gays and immigrants are taking over: how the use of polling data can distort reality and perpetuate inequality among immigrants. Ethn Racial Stud. 2014;37(5):731–7.
39. Miles R, Brown M. Racism. 2nd ed. London: Routledge; 2003.
40. United Nations High Commissioner for Refugees (UNHCR). Asylum in the industrial world, State of the World's Refugees, Chapter 7: pp. 55–185. 2000. http://www.unhcr.org/3ebf9bb87.html. Accessed 13 Mar 2015.
41. Blinder S. UK public opinion toward immigration: overall attitudes and level of concern. The Migration Observatory at the University of Oxford [Online]. 2014. www.migrationobservatory.ox.ac.uk. Accessed 9 Apr 2015.
42. Martin A, Stevens J. Sold out! Flights and buses full as Romanians and Bulgarians head for the UK. The Daily Mail [Online]. 2013. http://www.dailymail.co.uk/news/article-2531440/Sold-Flights-buses-Romanians-Bulgarians-head-UK.html. Accessed 14 Feb 2014.

43. Okojie I. You say bongo-bongo, I say bigot. The Observer [Online]. 2013. http://www.observer.co.uk/comment. Accessed 12 Aug 2013.
44. Masocha S. Asylum seekers in media and parliamentary discourses. In: Asylum seekers, social work and racism. Basingstoke: Palgrave Macmillan; 2015. p. 40–69.
45. Thomas P. The silent majority? White people, multiculturalism and the challenge of 'Englishness. In: British Sociological Association Annual Conference, 3rd–5th April 2013, London, 2013.
46. Reese SD, Lewis SC. Framing the war on terror: the internalization of policy in the US press. Journalism. 2009;10(6):777–97.
47. Legault L, Green-Demers I, Eadie AL. When internalization leads to automatization: the role of self-determination in automatic stereotype suppression and implicit prejudice regulation. Motiv Emot. 2009;33(1):10–24.
48. McCroskey JC. An introduction to rhetorical communication: a Western rhetorical Perspective. 9th ed. Boston: Allyn and Bacon; 2006.
49. Papadopoulos I. Transcultural health and social care: development of culturally competent practitioners. London: Churchill Livingstone; 2006.
50. Ramsden IM. Cultural safety and nursing education in Aotearoa and Te Waipounamu. Ph.D. Victoria University of Wellington, New Zealand; 2002.
51. World Health Organization. WHO Commission on Social Determinants of Health and World Health Organization: closing the gap in a generation: health equity through action on the social determinants of health [Online]. Commission on Social Determinants of Health final report. 2008. Accessed 12 Jan 2017.
52. Yigwana N. Intersectionality of sexuality, inequality and poverty. Institute of Development Studies [Online]. 2015. http://www.ids.ac.uk/opinion/intersectionality-of-sexuality-inequality-and-poverty. Accessed 5 Jan 2016.
53. Scollon R, Scollon SW, Jones RH. Intercultural communication: a discourse approach. Malden: Wiley; 2012.
54. McIntosh I, Sim D, Robertson D. Anti-immigration hostility in Britain. Political Stud. 2004;55(4):709–32.
55. Samovar LA, Porter RE, McDaniel ER, Roy CS. Communication between cultures. Wadsworth: Cengage Learning; 2014.
56. Lindgren SA. Michel Foucault. In: Andersen H, Kaspersen LB, editors. Classical and modern social theory. Oxford: Blackwell Publishers; 2000. p. 294–308.
57. Pearce S, Pickard H. Finding the will to recover: philosophical perspectives on agency and the sick role. J Med Ethics. 2010;36(12):831–3.
58. Reimer-Kirkham SM. Making sense of difference: the social organization of intergroup relations in healthcare provision. Ph.D. University of British Columbia, Canada; 2000.
59. Briscoe L. Becoming culturally sensitive: a painful process? Midwifery. 2013;29(6):559–65.
60. Legault A, Ducharme F. Advocating for a parent with dementia in a long-term care facility: the process experienced by daughters. J Fam Nurs. 2009;15(2):198–219.
61. Lalwani AK, Shrum LJ, Chiu CY. Motivated response styles: the role of cultural values, regulatory focus, and self-consciousness in socially desirable responding. J Pers Soc Psychol. 2009;96(4):870.
62. Stocké PV. "Good farmers" as reflexive producers: an examination of family organic farmers in the US Midwest. Sociol Rural. 2007;47(2):83–102.
63. Duffy ME. A critique on cultural education in nursing. J Adv Nurs. 2001;36(4):487–95.
64. Jirwe M, Gerrish K, Emami A. Student nurses' experiences of communication in cross-cultural care encounters. Scand J Caring Sci. 2010;24:436–44.
65. Nambiar-Greenwood G. Culturally appropriate care: a qualitative exploration of service users perspective of nursing care. PhD Thesis. Manchester Metropolitan University; 2016.
66. Hong Y, Coleman J, Chan G, Wong RYM, Chiu C, Hansen IG. Predicting intergroup bias: the interactive effects of implicit theory and social identity. Personal Soc Psychol Bull. 2004;30:1035–47.

67. Wrench JS, Corrigan MW, McCroskey JM, Punyanunt-Carter NM. Religious fundamentalism and intercultural communication: the relationships among ethnocentrism, intercultural communication apprehension, religious fundamentalism, homonegativity, and tolerance for religious disagreements. J Intercult Commun Res. 2006;35(1):23–44.
68. Van Boven L. Pluralistic ignorance and political correctness: the case of affirmative action. Polit Psychol. 2000;21(2):267–76.
69. Prentice D. Pluralistic ignorance. In: Baumeister R, Vohs K, editors. Encyclopaedia of social psychology. Thousand Oaks: Sage; 2007. p. 674–5.
70. Jeffreys MR. Teaching cultural competence in nursing and health care: inquiry, action, and innovation. New York: Springer; 2015.
71. Hamilton J. Multicultural health care requires adjustments by doctors and patients. Can Med Assoc J. 1996;155(5):585–7.
72. Ely RJ, Meyerson D, Davidson MN. Rethinking political correctness. Harv Bus Rev [Online]. 2006. https://hbr.org/2006/09/rethinking-political-correctness. Accessed 15 June 2015.
73. Marques I. Transnational discourses on class, gender and cultural identity. Lafayette: Purdue University Press; 2011.
74. Taylor SE, Welch WT, Kim HS, Sherman DK. Cultural differences in the impact of social support on psychological and biological stress responses. Psychol Sci. 2007;18(9):831–7.

Being Human: Cultivating Mindfulness and Compassion for Daily Living

Kathleen Neenan

Abstract

Mindfulness practises are useful in allowing us a way to connect with ourselves, while developing an awareness of our physical self which can be a useful way of telling us what is going on in our life. Mindfulness can also enable us to be more connected with people around us and the environment in which we find ourselves.

The mindfulness and compassion practices presented will allow us to develop awareness, which will facilitate us to notice our experiences, patterns and habits. This increased awareness allows us to make choices of where we can focus our attention. The ability to stand back and see situations from a different perspective gives us the chance to choose how we react or respond to situations. It also gives us space to realise that we may be contributing to our distress and discomfort by how we react to situations.

The body may be used as an anchor for our mindfulness practice, for example, using the breath or soles of the feet while walking. The availability of these tools can help facilitate a daily mindfulness practice which can help lower stress and enhance daily living if practiced regularly. Daily meditation can become a ritual like bathing or brushing our teeth. Mindfulness can allow us to feel a greater connection with ourselves and with experiences in our bodies and our minds.

These mindfulness practices can be carried out with an attitude of kindness and gentleness which can bring us peace and clarity when we are in difficult situations and in relationships with others. These tools may also enable us to enhance our joy, compassion, peace, gratitude and forgiveness.

Neuroscientists have published thousands of papers over the last two decades showing the benefits of mindfulness and compassion practises. They have described how positive epigenetic and brain changes can happen even after eight hours of mindful loving-kindness training.

K. Neenan (✉)
School of Nursing and Midwifery, Trinity College, Dublin, Ireland
e-mail: kaneenan@tcd.ie

13.1 Introduction

The aim of this chapter is to explore the practices of mindfulness and compassion, what these practices are and how they can contribute to our own wellbeing and others and who we work with and for. This chapter offers a discussion on the concept of meditation, mindfulness and self-compassion, and some practical tools will be presented that you can try to use at work or at home to live more skilfully. These practices are powerful and can enhance mental health and wellbeing and reduce stress and burnout [1]. Providing access to these practices will hopefully encourage you to try out the practices for yourself, make mindfulness part of your daily life, and see if you can enjoy living more and improve your own life.

Groundbreaking neuroscience research is presented that provides evidence of the changes that can occur in our brain when we practice these skills which helps practitioners to cultivate resilience and therapeutic presence and revitalise their interactions with others. All healthcare professionals and indeed all workers can benefit from these practices which provide a tool kit of resources that they can dip into to replenish themselves. Throughout the chapter, mindfulness practices will be given to allow the reader to test from themselves the practices and to develop and practice some mindfulness and compassion skills that may complement themselves and their practice.

Cultivating mindfulness can put us in touch with our humanity and allow us to draw from the reservoirs of our life. Life's interior resources like learning, growing, healing and transformation can be tapped and brought to the fore by practising meditation. This then has the capacity to allow us live more fully with the present moment [2].

13.2 Meditation

Meditation is nothing new; it has been practised for thousands of years by all the major spiritual traditions. Meditation is a practice that makes it possible to cultivate and develop certain basic positive human qualities in the same way as other forms of training make it possible to acquire any other skill or play the piano. Meditation helps us to familiarise ourselves with a clear and accurate way of seeing things and to cultivate wholesome qualities that remain dormant within us unless we make an effort to draw them out [3]. Generations of meditators have devoted much of their lives to observing the automatic mechanical patterns of thought and nature of consciousness. Practising meditation allows us to discover for ourselves the value and benefits of these experiences in our practice which may allow us to integrate them in ourselves and our lives. This fruition of meditation may be described as an optimal way of being [4].

Meditation is attempting to cultivate a way of being and to free us from habitual behaviours and setting a course towards a chosen destination. It is not a form of escape and it attempts to allow us to see a clearer view of reality. The mind is simultaneously confused, agitated, rebellious and subject to innumerable conditioned and automatic patterns. The object of meditation is the mind, and the goal of meditation is not to shut down the mind or anesthetise it but to make it free, lucid and balanced [5].

Most aspects of spirituality generally involve a degree of mindfulness. However, many people also practise it in a nonspiritual way today. Meditation is nothing new; it is part of the major religions for centuries. Although mindfulness is best known now, as deriving from it is not exclusively a Buddhist practise, it forms part of many traditions and religions. Anthony de Mello's discusses and applies mindfulness using a Christian perspective [6].

13.3 The Art of Meditation

The ultimate reason for meditation is to transform our experiences of the world alongside its health benefits. Experienced long-term meditators have been able to maintain concentration on a particular task for 45 min which are both enduring and powerful. Major US universities like the University of Wisconsin, Princeton University, Harvard University, and the University of California and research centres in Zurich have studied the long-term effect of meditation on the brain. These discoveries have demonstrated that certain human qualities can be cultivated through mental training that was not previously thought possible. We now know that neurons are produced right through life and neuroplasticity which is a term that takes into account the fact that the brain evolves continually in relation to our experience and that particular training like learning to play the violin can bring about profound changes in the brain. Mindfulness and compassion can be cultivated in the same way, and modifications of our neuronal system of the brain can be observed even after 4 weeks of regular practice.

Much of this evidence is gleaned from functional magnetic resonance imaging (fMRI) and sophisticated electroencephalograms (EEG) which has given support for our capacity to transform and change actions, thoughts and behaviours. Functional magnetic resonance imaging (fMRI) takes pictures of the brain and records brain activity occurring during the scan. This understanding of our mind and the possibility of developing our inner resources gives us the capacity to successfully face the high and low challenges that we may encounter in life. Mindfulness practice provides benefits for improving one's life, and in dealing with difficult challenges, one often encounters throughout life. We all have certain character traits, and they remain the same if we do nothing to change these habits and patterns. Neuroscience is teaching us that positive experiences can change the architecture of our brains and, through that, improve the health of our bodies [7].

Our minds do not wander in a haphazard way; if we pay attention, we will notice that they often travel along familiar pathways [8]. When we begin to notice these grooves, we realise that our emotions and our thoughts usually are circular and repetitive, and this may be our pattern over many years or even decades. By actually becoming aware of this, we can actually begin to take action on our unhelpful patterns, and we can make changes for the better [9]. We can begin to notice that we habitually react in a similar way over and over again, and these can be viewed as events in the mind, which are our thoughts. We don't even put word on these thoughts; it is a continual physical response which is below our awareness [3]. Meditation is often associated with various religious or spiritual groups, whereas mindfulness is more distinctly secular in modern Western societies.

13.4 Mindfulness: What Is It

As Hasenkamp and Barsalou [10] suggest, mindfulness is a form of meditation which is helpful. When practising mindfulness, you focus on one thing (say, your breath), and as your mind wanders off, you shift attention gently back to that one thing again. This deliberate act of bringing one's attention back to the present after it wanders off can be thought of as "building the mindfulness muscle" [11].

13.5 Formal and Informal Practices

Mindfulness practice typically involves the deliberate effort to stabilise one's attention on specific physical sensations and environmental stimuli while continually trying to attempt to re-establish an anchor and repeating this practice each time the mind begins to wander [12]. Mindfulness of breathing is the most popular way, but other objects, or parts of the body, can be used, for example, you can also be mindful of the feeling of your feet against the soles of your shoes, your hands, your posture and your walking, or the sense of energy in your entire body, or a breeze on your face, city or country sounds, scents, beautiful images, physical work and many more. You try experimenting with these and notice what feels best for you.

The beauty of mindfulness meditation is that you need no equipment; you can practice anywhere (in the shower, eating a meal, gardening, walking); it can be easily incorporated into your day. The practice is "dose-dependent"; the more you practice, the better you get at it and reap the benefits and learn to watch your thoughts and not get caught up with your thinking [13].

Two main categories of mindfulness practice have been described, either formal or informal, and the main difference is the length of time and the purpose for the practice. Formal is when we have a sustained period of focused attention of what we are sensing, feeling and thinking with in a fixed period of time, for example, 20 min. Whereas informal practice is when we take short mindful moments in our everyday routine, which includes observing the surroundings on the bus ride to work, listening intently to people during conversation or having awareness of the texture of food while chewing lunch.

How to practice informally try one of the following:

- Take a few calm breaths in awareness.
- When you realise you are going over and over a negative thought, bring your attention back into the present moment by choosing an anchor, e.g. notice your breath or your left foot.

- Bring your awareness into your walking, and notice what your senses are telling you and what do you hear, smell and see.
- Choose drinking tea or coffee, walking along the street, showering, brushing your teeth, starting the car and cycling with awareness.

Formal practice will uncover richer insights into our minds and our conditioning, and this type of self-monitoring is more likely to yield more self-compassionate responses during the day, and when challenges arise, it also has the possibility of allowing us to live with discomfort which may give us the freedom to respond rather than react and make wise choices about situations as they arise [13].

13.5.1 Exercise How to Practice Formal Sitting for Short Period

13.5.1.1 Preparation
Sit or lie in a comfortable position. You may choose to keep your eyes open or closed. If you are feeling tired, it may be useful to leave your eyes open or cast your gaze gently to the floor.

13.5.1.2 The Breath
Begin by gently moving your attention onto the process of breathing. Notice the sensations of each breath as it happens, whether you focus on the rise and fall of your chest or abdomen or on the feeling of the breath at the nostrils. Really feel what it is like to breath, just observing it as it happens.

As you engage in this exercise, you may find that your mind wanders, caught by thoughts or by noises in the room or bodily sensations. When you notice that this happens, know that this is okay, and simply notice the distraction but gently bring your attention back to the breath.

13.5.1.3 Ending the Exercise
Take a few moments to yourself, connecting with your experience in the present moment. Expand your awareness from the breath into the space around you, and as you feel comfortable to do so, open your eyes and bring the exercise to a close.

13.6 Secular Mindfulness

Jon Kabat-Zinn [2] popularised meditation in the west in the 1970s, and he founded the University of Massachusetts Centre for Mindfulness in Medicine, Healthcare, and Society. He developed mindfulness-based stress reduction training (MBSR), a secular mindfulness programme as an alternative therapy for a variety of often difficult-to-treat conditions. This is an 8-week training programme of 2.5 h/week and a daylong retreat and also 45 min of daily work on one's own, designed to help participants cultivate mindfulness. The MBSR programme offers a framework to navigate difficult territories. It is difficult to explain why it is necessary to practise to become aware of what is right with us and to allow us to waken up to our own body, mind, heart and life and to much of what we take for granted every day. Mindfulness means seeing things as they are without trying to change them. Practising mindfulness seems easy, but it requires commitment and supporting factors [14].

While engaging with this practice, Kabat-Zinn [2] encourages practitioners to cultivate the seven attitudinal factors of mindfulness: (1) non-judging, (2) patience, (3) beginner's mind, (4) trust, (5) non-striving, (6) acceptance and (7) letting go, all of which are necessary conditions to help us to live mindfully. The practice of mindfulness will flourish when these certain conditions are present and maintained. By continually maintaining an open non-judgemental awareness and maintaining a connection with the present moment, most thoughts and strong emotions will pass without being evaluated cognitively. While holding, reflecting and cultivating these qualities in the mind, it will nourish, support and strengthen one's own mindfulness practice. Developing these qualities is a way of channelling one's energies into the process of healing and growth. The ultimate aim of the practise is to dissolve our reactions to disturbing emotions while not burying or rejecting the emotion itself [11].

Mindfulness-based cognitive therapy (MBCT) is an adaption of the MBSR programme developed by Siegel et al. [15], which has emerged as a popular therapeutic intervention to prevent relapse in recurrent depression. This course contains many similarities, the formal practices of body scan movement and exercises with CD and course manual with the addition of psychoeducational and cognitive behavioural therapeutic material with a specific focus on vulnerability to depression [16].

13.7 Research

The MBSR and MBCT mindfulness programs have been the most researched mindfulness intervention. There is some evidence that mindfulness practices are helpful in reducing anxiety, depression and stress-related conditions. Several trials have been conducted that support mindfulness practices. They have found mindfulness-like attention training which reduces self-perceived stress, but not levels of the hormone cortisol, a commonly used biological gauge of stress levels. The other trial links mindfulness-like attention training to increase in thickness of the prefrontal cortex, a brain region associated with complex behaviour, decision-making and shaping personality. Other smaller experimental studies have shown positive several benefits in a number of illness including irritable bowel syndrome, fibromyalgia [17], psoriasis, anxiety [18], depression [19] and post-traumatic stress disorder. Desbordes et al. [20] demonstrated with fMRI that changes in brain activity in subjects who have learned to meditate hold steady even when they're not meditating. Desbordes et al. [20] took before and after scans of subjects who learned to meditate over the course of 2 months. She scanned them while they were performing everyday tasks and not meditating. The scans detected change in the subjects' brain activation patterns from the beginning to the end of the study, the first time such a change in a part of the brain called the amygdala had been detected.

Among the challenges researchers face is defining mindfulness itself. The word has come to describe a meditation-based practice whose aim is to increase one's sense of being in the present, but it has also been used to describe a non-meditative state in which subjects set aside their mental distractions to pay greater attention to the here and now, as in the work of Harvard psychologist [21]. Another challenge involves sorting through the many variations of meditative practice. However it is difficult to ascertain consistencies with the study outcomes as many of the studies had small sample sizes and had variable experimental designs. However, in the main mindfulness, interventions have demonstrated benefits comparable with other therapeutic benefits in participants with depression, chronic pain and anxiety.

Recent scientific exploration has largely focused on the secular practice of mindful meditation, but meditation is also a component of several ancient religious traditions, with variations. Even within the community, practising secular mindful meditation, there are variations that may be scientifically meaningful, such as how often one meditates and the duration of the meditation sessions. Desbordes et al. [20] has a specific interest in compassion meditation, whose aim is to increase caring for those around us.

13.8 Compassion

Compassion comes from the Latin word compati meaning "to suffer with" and to feel the pain of the other person and be motivated to relieve it. Compassion is a warm and loving emotion, while one may acknowledge others' pain, and suffering, it does not become your suffering, and you feel positive caring emotions [22]. Many practices can activate warm nurturing feelings when you are faced with difficulties within yourself and others. Compassion can help you move into a deeply positive and empowering mode. This supportive loving compassion can be the softer element to support you in difficulties. Very often in difficult circumstances, the deep shared embrace of meditation of a carer and the person in pain can be held in intimate silence. Halifax [23] states that being compassionate can mean being truly present for the person who is in difficult circumstances which can be very powerful.

Gilbert and Choden [24] have identified six key attributes of compassion: motivation, sensitivity, sympathy, non-judgement, empathy and distress tolerance. These emotional qualities are essential for you to engage your compassion when you feel the pain of others. Mindfulness facilitates compassion by developing a sense of interconnectedness and establishing emotional control, mindfulness practice nourishes the development of these six compassion attributes by cultivating non-judgement, and mindfulness can also help to attend to whatever is necessary to take compassionate action. The benefits of having the practice of mindfulness are that you will have the ability not to get taken over or overwhelmed by another person's pain but be able to stand back and keep your mind stable while you decide what the other person needs right now. Research shows that mindfulness helps improve your compassion capacity by helping you feel more interconnected, empathic and focused [25].

13.9 Why the Need for Self-Compassion

Gilbert [21] states that for someone to develop genuine compassion to others, first he or she must have a basis upon which to cultivate compassion and that basis is the ability to connect to one's own feelings and to care for one's own welfare we need to be able to learn to be compassionate to ourselves first. Cultivating self-compassion involves deliberately treating yourself, with your mixture of faults and virtues, with kindness and understanding and accepting that you share your painful experiences and your failings with many millions of others while underpinning it with the practice of mindfulness [13]. Self-compassion is the capacity for healthy nurturing of the self, helps recognise and soothes painful thoughts and emotions [26]. When you identify and relate to your emotions with kindness instead of harshness, you can tap into your biological caregiving system, and oxytocin is released which helps one feel calm, comforted and secure. With practice you can relate to your own fears and anxieties with compassion and understanding just as you might relate to another person [25]. The attributes of compassion help us to tune into suffering and learn ways to understand it and tolerate it. The seeds of self-compassion already lie within all of us allowing us the possibility to nurture and transform our lives by using and growing these skills. Compassion for others begins with kindness to ourselves, and self-compassion is always available to tap into [27].

13.10 Self-Compassion

"Self-compassion, therefore, involves being touched by and open to one's own suffering, not avoiding or disconnecting from it, and generating the desire to alleviate one's suffering and to heal oneself with kindness" ([22], p. 22). Compassion is a feeling of concern for the suffering of others, and compassion and mindfulness have the ability to interact and transform suffering [25].

According to Neff [22] the three components of self-compassion are self-kindness, a sense of common humanity and a balanced mindful awareness. Kindness opens us to give ourselves what we need. Common humanity opens us up to our interrelatedness, and we don't have to feel alone. Mindfulness allows us to become aware of the present moment, so we can accept ourselves and our experiences with greater ease. These three facets allow us to experience a combined sense of warmth, connectedness and presence.

13.10.1 Informal Exercise in Compassion

- Think of something nice you can do for yourself, which perhaps you may have postponed several times because you are too busy.
- Taking a walk and savouring the sights, smells and textures, reading a short story, having lunch in a café, sitting and being still.

When you've thought of your treat, work out when you're going to do it, and savour and enjoy the moment, and this in turn allows your positive experiences turn into lasting inner strengths like resilience, balance and positive emotions [28].

13.10.2 Research

There is a growing body of evidence of the benefits of mindfulness and self-compassion training as a way to build resilience [25]. The evidence from neuroscience, from the work of pioneers such as psychologists Paul Gilbert and Kristin Neff, is now beginning to build a body of evidence on the value of cultivating self-compassion and how this can contribute to our wellbeing. Neff [22] suggests that self- compassion can be applied to many different situations including the workplace environment, by incorporating it as a leadership style which may have positive knock-on benefits for all staff.

Neff [22] pioneered the research into self-compassion and has developed a tool to measure self-compassion that has been used widely in research. Much research has demonstrated that self-compassion supports emotional wellbeing; decreases anxiety, depression and stress; and helps in maintaining healthy habits such as diet [29] and exercise [30] and more satisfying personal relationships [31]. Engaging in mindfulness and compassion practices can increase wellbeing, reduce stress and boost moods. Self-compassion practice is also associated with greater emotional intelligence [32, 33]. Self-compassionate people have been found to ruminate less, and they are less likely to keep repeating and repeating negative thoughts to themselves.

People who are compassionate towards themselves have lower levels of depression, anxiety and stress [31]. Self-compassionate people feel less negative about the past even though they are more likely to take personal responsibility for what has gone wrong in the past. When self-compassionate people fail, they are more likely to try again. This might be because they know that if they fail again, they won't subject themselves to fierce criticism. Self-compassionate people are more likely to stick to their diets, to exercise and to succeed in reducing their alcohol use. Why this should be is not entirely clear, but it may be that a self-compassionate motivation is more helpful than a self-critical one.

Neff and Germer [34] have devised a Mindful Self-Compassion (MSC) systematic training programme with one to two different themes in each session. It designed similar to the MBSR programme, 8 weeks of 2.5 h with a 1-day silent retreat. The programme is presented in an experimental way, and participants are invited to meet their experiences with curiosity and kindness. This programme offers participants a tool kit to build emotional strength while helping them to relate to distress differently. The programme has a combination of formal sitting and informal practices but the focus is on learning and developing the habit of self-compassion. Van den Brink and Koster [26] have developed a similar type of programme called Mindfulness-Based Compassionate Living (MBCL) that has been developed for people with various types of chronic or recurring mental health problems as an effective method of coping with low self-esteem and shame and empowering participants to bring more warmth, acceptance and connection into their lives. Gilbert [25] has developed compassion focused therapy and various compassion training programmes for individuals and various patient groups.

13.11 Exercise in Compassion

- Observe your breathing calmly for short while.
- Now imagine that somebody has sat down in front of you, facing you. This is someone you like or love or admire. Imagining that person sitting in front of you, try to generate a feeling of goodwill and well-wishing towards them.
- Silently, say "May you be happy, may you be safe, may you be well". Repeat this slowly as many times as you like.
- Now imagine that this person is replaced by a second person. That second person is yourself, with all your present faults and virtues.
- Observe yourself sitting there, and try to generate the same feeling of goodwill and well-wishing towards yourself that you did towards the person you like or love or admire.
- Repeat the phrase "May I be happy, may I be safe, may I be well". Repeat this as many times as you like. Bring the practice to an end, and open your eyes if they're closed.

13.11.1 A Body Scan with Compassion

- Bring awareness to the top of your head. Now move your awareness down along your head to your shoulders, down your chest and tummy and back, arms and hands, hips, thighs, knees, calves and feet.
- Try to generate a sense of compassion towards your body.
- If you encounter tension or pain in your body or if you encounter parts of your body that you are not happy with, do so with compassion.
- Approach them, at least during the body scan, with a sense of kindness towards yourself and towards each part of your body.
- If you find it difficult to generate a feeling of kindness, do the body scan with the intention of being kind to your body?

13.11.2 Softening the Internal Tone of Voice

- When we are critical of ourselves, we often speak to ourselves harshly. One way to begin to work with this is to soften the tone of voice with which you speak to yourself and that changes the experience. If you criticise yourself with an internal tone of voice that is hard and harsh, pause and restate the point in a softer tone of voice.

Transformation is possible when we bring some elements of mindfulness and self-compassion into our daily lives even if we are very busy and don't have time for long formal meditation practices. It can be a combination of some reminders to incorporate into daily practices and routines.

13.11.3 Exercise to Implement Mindful Self-Compassion for Personal Transformation

How can you cultivate these qualities of mindfulness and self-compassion to transform yourself? Make aims for your self tomorrow and build the practices into your daily life while also being kind to yourself.

- Remind yourself every morning. as you get out of bed, or immediately after you wake up, allow yourself to take one mindful breath.
- Locate your anchor body. What can you use as your anchor and to return to easily at intervals during the day? Take your pick, breath part of the body, a silent word, and try and anchor yourselves at various points throughout the day.
- If you work in an office, maybe download the mindfulness bell, and set an alarm to take a mindful moment at various periods throughout the day, and each time your mind wanders, bring your attention back to the sound of the bell.
- If you have difficulty sleeping, try doing a short body scan where you systematically bring your awareness to your body working all the way up from your feet.
- Try to bring awareness to your breath, and take three deep in-breaths and count for three slow breaths.
- Mindful eating and drinking. Try having the first bite of your food at each meal of the day when you become aware of the colour and texture of your food. Try and begin to eat slower and savour your food.
- Be with your experiences pleasant or unpleasant in an accepting way during the day.
- If you catch yourself ruminating or problem solving, let it go and bring your attention to the present moment.

13.12 Conclusion

In this chapter, mindfulness, compassion and self-compassion have been explored. The practice of mindfulness and self-compassion has been presented with some practical exercises that you choose to practise to allow you to experience for yourself the effects of the practice. Mindfulness is a rich spiritual concept, and it can be difficult to transfer this into a standardised framework for testing and advising people to take on board and practice. It can sometimes too difficult to take on something else on an already packed schedule; however Gilbert [25] suggests that we all need compassion training as life is difficult.

Over the last two decades, scientific research has documented the long-term effects of meditation practice on the brain and on our behaviours. It is possible to develop and cultivate qualities such as attention, emotional balance, altruism and inner peace. Short periods of meditation can include reduced stress levels and reduction in anxiety and in vulnerability to pain and reduce the tendency towards anxiety and depression and anger as well as strengthening our attention, immune system and our general wellbeing. We all possess the potential to find inner peace and contribute to the welfare of others.

Meditation can contribute to enable us to live a balanced life, rich in meaning. Mindfulness practice can open us to a rich source of information [9]. The research evidence and neuroscience have been presented that gives weight to these practices. You are invited to try to practice mindfulness and compassion training by trying to live in the moment, notice what is happening and make choices about how you respond to your experience rather than being driven by habitual reactions. As a result of loving and accepting yourself a little bit more, you will improve your relationships with yourself and others, and start to become a more compassionate and happier human being. Mindfulness practice is suitable for all ages from the very young to the older person.

References

1. Wax R. How to be human; the manual. London: Penguin Life; 2018.
2. Kabat-Zinn J. Full catastrophe living: how to cope with stress, pain and illness using mindfulness meditation. London: Piatkus; 2013.
3. Nhat Hanh T. The miracle of mindfulness. New York: Beacon press; 1975.
4. Ricard M. The art of meditation. London: Atlantic Books; 2010.
5. Chah A. It's like this. London: Amaravati Publications; 2013.
6. De Mello A. Awareness. New York: Crown Publishers; 1987.
7. Lutz J, Herwig U, Opialla S, Hittmeyer A, Jäncke L, Rufer M, Martin M, Holtforth G, Brühl A. Mindfulness and emotion regulation—an fMRI study. Soc Cogn Affect Neurosci. 2014;9(6):776–85. https://doi.org/10.1093/scan/nst043.
8. Amaro A. Finding the missing peace. London: Amaravati Publications; 2012.
9. Silverstone S. The mindfulness breakthrough. London: Watkins; 2012.
10. Hasenkamp W, Barsalou WB. Effects of meditation experience on functional connectivity of distributed brain networks. Front Hum Neurosci. 2012;6:38.
11. Goleman T. Emotional alchemy: how the mind can heal the heart. New York: Harmony Books; 2001.
12. Hughes L. The art of allowing the breath in meditation and in life. Dublin: Columba; 2010.
13. Germer C. The mindful path to self compassion freeing yourself from destructive thoughts and emotions. New York: Guilford; 2009.
14. Williams M, Teasdale J, Segal ZV, Kabat-Zinn J. The Mindful way through depression: freeing yourself from chronic unhappiness. New York: Guilford; 2007.
15. Segal ZV, Williams M, Teasdale J. Mindfulness-based cognitive therapy for depression second edition. London: Guilford Press; 2018.
16. Crane R. Mindfulness based cognitive therapy. New York: Routledge; 2009.
17. Kozasa EH, Tanaka L, Monson C, Stephen Little S, Leao FC, Peres M. The effects of meditation-based interventions on the treatment of fibromyalgia. Curr Pain Headache Rep. 2012;16(5):383–7.

18. Bohlmeijer E, Prenger R, Taal E, Cuijpers P. The effects of mindfulness-based stress reduction therapy on mental health of adults with a chronic medical disease: a meta-analysis. J Psychosom Res. 2010;68(6):539–44. https://doi.org/10.1016/j.jpsychores.2009.10.005.
19. Chiesa A, Serretti A. Mindfulness based cognitive therapy for psychiatric disorders: a systematic review and meta-analysis. Psychiatry Res. 2011;187(3):441–53. https://doi.org/10.1016/j.psychres.2010.08.011.
20. Desbordes G, Negi LT, Pace TWW, Wallace BA, Raison CL, Schwartz EL. Effects of mindful-attention and compassion mediation training on amygdala response to emotional stimuli in an ordinary, non-meditative state. Front Hum Neurosci. 2012;6:Article ID 292.
21. Paginini F, Bercovitz K, Langer E. Perceived control and mindfulness: implications for clinical practice. J Psychother Integr. 2016;26(2):91–102.
22. Neff K. Self-compassion: the proven power of being kind to yourself. New York: Harper Collins; 2011.
23. Halifax J. The precious necessity of compassion. J Pain Symptom Manage. 2010;41(1):146–53.
24. Gilbert P, Choden M. Mindful compassion. London: Constable Robinson; 2013.
25. Gilbert P. Compassion: concepts, research and applications. London: Routledge; 2017.
26. Van den Brink E, Koster F. Mindfulness based compassionate living. New York: Routledge; 2015.
27. Chodon M. Start where you are: a guide to compassionate living. Boston: Shambhala Publications; 2001.
28. Hanson R. Hardwiring happiness. London: Rider; 2013.
29. Adams CE, Leary MR. Promoting self-compassionate attitudes toward eating among restrictive and guilty eaters. J Soc Clin Psychol. 2007;26:1120–44.
30. Berry KA, Kowalski KC, Ferguson LJ, McHugh TF. An empirical phenomenology of young adult women exercisers body self-compassion. Qual Res Sport Exerc. 2011;2:293–312.
31. MacBeth A, Gumley A. Exploring compassion: a meta-analysis of the association between self-compassion and psychopathology. Clin Psychol Rev. 2012;32:545–52.
32. Heffernan M, Griffin M, McNulty S, Fitzpatrick JJ. Self-compassion and emotional intelligence in nurses. Int J Nurs Pract. 2010;16:366–73.
33. Neff KD, Rude SS, Kirkpatrick K. An examination of self-compassion in relation to positive psychological functioning and personality traits. J Res Pers. 2007;41:908–16.
34. Neff K, Germer C. The mindful self compassion workbook: a proven way to accept yourself build inner strength and strive. New York: Guilford; 2018.

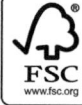

If you have any concerns about our products,
you can contact us on
ProductSafety@springernature.com

In case Publisher is established outside the EU,
the EU authorized representative is:
**Springer Nature Customer Service Center GmbH
Europaplatz 3, 69115 Heidelberg, Germany**

Printed by Libri Plureos GmbH
in Hamburg, Germany